ACSM'S

Certification Review

Sixth Edition

SENIOR EDITOR

Peter M. Magyari, PhD, FACSM, ACSM-EP
Brooks College of Health
University of North Florida
Jacksonville, Florida

ASSOCIATE EDITORS

Christopher G. Berger, PhD, ACSM-EP
University of North Texas
Denton, Texas

Samuel A. Headley, PhD, FACSM, ACSM-CEP, EIM3
Springfield College
Springfield, Massachusetts

Nicole Nelson, MSH, LMT, ACSM-EP
Brooks College of Health
University of North Florida
Jacksonville, Florida

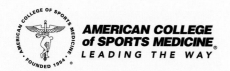

**AMERICAN COLLEGE
of SPORTS MEDICINE**®
LEADING THE WAY

ACSM'S
Certification Review

Sixth Edition

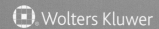
. Wolters Kluwer

Philadelphia · Baltimore · New York · London
Buenos Aires · Hong Kong · Sydney · Tokyo

Acquisitions Editor: Lindsey Porambo
Senior Development Editor: Amy Millholen
Senior Editorial Coordinator: Lindsay Ries
Marketing Manager: Phyllis Hitner
Senior Production Project Manager: Sadie Buckallew
Design Coordinator: Stephen Druding
Manufacturing Coordinator: Margie Orzech
Prepress Vendor: Lumina Datamatics Ltd.
ACSM Committee on Certification and Registry Boards Chair: Christie Ward-Ritacco, PhD, ACSM-EP, EIM2
ACSM Publications Committee Chair: Jeffrey Potteiger, PhD, FACSM
ACSM Certification-Related Content Advisory Committee Chair: Dierdra Bycura, EdD, ACSM-CPT, ACSM-EP
ACSM Chief Operating Officer: Katie Feltman
ACSM Development Editor: Angie Chastain

Sixth edition

9 8 7 6 5 4 3 2 1

Printed in China

Library of Congress Cataloging-in-Publication Data
Names: Magyari, Peter, author.
Title: ACSM's certification review / Peter Magyari, senior editor, Peter M.
  Magyari, Ph.D., FACSM, ACSM-EP Brooks College of Health, University of
  North Florida, Jacksonville, Florida ; associate editors, Christopher G.
  Berger, Ph.D., ACSM-EP University of North Texas Denton, Texas, Samuel
  A. Headley, Ph.D., FACSM, ACSM-CEP, EIM3, Springfield College,
  Springfield, Massachusetts, Nicole Nelson, MSH, LMT, ACSM-EP Brooks
  College of Health University of North Florida Jacksonville, Florida.
Description: Sixth edition. | Philadelphia : Wolters Kluwer, [2022]
Identifiers: LCCN 2021028352 | ISBN 9781975161910 (hardback) | ISBN
  9781975161941 (ebook)
Subjects: LCSH: Sports medicine--Outlines, syllabi, etc. | Sports
  medicine--Examinations, questions, etc. | Personal trainers--Outlines,
  syllabi, etc. | Personal trainers--Examinations, questions, etc. |
  BISAC: MEDICAL / Sports Medicine
Classification: LCC RC1213 .A268 2022 | DDC 617.1/027--dc23
LC record available at https://lccn.loc.gov/2021028352

shop.lww.com

Preface

This sixth edition of the *ACSM's Certification Review* has been extensively revised from previous editions of this text. This edition covers all the current knowledge and skills for the certifications of the ACSM Certified Personal Trainer® (ACSM-CPT®), the ACSM Certified Exercise Physiologist (ACSM-EP®), and the ACSM-Certified Clinical Exercise Physiologist (ACSM-CEP®).

TEXT ORGANIZATION

This text is organized into parts by certification level and is further subdivided into four main sections in each part:

- **What You Need to Know and Multiple Choice Practice Questions Divided by Subdomain**
  - **What you need to know:** Statements are based on the knowledge and skill statements provided in the exam content outline for each certification, provided in a format appropriate for the certification level.
  - **Multiple-choice questions:** Have been organized by Domain and Subdomain. As the subdomains are interconnected, questions may correspond to multiple domains. In an effort to avoid duplicating questions, a few subdomains have fewer multiple choice questions.
- **Answers to the Multiple Choice Practice Questions:** Include an explanation and list the resources where appropriate.
- **Case Study Challenges:** Include both multiple-choice questions and open-ended discussion questions. The ACSM-CEP case study section also includes a number of ECG case studies.
- **Answers to the Case Study Challenges:** Include an explanation and lists the resources where appropriate.

STUDYING FOR A CERTIFICATION EXAM

The many individuals involved in the preparation of this text in the current and previous editions intend that it be used as a review aid for the certification exams and assume that the reader is actively preparing to sit for one of the three ACSM certifications covered. This text represents one of many study tools available and should not be viewed as the sole source of information to use in preparing to take one of these three certification exams.

As a study or review tool, this text may help you clarify areas of strengths and weaknesses. Your individual weaknesses should be eliminated by further study. This text should be viewed as part of a study kit that each of you needs to identify for yourself. Certainly, *ACSM's Guidelines for Exercise Testing and Prescription, Eleventh Edition (GETP11)* must be considered as part of that package.

ACSM certification levels build upon one another. For instance, the ACSM-CEP certification encompasses all ACSM-EP and ACSM-CPT knowledge and skill statements. Thus, individuals who intend to use this book to review for the ACSM-CEP certification are responsible for all knowledge and skill statements covered in the ACSM-EP and ACSM-CPT sections as well as all knowledge and skill statements covered in the ACSM-CEP section. Similarly, individuals preparing for the ACSM-EP certification are responsible for all knowledge and skill statements covered in the ACSM-CPT section.

We are aware that facts, standards, and guidelines change on a regular basis in this ever-growing field of knowledge. Hence, in the event that conflict may be noted between this book and the *GETP11*, the latter text should be used as **the definitive and final resource**. In such cases, where an update is needed or where a conflict or error is identified, we will make every effort to provide further explanations or corrections online.

The web address for any corrections is https://www.acsm.org/get-stay-certified/get-certified/prepare-for-exams/acsm-book-updates.

ADDITIONAL RESOURCES

This edition of the *ACSM's Certification Review* includes additional online resources for students and instructors.

Students

■ Supplemental figures, tables, and boxes from related ACSM titles

Instructors

Approved adopting instructors will be given access to the following additional resource:

■ Image bank

Acknowledgments

I must have made over a thousand edits to produce this book chapter. Each one was composed with care so that certification candidates have the confidence to take an ACSM exam and the knowledge to serve their clients well. My efforts are dedicated to each new ACSM-certified fitness professional who uses this book. Your services are needed now more than ever—enjoy this new dimension to your professional development!

— Christopher G. Berger

I would like to thank my wife, Dawn, and my family for their continued love and support in all of my professional endeavors. I would also like to acknowledge the great work of Catherine M. Griswold, who ably assisted with the editing of Part 3 of the book.

— Samuel A. Headley

I could not have completed this project without the work of my associate editors Chris Berger, Sam Headley, and Nicole Nelson. I give a well-deserved thank you to Walt Thompson for all he has done for me professionally over the years and his leadership in ACSM. A special "Thank you" to the publishing staff at ACSM (Angela Chastain and Katie Feltman) for stepping in to provide much needed assistance when I needed it most and at Wolters Kluwer (Lindsey Porambo, Amy Millholen, and Lindsay Ries) whose input was always both needed and appreciated. Finally, to my mom and dad (Judy and Don Magyari), my siblings (Trish, Don, and Tom), and my sons Myo and Rox, who have supported me throughout, I simply wish to acknowledge that "I love you."

— Peter M. Magyari

First and always, thanks to my parents for being the most amazing life teachers and constant source of love and support.

Thanks to Pete Magyari for being open to new ideas and thinking I actually had enough expertise and talent to contribute to this book.

Special thanks to Angie Chastain for her patience and understanding during an unexpectedly wacky COVID year.

I'd also like to thank James Churilla; his graduate Exercise Science program at the University of North Florida taught me there is always room to raise the bar.

Finally, thanks to my bulldog Maggie for being the best sounding board.

— Nicole Nelson

Contributing Authors to the Sixth Edition*

Jasmin C. Hutchinson, PhD, ACSM-EP
Professor, Exercise Science and Athletic Training
Springfield College
Springfield, Massachusetts
Section 11, Case Studies

Hayden Riley Madera, MS, ACSM-CEP, TTS
Senior Clinical Exercise Physiologist & Tobacco
    Treatment Specialist
The Miriam Hospital
Providence, Rhode Island
Section 11, Case Studies

Emily M. Miele, PhD, ACSM-CEP, EIM3
Senior Clinical Research Scientist
Detect, Inc.
Guilford, Connecticut
Section 11, Case Studies

*See Appendix B for a list of contributors to the previous two editions.

Reviewers for the Sixth Edition

Daniel L. Carl, PhD, FACSM
University of Cincinnati
Cincinnati, Ohio

Garett Griffith, MS, MPH, ACSM-CEP, EIM3
Feinberg School of Medicine,
    Northwestern University
Chicago, Illinois

M. Allison Murphy, PhD, FACSM, ACSM-EP
Mercy College
Dobbs Ferry, New York

Ben Thompson, PhD, FACSM, ACSM-EP, EIM2
Metropolitan State University of Denver
Denver, Colorado

Contents

PART 1   ACSM CERTIFIED PERSONAL TRAINER® (ACSM-CPT®) CERTIFICATION

Associate Editor: Christopher Berger, PhD, ACSM-EP, CSCS

PART 2   ACSM CERTIFIED EXERCISE PHYSIOLOGIST (ACSM-EP) CERTIFICATION

Associate Editor: Nicole Nelson, MSH, LMT, ACSM-EP

PART 3 ACSM CERTIFIED CLINICAL EXERCISE PHYSIOLOGIST® (ACSM-CEP®) CERTIFICATION
Associate Editor: Samuel A. Headley, PhD, FACSM, ACSM-CEP, EIM3

ACSM Certified Personal Trainer® (ACSM-CPT®) Certification

Christopher Berger, PhD, ACSM-EP, CSCS
Associate Editor

DOMAIN NUMBER	I	II	III	IV
DOMAIN NAME	INITIAL CLIENT CONSULTATION AND ASSESSMENT	EXERCISE PROGRAMMING AND IMPLEMENTATION	EXERCISE LEADERSHIP AND CLIENT EDUCATION	LEGAL AND PROFESSIONAL RESPONSIBILITIES

OUTLINE OF THIS PART:

WHAT YOU NEED TO KNOW AND MULTIPLE CHOICE PRACTICE QUESTIONS DIVIDED BY SUBDOMAIN

DOMAIN I: INITIAL CLIENT CONSULTATION AND ASSESSMENT

A. PROVIDE DOCUMENTS AND CLEAR INSTRUCTIONS TO THE CLIENT IN PREPARATION FOR THE INITIAL INTERVIEW

Domain I Subdomain A: What You Need to Know

- The components of and preparation for the initial client consultation
- The necessary paperwork to be completed by the client prior to the initial client interview
- Effective communication
- Utilizing multimedia resources (*e.g.*, email, phone, text messaging)

Domain I Subdomain A: Multiple Choice Questions

1. Which is *not* part of the initial client consultation?
   A) Discussion of health history
   B) Health and fitness assessments
   C) Informed consent document
   D) Client feedback about goal progression

2. During motivational interviewing, an example of "change talk" employed by the ACSM-CPT to ask an evocative question is best exemplified by which of the following questions to the client?
   A) "What do you intend to do?"
   B) "Are there disadvantages of being physically inactive?"

   C) "What would it take for you to increase the importance of exercise?"
   D) "You mentioned that you used to walk regularly. What was that like?"

3. Which of the following was *not* identified as a "multimedia" resource example in the ACSM-CPT Job Task Analysis?
   A) Email
   B) Personal conversation
   C) Phone
   D) Text message

B. INTERVIEW THE CLIENT TO GATHER AND PROVIDE PERTINENT INFORMATION PRIOR TO FITNESS TESTING AND PROGRAM DESIGN

Domain I Subdomain B: What You Need to Know

- The components and limitations of a health/medical history, preparticipation screening, informed consent, trainer–client contract, and organizational policies and procedures
- The use of medical clearance for exercise testing and program participation
- Health behavior modification theories and strategies
- Orientation procedures, including equipment utilization and facility layout
- Obtaining a health/medical history, medical clearance, and informed consent

Domain I Subdomain B: Multiple Choice Questions

1. The preparticipation health screening process is based upon _____.
   A) how long the client has been physically active; presence of signs or symptoms and/or known metabolic, renal, or cardiovascular disease (CVD); and exercise intensity at which individual desires to exercise
   B) individuals' current physical activity level; presence of signs or symptoms and/or known metabolic, renal, or CVD; and exercise intensity at which individual desires to exercise
   C) how long the client has been exercising, number of CVD risk factors, and how long the individual has been physically active
   D) the current level of physical activity the individual is engaging in; how long client has been physically active; and presence of signs or symptoms and/or known metabolic, renal, or CVD

2. The informed consent document provides all of the following *except* _____.
   A) the opportunity to choose to withdraw involvement at any point
   B) information regarding risks and benefits of participation
   C) the opportunity for potential client to ask questions
   D) protection of personal trainer against lawsuits of negligence

3. During the preparticipation screening process, you learn that your new client has previously had a stent and also has diabetes. You also learn that he has been regularly physically active for the previous 2 yr, asymptomatic, and compliant with medication use as prescribed by his physician. Your client would like to engage in vigorous-intensity exercise. How do you advise your new client?

   A) Advise the new client to halt all exercise and seek medical clearance before resuming activity.
   B) Advise the new client to pursue medical clearance, and once obtained, your client may then begin adding in bouts of vigorous-intensity exercise.
   C) Advise the new client to begin vigorous-intensity exercise (*i.e.*, rating of perceived exertion [RPE] ≥14% or ≥60% heart rate reserve [HRR]) without medical clearance.
   D) Advise the new client not to engage in vigorous-intensity exercise for safety.

4. The informed consent document _____.
   A) is a legal document
   B) provides immunity from prosecution
   C) provides an explanation of the test to the client
   D) legally protects the rights of the client

5. In commercial settings, client screening should at least (minimally) include
   A) electrocardiography.
   B) cholesterol screening.
   C) medication review.
   D) personal medical history.

6. A new client is sedentary and has no known disease but does possess signs and symptoms that suggest presence of cardiovascular, metabolic, or renal disease. Is medical clearance recommended prior to beginning any intensity (*i.e.*, light, moderate, or vigorous) of exercise?
   A) Medical clearance is recommended prior to beginning any intensity exercise.
   B) Medical clearance is recommended for moderate- to vigorous-intensity but not light-intensity exercise.
   C) Medical clearance is recommended for vigorous-intensity exercise only.
   D) Medical clearance is not necessary.

7. Verbal encouragement, material incentives, self-praise, and use of specific contingency contracts are examples of ____.
   A) reinforcement
   B) shaping
   C) antecedent control
   D) setting goals

8. The health belief model assumes that people will engage in a behavior, such as exercise, when ____.
   A) external motivation is provided
   B) optimal environmental conditions are met
   C) there is a perceived threat of disease
   D) internal motivation outweighs external circumstances

9. Which of the following personnel is responsible for program design as well as implementation of that program?
   A) Administrative assistant
   B) Personal trainer
   C) Manager or director
   D) Health fitness specialist

10. If a client gets lost returning to the lab after a bathroom break, the ACSM-CPT most likely failed to
    A) assure the client that the fitness testing environment was safe for exercise.
    B) orient the client to the fitness testing environment.
    C) regulate the temperature of the testing environment.
    D) select a testing environment that was near a bathroom.

C. REVIEW AND ANALYZE CLIENT DATA TO IDENTIFY RISK, FORMULATE A PLAN OF ACTION, AND CONDUCT PHYSICAL ASSESSMENTS

Domain I Subdomain C: What You Need to Know

- Risk factors for CVD
- Signs and symptoms of chronic cardiovascular, metabolic, and/or pulmonary disease
- The process for determining the need for medical clearance prior to participation in fitness testing and exercise programs
- Relative and absolute contraindications to exercise testing
- Identifying modifiable risk factors for CVD and teaching clients about risk reduction
- Determining appropriate fitness assessments based on the initial client consultation
- Following protocols during fitness assessment administration

Domain I Subdomain C: Multiple Choice Questions

1. You have a new client, a 47-yr-old male who is a current smoker. He would like to quit smoking and adopt a more active lifestyle. He is currently not regularly exercising, has a blood pressure (BP) of 136/88 mm Hg, total cholesterol of 182 mg $\cdot$ dL^{-1}, waist circumference of 38 in., fasting plasma glucose of 92 mg $\cdot$ dL^{-1}, and no known family history of CVD. How many positive risk factors for CVD does he have?
   A) Two
   B) Three
   C) Four
   D) Five

2. According to the Adult Treatment Panel III, which of the following would be considered an optimal level of low-density lipoprotein cholesterol?
   A) 130 mg $\cdot$ dL^{-1}
   B) 105 mg $\cdot$ dL^{-1}
   C) 95 mg $\cdot$ dL^{-1}
   D) 120 mg $\cdot$ dL^{-1}

3. What is angina pectoris?
   A) Discomfort associated with myocardial ischemia
   B) Discomfort associated with hypertension
   C) Discomfort associated with heartburn
   D) Discomfort associated with papillary necrosis

4. A 62-yr-old obese factory worker complains of pain in his right shoulder on arm abduction; on evaluation, decreased range of motion (ROM) and strength are noted. You also notice that he is beginning to use accessory muscles to substitute movements and to compensate. These symptoms may indicate _____.
   A) a referred pain from a herniated lumbar disk
   B) rotator cuff strain or impingement
   C) angina
   D) advanced stages of multiple sclerosis

5. Studies designed to measure the success of a program based on some quantifiable data that can be analyzed examine _____.
   A) incomes
   B) outcomes
   C) client progress notes
   D) attendance records

6. You are conducting an initial client consultation. Your potential client has walked for $1 \text{ h} \cdot \text{d}^{-1}$, $6 \text{ d} \cdot \text{wk}^{-1}$ for the previous 10 yr. She informs you that 3 times over the previous 6 months she has been becoming dizzy during her walks and had one episode of syncope during a walk. She has not spoken with her physician about these episodes and attributes them to her not having eaten enough prior to her exercise bout. As her personal trainer, what would be the most prudent course of action?
   A) Explain the potential causes of dizziness before, during, and after exercise and continue with the consultation.
   B) Tell her it is nothing to be worried about but to mention it to her physician at her next appointment.
   C) Tell her to discontinue all exercise and make an appointment with her physician for medical clearance.
   D) Tell her to slow her walking pace and be sure to drink enough fluids.

7. Which condition is commonly associated with a progressive decline in bone mineral density and calcium content in postmenopausal women?
   A) Osteoporosis
   B) Epiphysitis
   C) Osteoarthritis
   D) Arthritis

8. Clients with ___ are no longer automatically referred for medical clearance.
   A) inactive lifestyles
   B) current chest pain
   C) sedentary lifestyles
   D) pulmonary disease

9. One relative contraindication to exercise testing is
   A) ongoing unstable angina.
   B) resting hypertension with systolic blood pressure >200 mm Hg or diastolic blood pressure >110 mm Hg.
   C) acute myocardial infarction within 2 days.
   D) symptomatic severe aortic stenosis.

D. EVALUATE BEHAVIORAL READINESS AND DEVELOP STRATEGIES TO OPTIMIZE EXERCISE ADHERENCE

Domain I Subdomain D: What You Need to Know

- Behavioral strategies to enhance exercise and health behavior change (*e.g.*, reinforcement, SMART goal setting, social support)
- Health behavior change models (*e.g.*, socioeconomic model, readiness to change model, social cognitive theory [SCT], theory of planned behavior) and effective strategies that support and facilitate behavioral change
- Setting effective client-oriented SMART behavioral goals
- Choosing and applying appropriate health behavior modification strategies based on the client's skills, knowledge, and level of motivation

Domain I Subdomain D: Multiple Choice Questions

1. Which of the following appropriately characterizes the "SMARTS" approach to goal setting?
   A) Specialized, meticulous, accurate, reasonable, total, scored
   B) Specific, measurable, achievable, realistic, temporary, sentimental
   C) Specialized, meticulous, achievable, realistic, time-oriented, standard
   D) Specific, measurable, action-oriented, realistic, timely, self-determined

2. A client is using a pedometer to measure the number of steps taken each day. He then logs that number in a daily journal. Doing this is an example of
   A) goal setting.
   B) self-monitoring.
   C) problem solving.
   D) goal measuring.

3. Which of the following is *not* an example of a social barrier?
   A) A single parent with no child care
   B) A friend encouraging you to skip your afternoon walk and have dinner with him instead
   C) Family members discouraging you to join a gym
   D) Gym membership costs that exceed your budget

4. The SCT posits which of the following as the most important factor relating to behavior change?
   A) Perception of risk of untoward health outcomes
   B) Self-efficacy and expectation of outcome related to behavior changes
   C) Belief that behavior change is worth the improvement in health
   D) Knowledge about exercise increases likelihood for nonadherence

5. A client has expressed to you that she has set a goal of wearing a particular dress size in time for the wedding of her son. This is an example of _____.
   A) intrinsic motivation
   B) self-efficacy
   C) extrinsic motivation
   D) self-worth

6. After 6 months of personal training and coaching sessions, your client expresses to you that she believes she can now implement what you have taught her and exercise on her own. This is an example of enhanced _____.
   A) self-worth
   B) self-esteem

C) self-regulation
D) self-efficacy

7. Which of the following statements is *false* about goal setting?
   A) Goals are most effective when the trainer selects them and the client agrees to them.
   B) Goal setting can help clients plan for potential barriers.
   C) Goal setting can increase motivation and effort to maintain positive behavior changes.
   D) It is an important tool that can help the client adhere to and maintain newly adopted behavior change.

8. Suppose you have a new client who tells you, "For the past three months, I've been walking after dinner on weekdays and I'm really enjoying it." This corresponds to the ___ stage of motivational readiness.
   A) action
   B) preparation
   C) contemplation
   D) precontemplation

9. Feeling good about being able to perform an activity or skill, such as finally being able to run a mile or to increase the speed of walking a mile, is an example of an _____.
   A) extrinsic reward
   B) intrinsic reward
   C) external stimulus
   D) internal stimulus

10. Which of the following transtheoretical model of behavior change stages is correctly defined?
    A) Action: Individual has been regularly active for less than 6 months.
    B) Preparation: Individual has begun to exercise regularly.
    C) Action: Individual has been regularly active and making positive behavior changes for more than 6 months.
    D) Maintenance: Individual is working on relapse prevention strategies.

E. ASSESS THE COMPONENTS OF HEALTH- AND/OR SKILL-RELATED PHYSICAL FITNESS TO ESTABLISH BASELINE VALUES, SET GOALS, AND DEVELOP INDIVIDUALIZED PROGRAMS.

Domain I Subdomain E: What You Need to Know

- The basic structures of bone, skeletal muscle, and connective tissue

- The basic anatomy of the cardiovascular and respiratory systems

- The definition of the following terms: anterior, posterior, proximal, distal, inferior, superior, medial, lateral, supination, pronation, flexion, extension, adduction, abduction, hyperextension, rotation, circumduction, agonist, antagonist, and stabilizer
- The sagittal, frontal (coronal), transverse (horizontal) planes of the body and plane in which each muscle action occurs
- The interrelationships among center of gravity, base of support, balance, stability, and proper spinal alignment
- The following curvatures of the spine: lordosis, scoliosis, and kyphosis
- The differences between the aerobic and anaerobic energy systems and the effects of acute and chronic exercise on each acute responses to cardiorespiratory exercise and resistance training
- Chronic physiological adaptations associated with cardiovascular exercise and resistance training
- Physiological responses related to warm-up and cool-down
- Physiological basis of acute muscle fatigue, delayed onset muscle soreness, and musculoskeletal injury/overtraining
- Physiological adaptations that occur at rest and during submaximal and maximal exercise following chronic aerobic and anaerobic exercise training
- Physiological basis for improvements in muscular strength and endurance
- Expected BP responses associated with postural changes, acute physical exercise, and adaptations as a result of long-term exercise training
- Types of muscle contraction, such as isotonic (concentric, eccentric), isometric (static), and isokinetic
- Major muscle groups (*e.g.*, trapezius, pectoralis major, latissimus dorsi, deltoids, biceps, triceps, rectus abdominis, internal and external obliques, erector spinae, gluteus maximus, hip flexors, quadriceps, hamstrings, hip adductors, hip abductors, anterior tibialis, soleus, gastrocnemius)

- Major bones (*e.g.*, clavicle, scapula, sternum, humerus, carpals, ulna, radius, femur, fibula, tibia, tarsals)
- Joint classifications (*e.g.*, hinge, ball and socket)
- The primary action and joint ROM specific to each major muscle group
- The following terms related to muscles: hypertrophy, atrophy, and hyperplasia
- Physiological basis of the components of health-related physical fitness (cardiovascular fitness, muscular strength, muscular endurance, flexibility, and body composition)
- Normal chronic physiologic adaptations associated with cardiovascular, resistance, and flexibility training
- Test termination criteria and proper procedures to be followed after discontinuing an exercise test
- Anthropometric measurements and body composition techniques (*e.g.*, skinfolds, plethysmography, bioelectrical impedance, infrared, dual-energy x-ray absorptiometry, body mass index [BMI], circumference measurements)
- Fitness testing protocols, including pretest preparation and assessments of cardiovascular fitness, muscular strength, muscular endurance, flexibility, and body composition
- Interpretation of fitness test results
- The recommended order of fitness assessments
- Appropriate documentation of signs or symptoms during an exercise session various mechanisms for appropriate referral to a physician.
- Locating/palpating pulse landmarks, accurately measuring heart rate (HR), and obtaining RPE
- Selecting and administering cardiovascular fitness assessments
- Locating anatomical sites for circumference (girth) and skinfold measurements
- Selecting and administering muscular strength and muscular endurance assessments
- Selecting and administering flexibility assessments for various muscle groups
- Recognizing postural deviations that may affect exercise performance and body alignment
- Delivering test and assessment results in a positive manner

Domain I Subdomain E: Multiple Choice Questions

1. ___ is characterized by a decreased bone mass with a prevalence rate in men as high as 4.2%.
   A) osteoarthritis
   B) osteochondritis
   C) osteomyelitis
   D) osteoporosis

2. All of the following are major agonist muscles involved in knee flexion *except* ____.
   A) gracilis
   B) gastrocnemius
   C) soleus
   D) popliteus

3. All of the following are major agonist muscles involved hip flexion *except* ____.
   A) quadratus lumborum
   B) sartorious
   C) rectus femoris
   D) iliopsoas

4. Which of the following terms represents an imaginary horizontal plane passing through the midsection of the body and dividing it into upper and lower portions?
   A) Sagittal
   B) Frontal
   C) Transverse
   D) Superior

5. Rotation of the anterior surface of a bone toward the midline of the body is called ____.
   A) medial rotation
   B) lateral rotation
   C) supination
   D) pronation

6. Which of the following is considered an abnormal curve of the spine with lateral deviation of the vertebral column in the frontal plane?
   A) Lordosis
   B) Scoliosis
   C) Kyphosis
   D) Morphosis

7. Regular chronic "aerobic" exercise is *not* associated with
   A) increased resting HR.
   B) decreased time for HR recovery.
   C) increased stroke volume at rest.
   D) decreased resting HR.

8. Cardiovascular adaptations to regular "aerobic" exercise include increases to all of the following *except*
   A) heart size.
   B) cardiac output.
   C) resting BP.
   D) red blood cell counts.

9. Which of the following is an adaptation to resistance training?
   A) Decreased capillary density
   B) Decreased lactate removal
   C) Increased resting HR
   D) Increased aerobic enzyme activity

10. Which of the following is an adaptation to aerobic conditioning?
    A) Maximal HR will decrease at maximal effort exercise.
    B) Total lung capacity will increase.
    C) Lactic acid production will decrease during submaximal effort exercise.
    D) Resting BP will increase.

11. Cool-down exercise reduces
    A) blood flow to the brain.
    B) maximal HR.
    C) blood flow to the heart.
    D) body temperature.

12. Which of the following exercise modes allows buoyancy to reduce the potential for musculoskeletal injury?
    A) Basketball
    B) Race walking
    C) Skiing
    D) Water exercise

13. If a client exercises without rest days or develops a minor injury and does not allow time for the injury to heal, what can occur?
    A) An overuse injury
    B) Deconditioning
    C) An impaired fasting glucose
    D) Sarcopenia

14. A method of strength and power training that involves an eccentric loading of muscles and tendons followed immediately by an explosive concentric action is called ____.
    A) plyometrics
    B) periodization
    C) supersets
    D) isotonic reversals

15. Within a skeletal muscle fiber, large amounts of calcium are stored in the ____.
    A) nucleus
    B) plasma membrane
    C) myosin
    D) sarcoplasmic reticulum

16. Which of the following BP readings is classified as "elevated" according to current standards?
    A) 126/80 mm Hg
    B) 124/72 mm Hg
    C) 144/94 mm Hg
    D) 156/92 mm Hg

17. Specifically, muscle shortening under a load is a type of muscle action referred to as a/n ___ action.
    A) concentric
    B) isometric
    C) eccentric
    D) dynamic

18. All of the following are isotonic resistance exercises *except*:
    A) Dumbbell biceps curls
    B) Pull-ups
    C) Box squat jumps
    D) The half-squat wall-sit

19. All of the following are rotator cuff muscles *except*
    A) infraspinatus.
    B) teres minor.
    C) subscapularis.
    D) trapezius.

20. Which of the following statements is *not* true about synovial joints?
    A) They are the least common type of joint found in the human body.
    B) The joint cavity is enclosed by the joint capsule.
    C) They are the most common type of joint found in the human body.
    D) A synovial membrane lines the joint cavity.

21. After 30 yr of age, skeletal muscle strength begins to decline primarily because of
    A) calcium deficiencies.
    B) increased sodium consumption.
    C) loss of muscle mass.
    D) neuromuscular junction defects.

22. Compared with running, swimming will result in a ___ even if exercise intensity is the same.
    A) higher HR
    B) lower HR
    C) lower CO
    D) higher CO

23. Your new client is 6 ft tall and weighs 275 lb. What is his BMI classification?
    A) 37.3 kg m^{-2}; class I obesity
    B) 40.0 kg m^{-2}; class III obesity
    C) 40.0 kg m^{-2}; class II obesity
    D) 37.3 kg m^{-2}; class II obesity

24. Which of the following BMI values would classify an individual as class I obesity?
    A) 29.9 kg m^{-2}
    B) 35.0 kg m^{-2}
    C) 32.5 kg m^{-2}
    D) 36.0 kg m^{-2}

25. An example or measure of muscular endurance is ___.
    A) number of curl-ups in 10 min
    B) one repetition maximum
    C) number of curl-ups in 1 min
    D) three repetitions maximum

26. The ___ valve of the heart is most responsible for preventing a backflow of blood from the right atrium to the right ventricle.
    A) bicuspid
    B) tricuspid
    C) mitral
    D) septal

F. DEVELOP A PLAN AND TIMELINE FOR REASSESSING PHYSICAL FITNESS, GOALS, AND RELATED BEHAVIORS

Domain I Subdomain F: What You Need to Know

- Developing fitness plans based on the information obtained in the client interview and the results of the physical fitness assessments
- Alternative health behavior modification strategies

- The purpose and timeline for reassessing each component of physical fitness (cardiovascular fitness, muscular strength, muscular endurance, flexibility, and body composition)

Domain I Subdomain F: Multiple Choice Questions

For this subdomain, mutliple choice questions for Domain I
Subdomains A–D should be reviewed.

DOMAIN II: EXERCISE PROGRAMMING AND IMPLEMENTATION

A. REVIEW THE CLIENT'S GOALS, MEDICAL HISTORY, AND ASSESSMENT RESULTS AND DETERMINE EXERCISE PRESCRIPTION

Domain II Subdomain A: What You Need to Know

- The risks and benefits associated with guidelines for exercise training and programming for healthy adults, older adults, children, adolescents, and pregnant women
- The risks and benefits associated with guidelines for exercise training and programming for clients with chronic disease who are medically cleared to exercise
- Health-related conditions that require consultations with medical personnel prior to initiating physical activity
- Components of health-related physical fitness (cardiovascular fitness, muscular strength, muscular endurance, flexibility, and body composition)

- Program development for specific client needs (*e.g.*, sport-specific training, performance, lifestyle, functional, balance, agility, aerobic and anaerobic)
- Special precautions and modifications of exercise programming for participation in various environmental conditions (*e.g.*, altitude, variable ambient temperatures, humidity, environmental pollution)
- Documenting exercise sessions and performing periodic reevaluations to assess changes in fitness status

Domain II Subdomain A: Multiple Choice Questions

1. Which of the following is an appropriate method of monitoring exercise intensity for a pregnant client?
   A) RPE
   B) Target $\dot{V}O_{2max}$
   C) Percentage of maximal HR
   D) Percentage of HRR

2. __ is a good reason for terminating an exercise bout in the pregnant female.
   A) Increased fetal movement
   B) Dyspnea prior to exertion
   C) Profuse sweating and flushed skin
   D) Elevated maternal HR

3. Which of the following statements about exercise prescription for children (age 6–17 yr) is correct?
   A) Children have a better tolerance for heat and humidity during heavy exercise.
   B) Resistance exercise is recommended for ≥3 days per week.
   C) Treadmill and cycle ergometry are poor modes of exercise when fitness testing children.
   D) Children are less physically active than their adult counterparts.

4. Which of the following is *not* an absolute aerobic exercise contraindication during pregnancy?
   A) Preeclampsia
   B) Restrictive lung disease
   C) Persistent third trimester bleeding
   D) Poorly controlled hyperthyroidism

5. Which of the following conditions refers to the loss of skeletal muscle mass typically observed with aging?
   A) Osteopenia
   B) Osteoporosis
   C) Sarcopenia
   D) Scoliosis

6. Which of the following statements about older adults and exercise is correct?
   A) Age may be accompanied by deconditioning and disease.
   B) Age predisposes the older adult to clinical depression and neurologic diseases.
   C) The older adult cannot be physically stressed beyond 75% of age-adjusted maximum HR.
   D) The older adult is not as motivated to exercise as a younger person.

7. Which of the following is a result of an older person participating in an exercise program?
   A) Overall improvement in the quality of life and increased independence
   B) No changes in the quality of life but an increase in longevity
   C) Increased longevity but a loss of bone mass
   D) Loss of bone mass with a concomitant increase in bone density

8. Older adults who have a mobility disability or are at increased risk for falls should incorporate neuromuscular exercise at least ____.
   A) $5 \, \text{d} \cdot \text{wk}^{-1}$
   B) $1-2 \, \text{d} \cdot \text{wk}^{-1}$
   C) $2-3 \, \text{d} \cdot \text{wk}^{-1}$
   D) $7 \, \text{d} \cdot \text{wk}^{-1}$

9. Uncoordinated gait, headache, dizziness, vomiting, and elevated body temperature are signs and symptoms of ____.

   A) acute exposure to the cold
   B) hypothermia
   C) heat exhaustion and heat stroke
   D) acute altitude sickness

10. Which physiologic response(s) would be expected to occur under conditions of high ambient temperature?
    A) Decreased maximal oxygen uptake
    B) Decreased HR at rest
    C) Increased HR at submaximal workload
    D) Decreased maximal HR

11. Which of the following is *not* a sign of exertional heat stroke?
    A) Hypoventilation
    B) Disorientation
    C) Hyperventilation
    D) Vomiting

B. SELECT EXERCISE MODALITIES TO ACHIEVE THE DESIRED ADAPTATIONS BASED ON THE CLIENT'S GOALS, MEDICAL HISTORY, AND ASSESSMENT RESULTS

Domain II Subdomain B: What You Need to know

- Selecting exercises and training modalities based on client's age, functional capacity, and exercise test results
- The principles of specificity and program progression
- The advantages, disadvantages, and applications of interval, continuous, and circuit training programs for cardiovascular fitness improvements
- Activities of daily living and their role in the overall health and fitness of the client
- Differences between physical activity recommendations and training principles for general health benefits, weight management, fitness improvements, and athletic performance enhancement
- Advanced resistance training programming (*e.g.*, super sets, Olympic lifting, plyometric exercises, pyramid training)
- The six motor skill-related physical fitness components: agility, balance, coordination, reaction time, speed, and power
- The benefits, risks, and contraindications for a wide variety of resistance training exercises specific to individual muscle groups (*e.g.*, for rectus abdominis, performing crunches, supine leg raises, and plank exercises)
- The benefits, risks, and contraindications for a wide variety of ROM exercises (*e.g.*, dynamic and passive stretching, Tai Chi, Pilates, yoga, proprioceptive neuromuscular facilitation, partner stretching)
- The benefits, risks, and contraindications for a wide variety of cardiovascular training exercises and applications based on client experience, skill level, current fitness level, and goals (*e.g.*, walking, jogging, running)

Domain II Subdomain B: Multiple Choice Questions

1. Which of the following fitness parameters is *not* specifically associated with motor- or skill-related physical fitness?
   A) Coordination
   B) Strength
   C) Power
   D) Speed

2. Suppose you observe a patron at your gym seated in front of a sit-and-reach box. In an effort to reach as far as possible, she reaches for the marker with multiple short, forward-jabbing stretches. This type of movement is most associated with ___ stretching.
   A) static
   B) passive
   C) tonal
   D) ballistic

C. DETERMINE INITIAL FREQUENCY, INTENSITY, TIME, TYPE, VOLUME, AND PROGRESSION (*i.e.*, FITT-VP PRINCIPLE) OF EXERCISE BASED ON THE CLIENT'S GOALS, MEDICAL HISTORY, AND ASSESSMENT RESULTS

Domain II Subdomain C: What You Need to Know

- The recommended FITT-VP principle for physical activity for cardiovascular and musculoskeletal fitness in healthy adults, older adults, children, adolescents, and pregnant women
- The recommended FITT-VP principle for development of cardiovascular and musculoskeletal fitness in clients with stable chronic diseases who are medically cleared for exercise
- Exercise modifications for those with physical and intellectual limitations (*e.g.*, injury rehabilitation, neuromuscular and postural limitations)
- Implementation of the components of an exercise training session (*e.g.*, warm-up, conditioning, cool down, stretching)
- Application of biomechanics and exercises associated with movements of the major muscle groups (*i.e.*, seated knee extension: quadriceps)

- Establishing and monitoring levels of exercise intensity, including HR, RPE, pace, maximum oxygen consumption, and/or metabolic equivalents
- Determining target/training HRs using predicted maximum HR and the HRR method (Karvonen formula) with recommended intensity percentages based on client fitness level, medical considerations, and goals
- Periodization for cardiovascular, resistance training, and conditioning program design and progression of exercises
- Repetitions, sets, load, and rest periods necessary for desired goals
- Using results from repetition maximum tests to determine resistance training loads

Domain II Subdomain C: Multiple Choice Questions

1. Which of the following components of the exercise prescription work inversely with each other?
   A) Intensity and duration
   B) Mode and intensity
   C) Mode and duration
   D) Mode and frequency

2. When using the original (6–20) Borg scale to estimate exercise intensity, a range of ___ is commonly associated with "moderate" exercise intensity.
   A) 10–11
   B) 12–13
   C) 14–16
   D) 17–19

3. Which of the following examples is correct regarding appropriate sequencing of resistance exercises?
   A) Perform exercises for strong areas before those for weak areas.
   B) Perform least intense exercises prior to most intense exercises.
   C) Perform small muscle group exercises prior to large group exercises.
   D) Perform multijoint exercises prior to single-joint exercises.

D. REVIEW THE PROPOSED PROGRAM WITH THE CLIENT, DEMONSTRATE EXERCISES, AND TEACH THE CLIENT HOW TO PERFORM EACH EXERCISE

Domain II Subdomain D: What You Need to Know

- Adaptations to strength, functional capacity, and motor skills
- The physiological effects of the Valsalva maneuver and the associated risks
- The biomechanical principles for the performance of common physical activities (*e.g.*, walking, running, swimming, cycling, resistance training, yoga, Pilates, functional training)
- The concept of detraining or reversibility of conditioning and effects on fitness and functional performance
- Signs and symptoms of overreaching/overtraining
- Modifying exercise form and/or technique to reduce musculoskeletal injury
- Exercise attire for specific activities, environments, and conditions (*e.g.*, footwear, layering for cold, light colors in heat)
- Communication techniques for effective teaching with awareness of visual, auditory, and kinesthetic learning styles.
- Demonstrating exercises designed to enhance cardiovascular endurance, muscular strength and endurance, balance, and ROM
- Demonstrating exercises for improving ROM of major joints
- Demonstrating a wide range of resistance training modalities and activities (*e.g.*, variable resistance devices, dynamic constant external resistance devices, kettlebells, static resistance devices)
- Demonstrating a wide variety of functional training exercises (*e.g.*, stability balls, balance boards, resistance bands, medicine balls, foam rollers)
- Proper spotting positions and techniques for injury prevention and exercise assistance

Domain II Subdomain D: Multiple Choice Questions

1. Attempting to decrease sweating via clothing insulation adjustments and use of clothing vents are recommended during exercise in what type of environment?

   A) High-altitude environment
   B) Cold weather environment
   C) Dry-heat environment
   D) Wet environment

E. MONITOR THE CLIENT'S TECHNIQUE AND RESPONSE TO EXERCISE, PROVIDING MODIFICATIONS AS NECESSARY

Domain II Subdomain E: What You Need to Know

- Normal and abnormal responses to exercise and criteria for termination of exercise (*e.g.*, shortness of breath, joint pain, dizziness, abnormal HR response)
- Proper and improper form and technique while using cardiovascular conditioning equipment (*e.g.*, stair-climbers, stationary cycles, treadmills, elliptical trainers)
- Proper and improper form and technique while performing resistance exercises (*e.g.*, resistance machines, stability balls, free weights, resistance bands, calisthenics/body weight)
- Proper and improper form and technique while performing flexibility exercises (*e.g.*, static stretching, dynamic stretching, partner stretching)
- Interpreting client comprehension and body language during exercise
- Effective communication, including active listening, cuing, and providing constructive feedback during and after exercise

Domain II Subdomain E: Multiple Choice Questions

1. A transient deficiency of blood flow to the myocardium resulting from an imbalance between oxygen demand and oxygen supply is known as ____.

   A) infarction
   B) angina
   C) ischemia
   D) thrombosis

2. Which of the following types of flexibility training involves alternating contraction and relaxation of a muscle group to improve joint ROM?
   A) Ballistic stretching
   B) Myofascial release
   C) Static stretching
   D) Proprioceptive neuromuscular facilitation

3. Nodding your head, clarifying what your client has told you, and making eye contact are all examples of _____.
   A) active listening
   B) appreciative inquiry
   C) rapport development
   D) motivational interviewing

F. RECOMMEND EXERCISE PROGRESSIONS TO IMPROVE OR MAINTAIN THE CLIENT'S FITNESS LEVEL

Domain II Subdomain F: What You Need to Know

- Exercises and program modifications for healthy adults, older adults, children, adolescents, and pregnant women
- Exercises and program modifications for clients with chronic disease who are medically cleared to exercise (*e.g.*, stable coronary artery disease, other CVDs, diabetes mellitus, obesity, metabolic syndrome, hypertension, arthritis, chronic back pain, osteoporosis, chronic pulmonary disease, chronic pain)

- Principles of progressive overload, specificity, and program progression
- Progression of exercises for major muscle groups (*e.g.*, standing lunge to walking lunge to walking lunge with resistance)
- Modifications to periodized conditioning programs to increase or maintain muscular strength and/or endurance, hypertrophy, power, cardiovascular endurance, balance, and ROM/flexibility

Domain II Subdomain F: Multiple Choice Questions

1. Limited flexibility of which of the following muscle groups increases the risk of low back pain?
   A) Quadriceps
   B) Hamstrings
   C) Hip flexors
   D) Gluteus maximus

2. For obese individuals, exercise programming is associated with
   A) reductions in lean body mass.
   B) increased sedentary behavior.
   C) decreased caloric expenditure.
   D) improved metabolic profile.

G. OBTAIN CLIENT FEEDBACK TO ENSURE EXERCISE PROGRAM SATISFACTION AND ADHERENCE

Domain II Subdomain G: What You Need to Know

- Effective techniques for program evaluation and client satisfaction (*e.g.*, survey, written follow-up, verbal feedback)

- Client goals and appropriate review and modification

Domain II Subdomain G: Multiple Choice Questions

For this subdomain, multiple choice questions for Domain II
Subdomains A-F should be reviewed.

DOMAIN III: EXERCISE LEADERSHIP AND CLIENT EDUCATION

A. OPTIMIZE PARTICIPANT ADHERENCE BY USING EFFECTIVE COMMUNICATION, MOTIVATIONAL TECHNIQUES, AND BEHAVIORAL STRATEGIES

Domain III Subdomain A: What You Need to Know

- Verbal and nonverbal behaviors that communicate positive reinforcement and encouragement (*e.g.*, eye contact, targeted praise, empathy)
- Learning preferences (auditory, visual, kinesthetic) and how to apply teaching and training techniques to optimize training session
- Applying health behavior change models (*e.g.*, socioecological model, readiness to change model, SCT, theory of planned behavior) and strategies that support and facilitate adherence
- Barriers to exercise adherence and compliance (*e.g.*, time management, injury, fear, lack of knowledge, weather)
- Techniques to facilitate intrinsic and extrinsic motivation (*e.g.*, goal setting, incentive programs, achievement recognition, social support)
- Strategies to increase nonstructured physical activity (*e.g.*, stair walking, parking farther away, biking to work)
- Health coaching principles and lifestyle management techniques related to behavior change
- Leadership techniques and educational methods to increase client engagement
- Applying active listening techniques
- Using feedback to optimize a client's training sessions
- Effective and timely uses of a variety of communication modes (*e.g.*, telephone, newsletters, email, social media)

Domain III Subdomain A: Multiple Choice Questions

1. According to sources cited in the 11th edition of the *ACSM's Guidelines for Exercise Testing and Prescription*, what model or theory can be applied if a client says, "There's nowhere for me to exercise," which is a common barrier to exercise?
   A) Health belief model
   B) Transtheoretical model
   C) Social ecological model
   D) SCT

2. Which of the following is an example of a biological barrier to exercise?
   A) Obesity
   B) Pregnancy
   C) Disease
   D) Injury

B. EDUCATE CLIENTS USING SCIENTIFICALLY SOUND RESOURCES

Domain III Subdomain B: What You Need to Know

- Influential lifestyle factors, including nutrition and physical activity habits
- The value of carbohydrates, fats, and proteins as fuels for exercise and physical activity
- The following terms: body composition, BMI, lean body mass, anorexia nervosa, bulimia nervosa, and body fat distribution
- The relationship between body composition and health
- The effectiveness of diet, exercise, and behavior modification as a method for modifying body composition
- The importance of maintaining hydration before, during and after exercise
- Dietary Guidelines for Americans
- The female athlete triad
- The myths and consequences associated with various weight loss methods (*e.g.*, fad diets, dietary supplements, overexercising, starvation diets)
- The number of kilocalories in 1 g of carbohydrate, fat, protein, and alcohol
- Industry guidelines for caloric intake for individuals desiring to lose or gain weight
- Accessing and disseminating scientifically based, relevant, fitness- and wellness-related resources and information

- Community-based exercise programs that provide social support and structured activities (*e.g.*, walking clubs, intramural sports, golf leagues, cycling clubs)

- Stress management and relaxation techniques (*e.g.*, progressive relaxation, guided imagery, massage therapy)

Domain III Subdomain B: Multiple Choice Questions

1. Calcium, phosphorus, magnesium, potassium, sulfur, sodium, and chloride are examples of ____.
   A) macrominerals
   B) microminerals
   C) proteins
   D) vitamins

2. Vitamins ___ and ___ can be manufactured by the body.
   A) E, K
   B) A, E
   C) C, D
   D) D, K

3. Hyponatremia is best defined as an
   A) imbalance of sodium and potassium caused by profuse sweating.
   B) excess of total body sodium that comes about because of exercise in the heat.
   C) underconsumption of water during exercise in any environmental condition.
   D) excess of total body water relative to total body sodium content.

4. Which of the following represents more than 90% of the fat stored in the body?
   A) Phospholipids
   B) Cholesterol
   C) Triglycerides
   D) Free fatty acids

5. How many kilocalories are contained in an "energy bar" that contains 5 g of fat, 30 g of carbohydrates (including 4 g of insoluble fiber), and 3 g of protein?
   A) 161 kcal
   B) 168 kcal
   C) 177 kcal
   D) 193 kcal

6. Which of the following is *not* an example of social support?
   A) Encouragement from a friend to join their walking group
   B) A family member requesting to join you on your daily walks
   C) Spouses synchronizing schedules so they can attend the same group fitness classes
   D) A friend inquiring why you have not been in exercise class lately

DOMAIN IV: LEGAL AND PROFESSIONAL RESPONSIBILITIES

A. COLLABORATE WITH HEALTH CARE PROFESSIONALS AND ORGANIZATIONS TO CREATE A NETWORK OF PROVIDERS WHO CAN ASSIST IN MAXIMIZING THE BENEFITS AND MINIMIZING THE RISK OF AN EXERCISE PROGRAM

Domain IV Subdomain A: What You Need to Know

- Reputable professional resources and referral sources to ensure client safety and program effectiveness
- The scope of practice for the Certified Personal Trainer and the need to practice within this scope
- Effective and professional communication with allied health and fitness professionals

- Identifying individuals requiring referral to a physician or allied health services (*e.g.*, physical therapy, dietary counseling, stress management, weight management, psychological and social services)

Domain IV Subdomain A: Multiple Choice Questions

1. Which of the following is *not* within the scope of practice of an ACSM Certified Personal Trainer?

    A) Determination of current level of client fitness through fitness assessment and testing

    B) Aiding clients in setting realistic goals

    C) Development of client exercise prescription

    D) Providing the client a written detailed dietary plan in conjunction with the exercise prescription

B. DEVELOP A COMPREHENSIVE RISK MANAGEMENT PROGRAM (INCLUDING AN EMERGENCY ACTION PLAN AND INJURY PREVENTION PROGRAM) CONSISTENT WITH INDUSTRY STANDARDS OF CARE

Domain IV Subdomain B: What You Need to Know

- Resources available to obtain basic life support, automated external defibrillator, and cardiopulmonary resuscitation certification
- Emergency procedures (*i.e.*, telephone procedures, written emergency procedures, personnel responsibilities) in a health and fitness setting
- Precautions taken to ensure participant safety (*e.g.*, equipment placement, facility cleanliness, floor surface)
- The following terms related to musculoskeletal injuries (*e.g.*, shin splints, sprain, strain, bursitis, fractures, tendonitis, patellofemoral pain syndrome, low back pain, plantar fasciitis)
- Contraindicated exercises/postures and risks associated with certain exercises (*e.g.*, straight-leg sit-ups, double leg raises, full squats, hurdler's stretch, cervical and lumbar hyperextension, standing bent-over toe touch)
- The responsibilities, limitations, and legal implications for the Certified Personal Trainer of carrying out emergency procedures
- Potential musculoskeletal injuries (*e.g.*, contusions, sprains, strains, fractures), cardiovascular/pulmonary complications (*e.g.*, chest pain, palpitations/arrhythmias, tachycardia, brady-cardia, hypotension/hypertension, hyperventilation), and metabolic abnormalities (*e.g.*, fainting/syncope, hypoglycemia/hyperglycemia, hypothermia/hyperthermia)
- The initial management and basic first-aid procedures for exercise-related injuries (*e.g.*, bleeding, strains/sprains, fractures, shortness of breath, palpitations, hypoglycemia, allergic reactions, fainting/syncope)
- The need for and components of an equipment service plan/agreement
- The need for and use of safety policies and procedures (*e.g.*, incident/accident reports, emergency procedure training) and legal necessity thereof
- The need for and components of an emergency action plan
- Effective communication skills and the ability to inform staff and clients of emergency policies and procedures
- Demonstrating and carrying out emergency procedures during exercise testing and/or training
- Assisting, spotting, and monitoring clients safely and effectively during exercise testing and/or training

Domain IV Subdomain B: Multiple Choice Questions

1. What is the purpose of agreements, releases, and consent forms?

    A) To inform the client of participation risks and outline rights of the client and the facility

    B) To articulate policies associated with litigation that may develop between clients and trainers

    C) To define the relationship between the facility operator and the personal trainer

    D) To ensure that facilities operate within the law and educate clients about such directives

2. Emergency procedures and safety planning should address which of the following?

    A) Metabolic calculations

    B) Common exercise scenarios

    C) Injury prevention

    D) Basic principles for exercise training

3. An important safety consideration for exercise equipment in a fitness center includes ____.
   A) ability of equipment to restrict ROM
   B) flexibility of equipment to allow for different body sizes
   C) affordability of equipment to allow for changing out equipment periodically
   D) mobility of equipment to allow for easy rearrangement

4. For the client with hypertension, ___ should be avoided.
   A) muscle-strengthening exercises that involve low resistance
   B) activities that involve the Valsalva maneuver
   C) emphasis on aerobic activities
   D) consuming antihypertensive medications during exercise testing meant to develop the exercise prescription

C. ADHERE TO ACSM CERTIFICATION'S CODE OF ETHICS BY PRACTICING IN A PROFESSIONAL MANNER WITHIN THE SCOPE OF PRACTICE OF AN ACSM CERTIFIED PERSONAL TRAINER

Domain IV Subdomain C: What You Need to Know

- The components of both the ACSM Code of Ethics and the ACSM Certified Personal Trainer scope of practice
- Appropriate work attire and professional behavior
- Conducting all professional activities within the scope of practice of the ACSM Certified Personal Trainer

Domain IV Subdomain C: Multiple Choice Questions

For this subdomain, multiple choice questions for Domain IV Subdomains A-B should be reviewed.

D. FOLLOW INDUSTRY-ACCEPTED PROFESSIONAL, ETHICAL, AND BUSINESS STANDARDS

Domain IV Subdomain D: What You Need to Know

- Professional liability and potential for negligence in training environments
- Legal issues for licensed and nonlicensed health care professionals providing services, exercise testing, and risk-management strategies
- Equipment maintenance to decrease risk of injury and liability (*e.g.*, maintenance plan, service schedule, safety considerations)

Domain IV Subdomain D: Multiple Choice Questions

1. Suppose that a new client is training at your facility and she injures herself when a dumbbell drops on her face while performing heavy incline presses. For you (the certified trainer) to be held liable for negligence in this case, this client and her attorney must show all of the following elements of negligence *except*
   A) damages.
   B) breach of duty.
   C) causation.
   D) intent.

2. Injury associated with a wet floor in your weight room that you failed to alert patrons about is best termed ___.
   A) "nonfeasance"
   B) "malpractice"
   C) "commission"
   D) "malfeasance"

3. A type of negligence action that involves claims brought against a described professional is referred to as ____.
   A) risk management
   B) liability
   C) malpractice
   D) assumption of risk

E. RESPECT COPYRIGHT LAWS BY OBTAINING PERMISSION BEFORE USING PROTECTED MATERIALS AND ANY FORM OF APPLICABLE INTELLECTUAL PROPERTY

Domain IV Subdomain E: What You Need to Know

- National and international copyright laws
- Referencing nonoriginal work

Domain IV Subdomain E: Multiple Choice Questions

1. Which of the following statements about intellectual property is correct?
   A) Work that you create is protected by copyright the moment that work is produced and made available.
   B) Sending an email copy to yourself of something you wrote is a legal substitute for registering your work with the U.S. Copyright Office.
   C) Registering work with the U.S. Copyright Office is required by law for your work to be protected as intellectual property.
   D) Work that you create in one country is automatically protected by law in another country.

F. SAFEGUARD CLIENT CONFIDENTIALITY AND PRIVACY RIGHTS UNLESS FORMALLY WAIVED OR IN EMERGENCY SITUATIONS

Domain IV Subdomain F: What You Need to Know

- Practices/systems for maintaining client confidentiality
- The importance of client privacy (*i.e.*, client personal safety, legal liability, client credit protection, client medical disclosure)
- The Family Educational Rights and Privacy Act and the Health Insurance Portability and Accountability Act (HIPAA) laws
- Rapidly accessing client emergency contact information

Domain IV Subdomain F: Multiple Choice Questions

1. Which of the following statements about confidentiality is *not* correct?
   A) All records must be kept by the program director/manager under lock and key.
   B) Data must be available to all individuals who need to see it.
   C) Data should be kept on file for at least 1 yr before being discarded.
   D) Sensitive identifying information needs to be protected.

2. Which of the following is *not* true regarding the HIPAA?
   A) The patient must provide written authorization prior to disclosure or use of information by a third party.
   B) It assures the individual will have access to the individual's own personal health information.
   C) Copies of the HIPAA privacy rule do not need to be provided to the individual.
   D) It provides protection of privacy of one's personal health care information.

3. The acronym "HIPAA" stands for _____.
   A) "Health Insurance Privacy and Accountability Association"
   B) "Health Insurance Portability and Accountability Act"
   C) "Health Insurance Privacy and Accountability Act"
   D) "Health Information Portability and Accountability Association"

SECTION 2

ANSWERS TO THE MULTIPLE CHOICE PRACTICE QUESTIONS

DOMAIN I

Domain I Subdomain A: Multiple Choice Answers

1. —D.

   Explanation: The initial client consultation consists of the assessment of health history, completion of relevant informed consent documentation, and fitness assessment(s) to be conducted that may include only simple measures such a resting heart rate and blood pressure. Discussion of goal progression with the client would occur following the exercise prescription and subsequent progression.

2. —A.

   Explanation: The 11th edition of the *ACSM's Guidelines for Exercise Testing and*

   Prescription (Chapter 12) describes motivational interviewing as a person-centered communication where the fitness professional and the client work together to help the client change their behavior. "Change talk" is most associated with the client's desire or reason to change.

3. —B.

   Explanation: The ACSM-CPT Job Task Analysis references email, phone, and text messaging as examples of "multimedia" intended to document and instruct clients in preparation for the initial interview.

Domain I Subdomain B: Multiple Choice Answers

1. —B.

   Explanation: Individual's current physical activity level; presence of signs or symptoms and/or known metabolic, renal, or cardiovascular disease; and exercise intensity at which individual desires to exercise. Please see Chapter 2 of the 11th edition of the *ACSM's Guidelines for Exercise Testing and Prescription* for details on the preparticipation health screen process.

2. —D.

   Explanation: The informed consent document does not provide protection against negligence lawsuits. It provides subjects with opportunities to withdraw from test involvement. More information about informed

   consent can be found in the current edition of the *ACSM's Resources for the Personal Trainer.*

3. —B.

   Explanation: Please refer to the algorithm in Chapter 2, Figure 2.2, of the 11th edition of the *ACSM's Guidelines for Exercise Testing and Prescription*. This individual would be clear to exercise at light- and moderate-intensity activity levels. Note that due to his history (stent placement and diabetes), it is recommended that he pursue medical clearance prior to engaging in vigorous-intensity physical activity.

4. —C.

   Explanation: Informed consent is not a legal document. It does not provide legal immunity to a facility or individual in the event of injury to a client nor does it legally protect the rights of the client. It simply provides evidence that the client was made aware of the purposes, procedures, and risks associated with the test or exercise program. Consent forms do not relieve the facility or individual of the responsibility to do everything possible to ensure the safety of the client. Negligence, improper test administration, inadequate personnel qualifications, and insufficient safety procedures all are items that are not expressly covered by informed consent. Because of the limitations associated with informed consent documents, legal counsel should be sought during the development of the document.

5. —D.

Explanation: Different types of health screenings are used for various purposes. In commercial settings, clients should be screened more extensively for potential health risks. At minimum, a personal medical history should be taken.

6. —A.

Explanation: Medical clearance is recommended for any sedentary individual with signs or symptoms suggestive of cardiovascular, metabolic, or renal disease independent of disease status. Following medical clearance, this individual should begin an exercise program of light-to-moderate intensity exercise, progressing as tolerated following ACSM guidelines.

7. —A.

Explanation: Reinforcement is the positive or negative consequence for performing or not performing a behavior. Positive consequences

are rewards that motivate behavior. This can include both intrinsic and extrinsic rewards. Intrinsic rewards are the benefits gained because of the rewarding nature of the activity. Extrinsic or external rewards are the positive outcomes received from others, which may include encouragement and praise or material reinforcements such as T-shirts and money.

8. —C.

Explanation: The health belief model assumes that people will engage in a behavior (such as exercise) when there exist a perceived threat of disease and a belief of susceptibility to that disease. This is true when the disease is severe. This model also incorporates cues to action as critical to adopting and maintaining behavior. The concept of self-efficacy (confidence) is also added to this model. Motivation and environmental considerations are not a part of the health belief model.

9. —C.

Explanation: Characteristics of a good manager or director include designing programs and monitoring their implementation. Directors and managers guide staff or clients through the program. Directors and managers are good communicators who also purchase equipment and supplies and monitor the safety of the program or facility.

10. —B.

Explanation: Fitness professionals have orientation obligations to their clients. Examples include facility introduction and layout explanation as well as equipment familiarization and utilization.

Domain I Subdomain C: Multiple Choice Answers

1. —C.

Explanation: Positive risk factors for this client include age, blood pressure, current smoker, and not regularly physically active. This client is also borderline for obesity. Table 2.2 in the 11th edition of the *ACSM's Guidelines for Exercise Testing and Prescription* lists each of the negative and positive risk factors for cardiovascular disease.

2. —C.

Explanation: An LDL level of <100 mg · dL^{-1} is considered optimal. For details, see Table 2.4 in the 11th edition of the *ACSM's Guidelines for Exercise Testing and Prescription.*

3. —A.

Explanation: Angina pectoris is heart-related chest pain caused by ischemia, which is insufficient blood flow through one or more coronary arteries. Angina-like symptoms often are felt in the chest, neck, shoulder, and/or arm regions of the body.

4. —B.

Explanation: The subdeltoid bursa, supraspinatus muscle, and nerves become impinged between the coracoid and acromion process with shoulder abduction. The resulting pain leads to decreased ROM, disuse, and muscle atrophy. Such impingement of the rotator cuff is common in assembly line workers performing repetitive overhead tasks.

5. —B.

Explanation: Outcomes are designed to measure the success of a program for the client. Outcome studies require quantifiable data that can be analyzed. Such data come from measures that include client satisfaction, level of change, length of time for change to occur, or percentage of clients who reach their goals. Outcomes can be very helpful in marketing programs as well as in comparing one facility with another.

6. —C.

Explanation: This client is expressing symptoms suggestive of metabolic, cardiovascular, or pulmonary disease, and medical clearance is needed prior to continuing with an exercise program prescription. Please refer to Chapter 2, Figure 2.2, in the 11th edition of the *ACSM's Guidelines for Exercise Testing and Prescription* for the full preparticipation screening algorithm.

7. —A.

Explanation: Every population that has been studied exhibits a decline in bone mass with aging. Therefore, bone loss is considered by most clinicians to be an inevitable consequence of aging. "Osteoporosis" refers to a condition characterized by a decrease in bone mass and density leading to susceptibility to fracture from minor trauma. Risk factors for age-related bone loss and development of clinical osteoporosis include being an Asian or Caucasian female, having a small skeletal frame, and having a family history of osteoporosis, premature or surgically induced menopause, alcohol abuse, cigarette smoking, sedentary lifestyle, and inadequate dietary calcium intake among others.

8. —D.

Explanation: In the 11th edition of the *ACSM's Guidelines for Exercise Testing and Prescription*, page 37 state that individuals with pulmonary disease are no longer automatically referred for medical clearance because pulmonary disease does not increase the risks of nonfatal or fatal cardiovascular complications in conjunction with exercise.

9. —B.

Explanation: In the 11th edition of the *ACSM's Guidelines for Exercise Testing and Prescription*, Box 4.1 lists eight relative contraindications to symptom-limited maximal exercise testing. Among these is the observance of resting hypertension with SBP >200 mm Hg or DBP >110 mm Hg.

Domain I Subdomain D: Multiple Choice Answers

1. —D.

Explanation: As discussed in the 11th edition of the *ACSM's Guidelines for Exercise Testing and Prescription*, SMART goal setting involve objectives that are specific, measurable, action oriented, realistic, and timely. Note too that the 11th edition of the *ACSM's Guidelines for Exercise Testing and Prescription* also suggests that goals should be self-determined (SMARTS) as well (see Chapter 12).

2. —B.

Explanation: The client is using the pedometer as a measurement device. He is self-monitoring daily steps. Other examples of self-monitoring include maintaining a daily food intake journal, accelerometer use, and tracking workout days in a journal.

3. —D.

Explanation: As described by the American Heart Associated, obligations that include work and other realities of daily life often interfere with plans to be more active. According to the U.S. Centers for Disease Control and Prevention, "social" barriers can be thought of as conditions in which people are born, grow, live, learn, work, and age that factor into health and physical activity decision-making.

4. —B.

Explanation: Social Cognitive Theory (SCT) employs the client's personal experiences, the actions of others, and environmental factors on health behaviors. SCT is particularly reliant on expectations, self-efficacy, reinforcements, and observational learning to achieve behavior change.

5. —C.

Explanation: Factors such as managing body weight and changing appearance extrinsic motivation. Clients in this example are pursuing activities in order to achieve an external result. Intrinsic motivation may include activities that clients pursue they enjoy the internal feeling as though they accomplished a goal or enjoyed participating in an activity. Self-efficacy refers to one's belief that one is capable and able to complete a given task or activity. Self-worth refers to how well a client may perceive that they are accomplishing or performing what was set out to do.

6. —D.

Explanation: What this client is expressing is that she now has a belief that she is able to competently implement the exercises you have taught her on her own. This is an example of self-efficacy. Self-worth better corresponds to how well she perceives herself carrying out the exercises you have taught her, and self-esteem simply refers to how one views themselves overall.

7. —A.

Explanation: Goals are most effective and adhered to when the client is the one to identify and set their own goals. It is the responsibility of the personal trainer to provide the client with the education and tools for success in how to reach those goals and identify potential barriers.

8. —A.

Explanation: As described by the Transtheoretical Model for understanding behavior change in Chapter 12 of the 11th edition of the *ACSM's Guidelines for Exercise Testing and Prescription*, this stage corresponds to "action" because your client has started to implement

changes and has been consistent but for less than 6 months.

Preparation is an individual who is planning for or irregularly exercising, whereas the stage of action represents a person who is currently exercising.

9. —B.

Explanation: Intrinsic rewards are associated with good feelings gained because of the rewarding nature of the activity. Extrinsic or external rewards are the positive outcomes received from others, which may include encouragement and praise or material reinforcements such as a paycheck bonus for wellness program participation.

10. —D.

Explanation: The Transtheoretical Model for understanding behavior change is summarized as follows:

Precontemplation: Client is neither intending on making behavior change nor considering the benefits the change may bring.

Contemplation: Client is weighing the pros and cons of behavior change and is considering implementing changes in <6 months.

Preparation: Client has developed a behavior change plan and intends to implement it within the next month.

Action: Client has been making positive activity and behavior changes for 6 months or less.

Maintenance: Individual is maintaining positive behavior changes for ≥6 months and is working on relapse prevention strategies.

Domain I Subdomain E: Multiple Choice Answers

1. —D.

Explanation: Osteoporosis is a condition in which bones become less dense and more likely to fracture. By contrast, osteoarthritis is a painful, degenerative disease that develops in joints subjected to overuse and high body weight.

2. —C.

Explanation: Hamstring, gracilis, sartorius, popliteus, and gastrocnemius muscle are all major agonist muscles involved in knee flexion.

3. —A.

Explanation: The quadratus lumborum is an agonist muscle involved in lateral flexion of the lumbar spine. The rectus femoris,

sartorius, and iliopsoas are all agonist muscles involved in hip flexion.

4. —C.

Explanation: The body has three cardinal planes and each is perpendicular to the other two. Movement occurs along these planes. The sagittal plane divides the body into right and left parts, and the midsagittal plane is represented by an imaginary vertical plane passing through the midline of the body, dividing it into right and left halves. The frontal plane is represented by an imaginary vertical plane passing through the body, dividing it into front and back halves. The transverse plane represents an imaginary horizontal plane passing through the midsection of the body and dividing it into upper and lower portions.

5. —A.

Explanation: Rotation is the turning of a bone around its longitudinal axis or around another bone. Rotation of the anterior surface of the bone toward the midline of the body is medial rotation whereas rotation of the same bone away from the midline is lateral rotation. Supination is a specialized rotation of the forearm that results in the palm of the hand being turned forward (anteriorly). Pronation is the opposite of supination and constitutes rotation of the forearm that results in the palm of the hand being directed backward (posteriorly).

6. —B.

Explanation: The vertebral column serves as the main axial support for the body. Scoliosis is an abnormal lateral deviation of the vertebral column. Kyphosis is an abnormal increased posterior curvature, especially in the thoracic region. Lordosis is an abnormal, exaggerated anterior curvature in the lumbar region.

7. —A.

Explanation: Regular chronic exercise is associated with decreased resting heart rates, increased cardiac output, increased stroke volume, and a faster heart rate recovery. For the latter adaptation, this means that the exercise heart rate returns to resting values much faster following aerobic-type exercise training.

8. —C.

Explanation: Cardiovascular adaptations to regular "aerobic" exercise include increases to heart size, cardiac output, and red blood cell counts. Resting blood pressure values fall with regular exercise and this is seen as an important benefit to hypertensive clients.

9. —D.

Explanation: Aerobic enzyme activity, capillary density, and lactate recycling all increase in response to chronic resistance training. Resting heart rate tends to decrease with regular "aerobic" exercise but may not necessarily decrease with long-term resistance training.

10. —C.

Explanation: Maximal heart rate does not change with maximal (or, for that matter, submaximal) exercise effort. Resting blood pressure and lactic acid production will decrease over time in response to training. Total lung capacity does not change with regular exercise.

11. —D.

Explanation: The cooldown phase of exercise allows blood to return to the heart and brain instead of pooling in the lower extremities, potentially causing hypotension and dizziness. Maximal heart rate is unchanged by cooldown. Body temperature will decrease in response to cooldown.

12. —D.

Explanation: Water exercise has gained in popularity because the buoyancy properties of water help to reduce the potential for musculoskeletal injury and may even allow injured clients an opportunity to exercise therapeutically. Various activities may be offered in a water-exercise class. Walking, jogging, and dance activity all may be adapted for water. Water-exercise classes typically should combine the benefits of the buoyancy properties of water with the resistive properties of water. In this regard, both an aerobic stimulus as well as activity to enhance muscular strength and endurance may be provided.

13. —A.

Explanation: Overuse injuries become more common when people participate in greater amounts of exercise by increasing time, duration, or intensity too quickly.

14. —A.

Explanation: Plyometric exercise is a method of strength and power training that involves an eccentric loading of muscles and tendons followed immediately by "explosive" concentric actions. This stretch-shortening cycle may allow an enhanced generation of force during the concentric (shortening) phase. Note that the high intensity of plyometrics may increase the risk for musculoskeletal injury in novices.

15. —D.

Explanation: Within skeletal muscle fibers, the endoplasmic (sarcoplasmic) reticulum is particularly well developed so that it can store large amounts of calcium. When the motor neuron excites the membrane (sarcolemma) of the fiber, calcium is released from the sarcoplasmic reticulum to bind to troponin.

16. —B.

Explanation:

Blood Pressure Categories

Blood Pressure Category	Systolic, mm Hg (upper number)		Diastolic, mm Hg (lower number)
Normal	<120	and	<80
Elevated	120-129	and	<80
High blood pressure (hypertension), stage 1	130-139	or	80-89
High blood pressure (hypertension) stage 2	140 or higher	or	90 or higher
Hypertensive crisis (consult your doctor immediately)	>180	and/or	>120

Source: American Heart Association https://www.heart.org/en/health-topics/high-blood-pressure/understanding-blood-pressure-readings

17. —A.

Explanation: Isometric (static) action is when a muscle attempts to shorten under load but is unable to overcome the resistance. Dynamic muscle actions encompass both concentric (muscle shortening under load) and eccentric (muscle lengthening under load) muscle actions.

18. —D.

Explanation: The half-squat wall-sit exercise is an example of an isometric exercise because skeletal muscle is developing tension in an effort to hold position without any movement. Biceps curls, pull-ups, and box squat jumps are all isotonic (dynamic) exercises involving both concentric and eccentric muscle actions.

19. —D.

Explanation: Rotator cuff muscles can be remembered using the "SITS" acronym. These muscles include the <u>s</u>ubscapularis, <u>i</u>nfraspinatus, <u>t</u>eres minor, and <u>s</u>upraspinatus muscles.

20. —A.

Explanation: Joints in the body can be classified from both structural and functional perspectives. Structural classifications include fibrous, cartilaginous, and synovial. Functional classifications include synarthrodial, amphiarthrodial, and diarthrodial. Synovial, diarthrodial joints are the most common joints in the human body.

21. —C.

Explanation: After 30 yrs of age, skeletal muscle strength begins to decline. However, the loss of strength is not linear, with most of the decline occurring after age 50. By 80, strength loss usually is in the range of 30%–40%. The loss of strength with aging is thought to occur mainly from a loss of muscle mass.

22. —B.

Explanation: At any given intensity, HR will be lower during swimming than exercise performed in a standing position, such as running, because of postural differences and gravity.

23. —D.

Explanation: BMI = weight (kg)/height (m)^2
Note that there are 2.2046 pounds to a kilogram and 2.54 centimeters to an inch.
Health Risk Classification According to Body Mass Index (BMI)

Classification	BMI Category (kg/m^2)	Risk of developing health problems
Underweight	<18.5	Increased
Normal Weight	18.5-24.9	Least
Overweight	25.0-29.9	Increased
Obese class I	30.0-34.9	High
Obese class II	35.0-39.9	Very high
Obese class III	≥40.0	Extremely high

Note: For persons 65 yrs and older, the "normal" range may begin slightly above BMI 18.5 and extend into the "overweight" range. Source: Health Canada. Canadian Guidelines for Body Weight Classification in Adults. Ottawa: Minister of Public Works and Government Services Canada; 2003. (https://www.canada.ca/en/health-canada/services/food-nutrition/healthy-eating/healthy-weights/canadian-guidelines-body-weight-classification-adults/body-mass-index-nomogram.html)

24. —C.

Explanation: BMI = weight (kg)/height (m)^2
Note that there are 2.2046 pounds to a kilogram and 2.54 centimeters to an inch.
Health Risk Classification According to Body Mass Index (BMI)

Classification	BMI Category (kg/m^2)	Risk of developing health problems
Underweight	<18.5	Increased
Normal Weight	18.5–24.9	Least
Overweight	25.0–29.9	Increased
Obese class I	30.0–34.9	High
Obese class II	35.0–39.9	Very high
Obese class III	≥40.0	Extremely high

Note: For persons 65 yrs and older, the "normal" range may begin slightly above BMI 18.5 and extend into the "overweight" range. Source: Health Canada. Canadian Guidelines for Body Weight Classification in Adults. Ottawa: Minister of Public Works and Government Services Canada; 2003. (https://www.canada.ca/en/health-canada/services/food-nutrition/healthy-eating/healthy-weights/canadian-guidelines-body-weight-classification-adults/body-mass-index-nomogram.html)

25. —A.

Explanation: Although the threshold for "endurance" is somewhat arbitrary, it is helpful to think about the primary energy system of the body being used to do the work of interest. Longer duration physical activity makes primary use of the oxidative system for ATP utilization. The remaining three answers in this question exemplify exercises that would be reliant on the phosphagen and/or glycolytic systems for energy.

26. —B.

Explanation: See Figure 2.1.

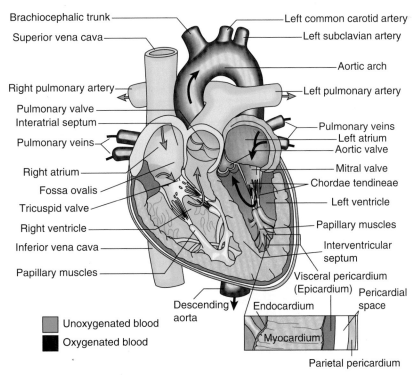

Figure 2.1 Anatomy of the heart and direction of blood flow. From Smeltzer SCO, Bare BG. *Brunner and Suddarth's Textbook of Medical–Surgical Nursing.* 9th ed. Philadelphia, PA: Lippincott Williams & Wilkins; 2002, with permission.

DOMAIN II

Domain II Subdomain A: Multiple Choice Answers

1. —A.

   Explanation: RPE (and the talk test) are both appropriate measures of exercise intensity for the pregnant individual. HR at rest and during maximal exertion can vary greatly over the course of a pregnancy and should not be used in as a method of monitoring exercise intensity.

2. —B.

   Explanation: Exercise should be stopped and medical counsel should be pursued if any of the following signs or symptoms are present: dyspnea prior to exertion, dizziness, vaginal bleeding, headache, muscle weakness, chest pain, preterm labor, calf pain or swelling, detection of decreased fetal movement, or amniotic fluid leakage.

3. —B.

   Explanation: Children have immature thermoregulatory systems and have a lower tolerance for heat and humidity during heavy exercise. Treadmill and cycle ergometry are appropriate modes of exercise when fitness testing children bearing in mind the cycle ergometry are less risky for injury, provided that the equipment is sized appropriately. Children are more physically active than their adult counterparts though it should be noted that most children who are 10 yrs of age or older do not meet most physical activity recommendations.

4. —D.

   Explanation: As listed in Box 6.3 of the 11th edition of the *ACSM's Guidelines for Exercise Testing and Prescription*, absolute contraindications for exercise during pregnancy include preeclampsia, restrictive lung disease, and persistent third trimester bleeding. Poorly controlled hyperthyroidism is classified as a relative contraindication.

5. —C.

   Explanation: Sarcopenia corresponds to an age-related, involuntary loss of skeletal muscle mass and strength. Osteopenia and osteoporosis pertain to reduced bone mineral density and fracture risk. Scoliosis is an abnormal lateral curvature of the spine often first seen during childhood or early adolescence.

6. —A.

   Explanation: Age is often accompanied by deconditioning and illness and these factors must be taken into consideration during fitness testing. Adaptations to specific workloads are often prolonged in older adults (a prolonged warm-up followed by small increments in workload is recommended).

7. —A.

   Explanation: Most older adults are not sufficiently active. This population can benefit greatly from regular participation in a well-designed exercise program. Benefits of such a program include increased fitness, improved health status (reduction in risk factors associated with various diseases), increased independence, and overall improvement in the quality of life.

8. —C.

   Explanation: Individuals who are at increased risk for falls or have a mobility disability are encouraged to participate in at least $2–3 \text{ d} \cdot \text{wk}^{-1}$ of exercise meant to improve muscular fitness.

9. —C.

   Explanation: Heat exhaustion and heat stroke are serious conditions that result from a combination of the metabolic heat generated from exercise accompanied by dehydration and electrolyte loss from sweating. Signs and symptoms include uncoordinated gait, headache, dizziness, vomiting, and elevated body temperature. If these conditions are present, exercise must be stopped. Attempts to rehydrate, perhaps intravenously, should be attempted, and the body must be cooled by any means possible. Victims should be placed in the supine position with the feet elevated.

10. —C.

    Explanation: Compared with a cool and dry environment, a higher metabolic cost exists at submaximal workloads when exercising in the heat and humidity. Thus, the exercise prescription should be altered by lowering the work intensity.

11. —A.

Explanation: Hypoventilation is an indication of heat syncope. Exertional heat stroke signs and symptoms include disorientation, dizziness, irrational behavior, apathy, headache, nausea, vomiting, hyperventilation, and wet skin.

Domain II Subdomain B: Multiple Choice Answers

1. —B.

Explanation: As listed in Box 1.1 of the 11th edition of the *ACSM's Guidelines for Exercise Testing and Prescription*, skill-related components of physical fitness include agility, balance, coordination, power, reaction time, and speed. Strength is most associated with health-related physical fitness.

2. —D.

Explanation: Ballistic stretching is a type of dynamic stretching associated with quick, low range of motion movements that increase risk for injury. Although many movements in sport practice and competition involve ballistic-type stretching, this type of stretching is generally not recommended over safer methods when flexibility fitness is part of exercise testing and prescription.

Domain II Subdomain C: Multiple Choice Answers

1. —A.

Explanation: Intensity and duration of exercise must be considered together and are inversely related. Similar improvements in aerobic fitness may be realized if a person exercises at a low intensity for a longer duration or at a higher intensity for less time.

2. —B.

Explanation: Once the fitness professional establishes a relationship between the client's exercise heart rate and the client's Borg RPE or "rating of perceived exertion," the RPE can stand in as an indicator of exercise intensity. The RPE is particularly useful when participants are incapable of monitoring their pulse accurately or when medications such as β-blockers alter the heart rate response to exercise.

3. —D.

Explanation: In general, exercising large muscle groups and performing multijoint exercises before working smaller muscle groups and employing single-joint exercises are recommended to manage fatigue. Clients will better manage heavy weights and more complex movements when sequencing resistance training exercises from large muscle groups to small or multi- to single-joint movements. Note that there may be good reasons to reverse this pattern (such as in rehabilitation) so fitness professionals should first consider the goals and needs of the client when sequencing a workout.

Domain II Subdomain D: Multiple Choice Answers

1. —B.

Explanation: To better insulate against colder temperatures, multiple light layers should be worn instead of one heavy layer. Multiple layers allow body heat generated during activity to be trapped between the layers of insulation. Clothing vents allow the body to dissipate heat from sweating and not to wet the clothing.

Domain II Subdomain E: Multiple Choice Answers

1. —C.

Explanation: Myocardial ischemia occurs when blood oxygen supply does not meet tissue oxygen demand. This comes about because of decreased blood flow to the myocardium. Atherosclerotic lesions reducing blood flow or coronary artery spasm angina (chest pain) or myocardial infarction (heart attack).

2. —D.

Explanation: Myofascial release makes use of devices such as a foam rollers to alleviate tension and improve joint range of motion by helping to relax the fascia or connective tissue that contains skeletal muscle. Ballistic stretching involves bouncing movements and is typically not recommended for improving joint flexibility. Static stretching involves performing a stretch and holding that position. Static stretches can be performed actively (by the client) or passively (with the help of a trainer). Proprioceptive neuromuscular facilitation (PNF) incorporates alternating contraction and relaxation of a muscle group to stimulate "autogenic inhibition," which is a neuromuscular adaptation leading to improved joint range of motion. PNF techniques are often performed actively and passively.

3. —A.

Explanation: Other examples of active listening include restating, repeating, and summarizing information your client has discussed with you.

Domain II Subdomain F: Multiple Choice Answers

1. —B.

Explanation: An adequate joint range of motion is requisite for optimal musculoskeletal health. Specifically, limited flexibility of the low back and hamstring regions may relate to an increased risk for development of chronic low back pain and disability. Activities that will enhance or maintain musculoskeletal flexibility should be included as a part of a comprehensive preventive or rehabilitative exercise program.

2. —D.

Explanation: One dimension of physical fitness is "physiologic" fitness, which corresponds to a range of body functions that are not necessarily performance related. Physiologic fitness has typically included measures of metabolic fitness that predict a client's risk for developing diabetes and cardiovascular disease. Clinically, these measures include blood work identified as a "comprehensive metabolic panel" that measures glucose, electrolyte levels, and other aspects of liver and kidney function. Regular exercise for lean and obese clients will improve many of these metabolic parameters of physiologic fitness.

DOMAIN III

Domain III Subdomain A: Multiple Choice Answers

1. —C.

Explanation: According to sources cited in the *11th edition of the ACSM's Guidelines for Exercise Testing and Prescription* (Specifically, Table 12.5), social ecological models relate the individual to their environment. By contrast, the health belief model suggests that the prospect of an illness or disease predicts behavior. The transtheoretical model explains decision-making as a continuous cyclical process. The SCT considers social influence and its importance for external and internal social reinforcement.

2. —B.

Explanation: Pregnancy is a biological barrier to exercise, whereas obesity, disease, and injury are all considered physical barriers to exercise.

Domain III Subdomain B: Multiple Choice Answers

1. —A.

Explanation: Minerals are inorganic substances that are necessary for a wide range of body functions. Minerals enable enzymes to catalyze biochemical reactions, help maintain electrical and water balance, facilitate the transmission of nervous system action potentials, and help bring about muscle tension. Minerals are considered to be either <u>macro</u> elements (needed in relatively large doses), such as calcium, phosphorus, magnesium, sodium, potassium, chloride, and sulfur, or <u>micro</u> elements (needed in very small amounts), such as iron, manganese, copper, iodine, zinc, cobalt, fluoride, and selenium.

2. —D.

Explanation: Humans can typically satisfy daily vitamin requirements from the foods we eat. Under normal circumstances, the body can manufacture the fat-soluble vitamins D and K.

3. —D.

Explanation: Hyponatremia is a serious condition associated with blood sodium that is low relative to total body water. Clients with hyponatremia may experience nausea, vomiting, headache, and muscle cramps. Although it is important to be adequately hydrated during exercise, excessive water consumption can generate hyponatremia, which may be life threatening if untreated.

4. —C.

Explanation: Dietary fats include triglycerides, phospholipids, and sterols. About 95% of the fat we eat comes from triglycerides, which subsequently account for 90% of the fat stored in the body.

5. —A.

Explanation: To answer this question, begin by associating carbohydrates with 4 kcal/g, fats with 9 kcal/g, and proteins with 4 kcal/g. By multiplying the respective energy content (kcal) by the quantity (g) of each macronutrient, we can estimate that this "energy bar" has a caloric content of 177 kcal. However, it must be noted that insoluble fiber (in this case, 4 g) is not able to be metabolized by the body for energy. Accordingly, we must subtract 4 g from the carbohydrate content of the bar meaning that there is really only 26 g of carbohydrate (or 104 kcal) in the bar available for energy use by the body. This bar then provides the body with approximately 161 kcal of energy.

6. —D.

Explanation: Encouragement to join a walking group by friends or family and spousal support for fitness class attendance are all examples of social support. If your friend was offering to pick you up and carpool to the exercise class, for example, we would see another example of social support. Simply asking why you are not attending class would not be an example of social support.

DOMAIN IV

Domain IV Subdomain A: Multiple Choice Answers

1. —D.

Explanation: All of the activities listed are within the scope of practice for the American College of Sports Medicine Certified Personal Trainer except for that associated with the development of a diet for the client. Trainers are permitted to talk with clients about healthy foods (such as those associated with current editions of the Dietary Guidelines for Americans). Trainers should also understand (state) laws regarding the practice of dietetics.

Domain IV Subdomain B: Multiple Choice Answers

1. —A.

Explanation: Agreements, releases, and consent documents describe what the client is participating in, the risks involved with that participation, and rights of the client and the facility. If signed by the client, they are accepting some of the responsibility and risk by participating in this program.

2. —C.

Explanation: Injury prevention is often overlooked, but it is an important part of a facility's emergency procedures and safety program. All exercise professionals should understand how to avoid emergencies. Basic principles for exercise training are important for general day-to-day operations but not for emergency procedures.

3. —B.

Explanation: Creating a safe environment in which to exercise is a primary responsibility for any fitness facility. In developing and operating facilities and equipment for use by exercisers, management and staff are obligated to meet a standard of care for exerciser safety. Equipment to be used includes not only testing, cardiovascular, strength, and flexibility pieces but also rehabilitation, pool, locker room, and emergency equipment. Fitness professionals must consider anatomic positioning and abilities to adjust to different body sizes when choosing equipment.

4. —B.

Explanation: For the client with hypertension, muscle-strengthening exercises that involve low resistance and emphasis on aerobic activities should be encouraged. Moreover, it is recommended that clients (continue to) take their usual anti-hypertensive medications during exercise testing when the test is intended to develop the exercise prescription. Hypertensive clients should be discouraged from inhaling and breath-holding during resistance training because doing so can lead to very high blood pressure, dizziness, and/or fainting.

Domain IV Subdomain D: Multiple Choice Answers

1. —D.

   Explanation: For the trainer to be held liable for negligence, the plaintiff must show four elements that include legal duty (a standard of care that the trainer owed the client), breach of duty (an error the trainer made), causation (proof the error made by the trainer caused the client harm), and damages (injury). Negligence is described as "unintentional". To establish negligence, the plaintiff would not have to prove that the trainer intended to harm her.

2. —A.

   Explanation: Injury associated with a wet floor in your weight room that you failed to alert patrons about relates to "nonfeasance". Nonfeasance is essentially the failure to fulfill an obligation. Malpractice is most associated with professional skill and some failure to employ that skill or ability correctly.

Malfeasance is worse than nonfeasance because it corresponds to intentional (and possibly unlawful) conduct. Commission corresponds to acting or allowing an individual to perform an act that causes harm. Omission is a failure to act responsibly. Acts of commission and omission exemplify negligence.

3. —C.

   Explanation: Negligence corresponds to a failure to conform to a generally accepted standard or obligation. Risk management is simply the identification of hazards and the implementation of procedures to reduce them. Assumption of risk is acknowledgement by a potential plaintiff to take the risk of injury onto themselves and release a potential defendant from liability. Malpractice is most associated with professional skill and some failure to employ that skill or ability correctly.

Domain IV Subdomain E: Multiple Choice Answers

1. —A.

   Explanation: The U.S. Copyright Office states that work you create is protected by copyright the moment that work is produced and made available. Sending an email copy to yourself of something you wrote is a not a legal substitute for registering your work with the U.S. Copyright Office. Registering work with the U.S. Copyright Office is not required by law for your work

to be protected as intellectual property but registration is required should you want to file an infringement complaint. Work that you create in one country may be protected by law in another country because of international copyright agreements but these relationships are country specific and no guarantee can be made that your work would be protected from infringement.

Domain IV Subdomain F: Multiple Choice Answers

1. —A.

   Explanation: There is no accepted minimal or maximal amount of time that data should be stored. Clearly, however, data must be stored in a confidential (lock-and-key) manner, and discretion must be used when sharing data.

2. —C.

   Explanation: Clients must provide written authorization prior to disclosure or use of health information by a third party. Clients

must be assured that they will have access to their own personal health information and copies of HIPAA rules and the policies that govern the use of health information must be provided to the client on request.

3. —B.

   Explanation: The acronym "HIPAA" stands for the U.S. Health Insurance Portability and Accountability Act of 1996.

SECTION

3

CASE STUDY CHALLENGES

There are five individual case studies in this section: Bill, Mary Lou, Carl, Beatrice, and Henry. This section also includes a sixth case study that covers brief scenarios on legal and professional responsibilities.

CASE STUDY 1: BILL
DOMAIN I: INITIAL CLIENT CONSULTATION AND ASSESSMENT
Author: M. Ryan Richardson, PhD
Author's Certifications: ACSM-EP, EIM2

You have been assigned a new client, Bill (62 years old). Bill would like to begin an exercise program focused on weight loss and becoming more active. During your initial assessment, you find the following:

Height	6 ft 2 in.
Weight	255 lb
Body mass index (BMI)	32.7 kg $\cdot$ m^{-2}
Resting blood pressure (BP)	136/86 mm Hg
Resting heart rate (HR$_{rest}$)	82 bpm
Lipids	High-density lipoprotein (HDL): 47; low-density lipoprotein (LDL): 128; triglycerides: 132 (all mg $\cdot$ dL^{-1})
Fasting blood glucose	114 mg $\cdot$ dL^{-1}
Family history	Bill informs you that his father had a coronary revascularization procedure at the age of 58 years; this procedure is referred to as a coronary artery bypass graft, often referred to as a coronary artery bypass graft. His mother died from cancer at 76 years of age and his younger brother had a myocardial infarction (heart attack) at age 56 years.
Smoking status	Never smoked
Current medications	Lipitor, a statin drug used to treat high-cholesterol Zestril, an angiotensin-converting enzyme (ACE) inhibitor used to treat high BP and heart failure. Prilosec, an antacid drug used to treat heartburn, stomach ulcers, and gastroesophageal reflux disease. Ibuprofen, a nonsteroidal anti-inflammatory drug Bill occasionally takes to treat back and joint pain.
Exercise history and/or sedentary lifestyle	Played golf, using a powered golf cart, two times per week until a back injury 5 years ago; played baseball and football in high school.
Surgeries	Bill had his gallbladder removed 2 years ago. He also had an endoscopic outpatient procedure to treat his stomach ulcer 1 year ago. He reports no orthopedic surgeries or active injuries other than occasional low back pain following activities like yard work.

(Continued)

CASE STUDY 1: BILL (Continued)

Bill is interested in lower-intensity exercise due to joint pain in his lower back and extremities. His stated goal is to lose a minimum of 30 lb. At the conclusion of the initial appointment, you decide on a combination of resistance training using machines and body weight exercises and aerobic exercise on the treadmill and recumbent bicycle. He will also begin a stretching program with a focus on the lower back and extremities.

Bill: Case Study 1 Questions

1. Bill should be characterized as meeting all defining criteria for American College of Sports Medicine (ACSM) risk factors for atherosclerotic cardiovascular disease, <u>except</u> for
   A) hypertension.
   B) obesity.
   C) sedentary lifestyle.
   D) family history.

2. According to his history and goals, your next session would occur when?
   A) Immediately, including high-intensity exercise
   B) Immediately, only for resistance training
   C) After meeting with the dietician
   D) After medical clearance has been obtained

3. Based on Bill's fasting glucose level, he would be classified as
   A) normal.
   B) prediabetic.
   C) hypoglycemic.
   D) diabetic.

4. What would be Bill's estimated maximum HR (using the formula 220—age)?

   A) 145 bpm
   B) 158 bpm
   C) 186 bpm
   D) Cannot be determined

5. Based on Bill's lipid profile, he would be classified as
   A) normal.
   B) hyperlipidemic.
   C) dyslipidemic.
   D) at risk for atherosclerosis.

Suppose now you have reviewed Bill's history and received his informed consent. Medical clearance has been obtained for the possible inclusion of vigorous-intensity exercise. Next, you perform a fitness assessment.

6. Identify appropriate fitness assessments and explain why these are appropriate protocols.

7. Use the Karvonen heart rate reserve (HRR) formula to calculate the training HR range for Bill during his initial training phase for aerobic exercise. Discuss the reasoning for choosing this training range.

CASE STUDY 2: MARY LOU
DOMAIN II: EXERCISE PROGRAMMING AND IMPLEMENTATION
Author: Brittany C. Montes, MSH
Author's Certifications: ACSM-CEP, ACSM-EP, EIM3

Suppose that you are a personal trainer at a local fitness center and have acquired a new client, Mary Lou, a fit young woman and expectant mother currently in her first trimester. She has recently joined your facility and feels that exercising in an environment with other people around would give her peace of mind. She informs you that she was a collegiate cross-country runner and prefers outdoor activity but would like an exercise prescription that includes aerobic, resistance, and balance activities modified for pregnancy.

Mary Lou expresses to you that although she hopes to maintain as much of her fitness as possible throughout her pregnancy, her main goals are to maintain her health and the health of her baby. She enjoys running in the morning with her husband for anywhere between 30 and 45 min (approximately 150–225 min · wk^{-1}) 5 d · wk^{-1} and performs additional full-body resistance training at 40%–60% of her one repetition maximum (1-RM). This has been her exercise routine for the previous 3 years. She hands you the bottom portion of the *PARmed-X for Pregnancy Health Evaluation Form* with her obstetrician's signature and comment reading, "No contraindications." You have the following information:

Age	27
Height	5 ft 7 in. (67 in.)
Weight	130 lb (59.1 kg)
BMI	20.4 kg · m^{-2}
Resting BP	110/60 mm Hg
HR$_{rest}$	62 bpm
LDL cholesterol (LDL-C)	86 mg · dL^{-1}
HDL cholesterol (HDL-C)	89 mg · dL^{-1}
Total cholesterol	175 mg · dL^{-1}
Fasting glucose	90 mg · dL^{-1}
Current medication use	None; daily vitamin supplements

Mary Lou: Case Study 2 Questions

1. Which of the following is an appropriate frequency, intensity, time, and type (FITT) exercise prescription for Mary Lou?
   A) Continue with current aerobic program of moderate-intensity running for 150–225 min · wk^{-1}. Use resistance bands, machines, and body weight exercises in place of free weights and perform high repetition sets (12–15 repetitions) to moderate fatigue at 40%–60% of estimated 1-RM. Include at least 10 min 2–3 d · wk^{-1} of flexibility exercise.
   B) Decrease current aerobic program to a maximum of 150 min · wk^{-1}. Include resistance exercises targeting large muscle groups at a frequency of 3 d · wk^{-1} and intensity of 50%–80% of estimated 1-RM; three sets of 8–10 repetitions using free weights should be performed. Include at least 10 min 2–3 d · wk^{-1} of flexibility exercise.
   C) Continue with current aerobic program of moderate-intensity running for 150–225 min · wk^{-1}. Include resistance exercises targeting large muscle groups at a frequency of 3 d · wk^{-1} and intensity of 50%–80% of estimated 1-RM; three sets of 8–10 repetitions using free weights should be performed. Include at least 10 min 2–3 d · wk^{-1} of flexibility exercise.
   D) Decrease current aerobic program to a maximum of 150 min · wk^{-1}. Use resistance bands, machines, and body weight exercises in place of free weights and perform high repetition sets (12–15 repetitions) to moderate fatigue at 40%–60% of estimated 1-RM. Include at least 10 min 2–3 d · wk^{-1} of flexibility exercise.

2. Which of the following would not be a safe exercise testing assessment for Mary Lou if she has an uncomplicated pregnancy?
   A) Submaximal cycle ergometer testing
   B) Maximal treadmill test using a Bruce protocol
   C) Submaximal treadmill test using a modified Balke protocol
   D) YMCA cycle ergometer protocol

3. All of the following are appropriate exercise modifications during pregnancy for Mary Lou except
   A) swim, cycle, or elliptical trainer if low back pain or joint pain occurs.
   B) transition from using free weights to weight machines and resistance bands.
   C) decrease aerobic activity from moderate–vigorous to light activity only.
   D) run on a treadmill or track instead of a sidewalk.

(Continued)

CASE STUDY 2: MARY LOU (Continued)

4. Which of the following is <u>not</u> an appropriate method of monitoring exercise intensity for Mary Lou?
   A) The talk test
   B) $\%\dot{V}O_2R$ (assuming $\dot{V}O_{2max}$ is estimated)
   C) Rating of perceived exertion
   D) $\%HR_{max}$ (assuming HR_{max} is measured during pregnancy)

5. All of the following are warning signs to terminate exercise during pregnancy <u>except</u>

   A) severe dizziness or headache.
   B) chest pain.
   C) calf pain or swelling.
   D) increased fetal movement.

6. What changes can Mary Lou expect in her fitness level over the duration of her pregnancy?

7. Why is it important that women not perform any exercises in the supine position after the first trimester?

CASE STUDY 3: CARL
DOMAIN II: EXERCISE PROGRAMMING AND IMPLEMENTATION
Author: Peter Ronai, MS, FACSM
Author's Certifications: ACSM-CEP, ACSM-EP, EIM3

Suppose that you are a personal trainer at a corporate fitness center and, Carl, a 50-year-old architect, is a new client who has recently joined your facility. He is seeking his initial fitness evaluation and first workout session. He is 5 ft 7 in. and weighs 220 lb (100 kg). His waist circumference is 40.5 in., and his hip circumference is 37 in. Carl is a nonsmoker with an HR_{rest} of 74 bpm, BP of 132/82 mm Hg, total cholesterol of 200 mg $\cdot$ dL^{-1}, HDL-C of 45 mg $\cdot$ dL^{-1}, LDL-C of 121 mg $\cdot$ dL^{-1}, triglycerides of 170 mg $\cdot$ dL^{-1}, and fasting glucose of 90 mg $\cdot$ dL^{-1}. His father and mother are in their 70s and are apparently healthy.

These are the results of his initial screening and fitness assessment with you:

Predicted $\dot{V}O_{2max}$ YMCA bike test	31.5 mL $\cdot$ kg^{-1} $\cdot$ min^{-1} or 9 metabolic equivalents (METs). Some low back and leg pain at the end of test which he alleviated by standing and gently leaning backward.
Flexibility/sit and reach with a ruler	15 in.; he experienced some low back and leg pain after the test, which he alleviated by standing and gently leaning backward (above average).
1-RM bench/chest press (selectorized machine)	150 lb; 40th percentile (fair).
1-RM leg press (selectorized machine)	300 lb; 35th percentile (below average).
Pull-ups/chin-ups	2 repetitions (poor).
Push-ups	9 repetitions (fair).
ACSM Abdominal Crunch Test	23 repetitions; he experienced some low back and leg pain after the test, alleviated by standing and gently leaning backward (above average).
Surgeries	None; occasional low back pain that his physician has defined as chronic and has cleared him to participate in a comprehensive exercise program.
Contraindications to exercise	None.

During additional preactivity screening, Carl had difficulty holding his extended arms directly overhead without arching his back, pushing his head and neck forward, and flexing at his waist when performing a series of overhead squats. He also seemed to become very knock kneed (genu valgus) during the descent phase of the overhead squat. He also stands with a forward head, rounded shoulders, and an anteriorly tilted pelvis. Carl does not currently have back pain; however, he did have some low back and leg pain after the bike test, sit-and-reach test, and the abdominal crunch test, which was alleviated by standing and gently leaning backward.

Upon discussing his medical history, Carl reports occasionally taking ibuprofen for low back pain. His physician told him that he has slight degeneration of a disc in his low back and metabolic syndrome. He wants him to get in shape and lose weight before he considers placing Carl on medications.

His current activity includes walking his energetic 5-mo-old black Labrador retriever, Midas, for about 2 miles (approximately 40 min) daily, a 3-MET activity. Additionally, he plays seasonal golf and softball, and he used to play three-on-three basketball 2 years ago, an activity he would like to be able to participate in again. He often feels "tired all over" after walking Midas and hopes that a structured exercise routine that combines endurance training and full-body strength training will help him lose weight and stay healthy, making walking Midas easier, improving his golf game, and enabling him to start playing basketball again.

Carl: Case Study 3 Questions

1. Based on Carl's profile, the initial phase of his resistance training program should include the following:
   (Note that rating of perceived exertion values correspond to 10-point scale.)
   A) Training each muscle group for 3–6 sets with 3–5 repetitions at a high intensity of ≥85% of 1-RM per set, with a rest interval of 5 min between sets at an RPE of 8–9.
   B) Training each muscle group for 2 sets with 15–25 repetitions at a low intensity of ≤50% of 1-RM per set, with a rest interval of 1 min between sets at an RPE of 3–4.
   C) Training each muscle group for 2–4 sets with 8–12 repetitions at a moderate-to-high intensity of >60%–80% of 1-RM per set, with a rest interval of 3–5 min between sets at an RPE of 7–8.
   D) Training each muscle group for ≥1 set with 10–15 repetitions at a moderate intensity of 60%–70% of 1-RM per set, with a rest interval of 2–3 min between sets at an RPE of 5–6.

2. During the first 4 wk, Carl's aerobic exercise program should include everything below except
   A) ≥5 d · wk^{-1} at an intensity of 40%–75% of $\dot{V}O_2R$ or HRR.
   B) exercises performed primarily in an upright or standing position.
   C) an initial exercise HR and MET range of approximately 146–170 bpm and 7–7.8 METs, respectively (using the HRR and $\dot{V}O_2R$ methods).

   D) a gradual weekly increase in exercise volume.

3. Carl wants to achieve an exercise volume of 1,000 MET-min · wk^{-1}. How long must each of his aerobic exercise sessions last if he is working at an exercise intensity of 5 METs five times per week? How many kilocalories would he expend at the end of a week if he did this?
   A) 20 min · session^{-1}; equivalent to 831 kcal · wk^{-1}
   B) 40 min · session^{-1}; equivalent to 1,670 kcal · wk^{-1}
   C) 60 min · session^{-1}; equivalent to 2,494 kcal · wk^{-1}
   D) 80 min · session^{-1}; equivalent to 3,325 kcal · wk^{-1}

4. Which initial resistance training workout will best enable Carl to safely enhance his muscle function and perform better during his follow-up fitness assessments?
   A) Bicep curls, triceps pushdowns, knee extensions, chest flys, sit-ups, lateral shoulder raises, front shoulder raises, straight-leg raises and reverse sit-ups, weighted side bends, accompanied by posterior shoulder and standing floor touch stretches
   B) Straight-leg deadlifts, barbell rows, barbell squats, roman chair sit-ups, barbell bench press, bent-over rear shoulder dumbbell raises, standing barbell bicep curls, overhead dumbbell triceps extensions, Russian twists, accompanied by posterior shoulder and standing toe touch stretches

(Continued)

CASE STUDY 3: CARL (Continued)

C) Machine hack squats, prone hamstring curls, seated machine trunk rotation, seated machine back extensions, seated machine scapular rows (cable), standing barbell shoulder press, barbell lunges, lying barbell triceps press, decline barbell press, preacher barbell biceps curl, accompanied by prone trunk rotation and knee hug and supine double knee hug stretches

D) Wall squats, body weight lunges, supine stability ball hamstring curls, standing cable chest press, cable scapular row in standing, machine shoulder press, latissimus dorsi pull-downs, opposite arm-leg raises (bird-dogs) in quadruped position, modified side bridges (side plank) with knees flexed, prone planks from the knees, accompanied by hip flexor and pectoral stretches

5. Carl wants to begin playing competitive three-on-three basketball (approximately an 8-MET activity) as an enjoyable means of attaining some of his goals. His maximal aerobic capacity is approximately 9 METs and his initial training intensity range will be between 60% and 80% of $\dot{V}O_2$ reserve ($\dot{V}O_2R$) or HRR. What is the corresponding MET range for him as he begins his exercise program over the first 4 wks? Is basketball within this range?

A) Between 2.8 and 4.4 METs; no, basketball exceeds his current prescribed intensity range

B) Between 3.8 and 5.4 METs; yes, basketball is within his prescribed intensity range

C) Between 4.8 and 6.4 METs; yes, basketball is within his prescribed intensity range

D) Between 5.8 and 7.4 METs; no, basketball exceeds his current prescribed intensity range

6. In order to avoid dropping out due to busyness, boredom, burnout, and injury, Carl has requested a list of outdoor activities he can do occasionally to substitute and supplement his fitness center exercises. Where can he find a resource to help him locate appropriate physical activities based on effort levels and their corresponding MET levels and kilocalorie expenditure rates?

7. What seems to be Carl's exercise "directional preference" or "movement bias" and how should this guide the development of his comprehensive exercise program?

CASE STUDY 4: BEATRICE
DOMAIN III: EXERCISE LEADERSHIP AND CLIENT EDUCATION
Author: Angela Kvies, BS
Author's Certifications: ACSM-CEP

Beatrice is a 65-year-old female and a new client. At her last appointment, Beatrice's primary care physician reported that she needs to improve her lifestyle choices and recommended that she find a personal trainer to help her get started. You are eager to help her modify her cardiovascular disease risk factors and immediately set up an interview and evaluation.

Beatrice lives alone, near her son and grandson. She used to be very active in her community but has recently stopped attending church and many other activities. She has a history of depression but denies any current symptoms. You ask her about coping techniques when she feels stressed, and she explains that she prays and talks to her friends and family. Over the course of the interview, Beatrice shares that she enjoys social activities. Beatrice's father died of a myocardial infarction when he was 62 years old, but no other family members have had heart problems.

Beatrice reports being inactive for the last few years. She would like to increase her endurance and strength so that she can keep up with her grandson. She has trouble walking long distances due to knee pain but does not report any other orthopedic limitations. She would like to lose some weight but expresses that she becomes very discouraged when she doesn't see immediate results. Beatrice is very resistant to discuss her current nutritional habits and states that she tries to eat low-fat, low-sodium, and low-carbohydrate meals.

Beatrice brought a copy of her most recent blood test with her for your review. She is currently taking medication for high BP and a statin for abnormal cholesterol levels. Her lipid profile reads as follows:

Total cholesterol	143 mg · dL^{-1}
Triglycerides	63 mg · dL^{-1}
HDL-C	46 mg · dL^{-1}
LDL cholesterol (LDL-C)	84 mg · dL^{-1}

Over the course of several visits, her resting BP has ranged between 130/88 and 138/90 mm Hg. She is a nonsmoker, reports not having diabetes, weighs 203 lb, and is 5 ft 2 in. tall. Beatrice has never had a stress test and denies any symptoms of angina or dyspnea with exertion. You have all the necessary clearance to begin an exercise regime with Beatrice.

Beatrice: Case Study 4 Questions

1. What is her weight classification based on her calculated BMI?
   A) Overweight
   B) Class I obesity
   C) Class II obesity
   D) Class III obesity

2. Beatrice would like to lose the minimal amount of weight to achieve a BMI that puts her in the "normal weight" category. Approximately (~) how much weight will she need to lose to achieve this goal?
   A) ~42 lb
   B) ~68 lb
   C) ~75 lb
   D) ~86 lb

3. Beatrice calculated that she has reduced her caloric intake by 200 kcal · d^{-1}. At this rate, with no additional energy expenditure, how many pounds will she lose in 1 wk?
   A) 0.4 lb
   B) 0.6 lb
   C) 0.8 lb
   D) 1.0 lb

4. What would Beatrice's recommended caloric deficit (by combination of diet and exercise) each day need to be in order to meet ACSM's guidelines for weight loss?
   A) 150–300 kcal
   B) 250–500 kcal
   C) 500–1,000 kcal
   D) 750–1,250 kcal

5. Weight loss would be an example of what type of motivation for Beatrice? Keeping up with her grandson would be what type of motivation?
   A) Extrinsic motivation and intrinsic motivation, respectively
   B) Extrinsic motivation and extrinsic motivation, respectively
   C) Intrinsic motivation and intrinsic motivation, respectively
   D) Intrinsic motivation and extrinsic motivation, respectively

6. Beatrice looks at her long-term goals. She expresses to you that she is discouraged by the amount of time it will take her to reach her desired weight loss. She is still resistant to discussing her diet in detail. Describe the motivational strategies you would use to encourage Beatrice and keep her interested in the program.

7. Beatrice is willing enough to exercise at the gym with your guidance two times per week for 1 h. When you discuss additional activity, Beatrice expresses that she tries to exercise at home but often lacks motivation. What alternatives can you give Beatrice for additional physical activity to keep her engaged in the exercise program? What specific guidelines for cardiovascular exercise will you give her?

CASE STUDY 5: HENRY
DOMAIN III: EXERCISE LEADERSHIP AND CLIENT EDUCATION
Author: Melissa Conway-Hartman, MEd, LAT, ATC
Author's Certifications: ACSM-EP, EIM2

Henry is a sedentary 45-year-old male. He ran track in high school and ran recreationally in college, routinely competing in 5K races. He now works at a desk job 40 h · wk^{-1}. He is the father of three boys and has discovered he can no longer keep up with them. He gets winded playing touch football in the park with his friends and family. He wants to run 5K races with his boys who are at the age where they are playing organized sports.

Henry has come to you, his personal trainer, seeking guidance to help him get back in shape and he shares the results of a recent physical examination with you:

Height	6 ft 2 in. (187.9 cm)
Weight	250 lb (113.6 kg)
Percentage body fat	30%
Resting BP	138/86 mm Hg
Blood glucose	111 mg · dL^{-1}
Total cholesterol	209 mg · dL^{-1}
LDL-C	160 mg · dL^{-1}
HDL-C	45 mg · dL^{-1}
Triglycerides	150 mg · dL^{-1}
Three-day dietary recall results	Daily caloric intake: 2,600 kcal Simple or refined carbohydrates: 60% Complex carbohydrates: 40% Protein: 115 g Carbohydrates: 400 g Fat: 60 g He drinks two cups of coffee a day and consumes no alcohol.

Henry: Case Study 5 Questions

1. What is Henry's BMI?
   A) 35.4 kg · m^{-2}
   B) 28.1 kg · m^{-2}
   C) 31.8 kg · m^{-2}
   D) 22.2 kg · m^{-2}

2. What is his BMI classification?
   A) Normal
   B) Underweight
   C) Overweight
   D) Class I obesity

3. You evaluate Henry's readiness to change and according to the transtheoretical model of behavior change, what stage of readiness is Henry currently experiencing?
   A) Action
   B) Preparation
   C) Contemplation
   D) Maintenance

4. In order to help Henry become successful at his behavioral change, what strategy can you use to move Henry to the next stage of readiness?
   A) Make a list of activities Henry likes so he won't get bored with his exercise.
   B) Teach Henry about the benefits of regular exercise.
   C) Emphasize self-liberation by helping Henry make a firm commitment to a goal and a start date.
   D) Have Henry list the places around his home where he can be active (*i.e.*, the park).

5. What is Henry's daily energy intake of carbohydrates, fats, and proteins?
   A) 460 protein, 1,600 carbohydrate, 540 fat
   B) 1,600 protein, 460 carbohydrate, 540 fat
   C) 1,560 carbohydrate, 520 protein, 520 fat
   D) 1,040 carbohydrate, 780 protein, 780 fat

6. According to the socioecological model, the park close to Henry's house is an example of a/an
   A) microsystem.
   B) mesosystem.
   C) exosystem.
   D) macrosystem.

7. Henry sets a long-term goal of losing 20 lb at a rate of 1 lb · wk^{-1}. Assuming he will burn 2,000 kcal through exercise each week and assuming all his weight loss is fat mass, what is his target for daily caloric intake?

A) 2,386 kcal
B) 1,572 kcal
C) 984 kcal
D) 2,466 kcal

8. When examining the information provided by Henry, what barriers might he encounter to achieving his goal? How will you help him overcome those barriers?

9. Setting goals can help clients stay motivated. How will you help Henry set appropriate goals to ensure his success? List specific steps you will take and provide examples of goals you may set.

CASE STUDY 6: LEGAL & PROFESSIONAL RESPONSIBILITIES
DOMAIN IV: LEGAL & PROFESSIONAL RESPONSIBILITIES
Author: Melissa Conway-Hartman, MEd, LAT, ATC
Author's Certifications: ACSM-EP, EIM2

Suppose that you have just been hired as a fitness professional at the new fitness facility in your town. Most of your day is spent as a floor trainer. You orient new members to the facility while assisting current members with workouts, offering fitness advice, and keeping the fitness floor clean and safe. Part of your duty is to recruit new and current members to augment personal training clientele.

Legal & Professional Responsibilities: Case Study 6 Questions

1. During consultation with a new client, you are recording her health history and she tells you she has high BP and high cholesterol. Her doctor wants her to start exercising and that is why she joined the gym. She states her BP is 138/86 mm Hg and her total cholesterol is 220 mg · dL^{-1}. You would like to start her out walking or using the stationary bike and doing light resistance exercises; however, before this can begin, she must have a
   A) medically supervised maximal graded exercise test.
   B) submaximal test with a physician present.
   C) maximal graded exercise test without a physician present.
   D) physician consent form signed for your review.

2. While you are cleaning equipment, you notice a patron performing a lat pull-down by pulling the bar down behind her head and neck. What action should you take in response?
   A) Encourage her to reduce the weight lifted for this technique.
   B) Let her continue and note these exercises on her workout log.
   C) Explain to her that the risks do not outweigh the benefits of this technique.
   D) Suggest using ropes rather than a straightbar to perform lat pull-downs this way.

3. The facility manager has asked for help in promoting the gym to the neighboring communities. You suggest she
   A) use social media exclusively.
   B) put flyers up in the group fitness room.
   C) have the front desk staff greeters hand flyers out to each member.
   D) use direct mail and host a fitness activity in the neighborhood park.

(Continued)

4. A member comes to you and states he has a superior labral tear from anterior to posterior lesion in his right shoulder from years ago that he never had repaired. He wants you to show him exercises to help treat his shoulder. What should you do?
   A) Try to convert him to a client.
   B) Show him the close grip dumbbell bench press exercise but stay away from other free weights.
   C) Refer him to his physician or physical therapist.
   D) Teach him to work his biceps and triceps and not address the glenohumeral joint.

5. While walking on the treadmill, one of the members attempted to remove her sweatshirt without stopping the treadmill. She fell while the belt was still moving and was thrown off the treadmill. As you help her, you discover that she has a few abrasions but nothing serious. She wants to finish her workout. What should you do?
   A) Make her go home and rest for the day.
   B) Write an incident report describing what happened and have her sign it.
   C) Give her a few adhesive bandages and leave her alone.
   D) Try to convert her to be your client.

6. During an initial interview with a client, you review the informed consent form. The purpose of this form is to

A) protect you from any legal action on the part of the client.
B) provide information to the client regarding participation options and risks.
C) prove you are not negligent.
D) open a discussion about assessments.

7. One of the members sustained a grade 2 hamstring strain. Which of the following signs is most associated with this type of strain?
   A) Loss of function
   B) Ecchymosis
   C) More than 70% of fibers torn
   D) Soreness resulting from muscle spasm as opposed to compromised tissue

8. While working with your personal training client, she trips over a weight that was left on the floor. She says she felt a pop in her ankle. On observation, you notice swelling on the lateral aspect. What do you think her injury could be and how would you handle this situation?

9. The facility manager wishes to establish an hourly safety checklist of the fitness floor; this includes the cardio and flexibility areas, group fitness room, and locker rooms. She requests your assistance in completing the checklist. What tasks should be included in this list?

ANSWERS TO THE CASE STUDY CHALLENGES

BILL CASE STUDY 1: ANSWERS

1. —D. Family history

2. —D. After medical clearance has been obtained

3. —B. Prediabetic

4. —B. 158 bpm

5. —C. Dyslipidemic

Resource: Liguori G, senior editor. *ACSM's Guidelines for Exercise Testing and Prescription*. 11th ed. Philadelphia (PA): Wolters Kluwer; 2021.

Notes for Risk Factors (positive):

Age: Yes, he is male ≥45 years of age.

Family history: No, father and brother were older than 55 years of age when they suffer their respective

cardiovascular events.

Cigarette smoking: No, he reports never smoking.

Sedentary lifestyle: Yes, he is not meeting the minimum criteria of 30 min of moderate-intensity physical

activity on at least 3 d of the week during the past 3 months.

Obesity: Yes, based on his current height and weight, his BMI exceeds 30 kg · m^{-2}.

Hypertension: Yes, he currently takes an ACE inhibitor, which is an antihypertensive medication.

Dyslipidemia: Yes, he currently takes a statin medication for his cholesterol.

Prediabetes: Yes, his current fasting glucose meets the criteria for impaired (100–125 mg · dL^{-1}).

Notes for Risk Factors (negative):

HDL: No, his HDL concentration does not meet this criterion (≥60 mg · dL^{-1}).

Bill is asymptomatic but has ≥2 cardiovascular disease risk factors including a history of hypertension that he currently takes an ACE inhibitor to treat. He will require a medical exam prior to vigorous exercise.

Resources: Hargens T, senior editor. *ACSM's Resources for the Personal Trainer*. 6th ed. Philadelphia (PA): Wolters Kluwer; 2021.

Liguori G, senior editor. *ACSM's Guidelines for Exercise Testing and Prescription*. 11th ed. Philadelphia (PA): Wolters Kluwer; 2021.

(Continued)

BILL CASE STUDY 1: ANSWERS (Continued)

6. Following physician clearance, Bill can begin an exercise program. Submaximal tests are appropriate. For estimation of cardiorespiratory fitness, tests may include submaximal cycle ergometer tests (*e.g.*, Åstrand-Ryhming bike test for unconditioned men, YMCA bike test), step tests (*e.g.*, Queens College, 3-min YMCA, Astrand-Rhyming), submaximal treadmill protocols (shown to produce the highest $\dot{V}O_{2peak}$ in individuals with low back pain), and track tests (*e.g.*, 6-min walk, Rockport). For muscular strength assessment, a 10- to 15-RM is recommended for those considered higher risk. Muscular endurance tests may include the push-up or YMCA bench press test, and partial curl-up depending on Bill's back pain. Maximal testing would not be appropriate in a gym setting due to his moderate risk classification

   Resources: Hargens T, senior editor. *ACSM's Resources for the Personal Trainer*. 6th ed. Philadelphia (PA): Wolters Kluwer; 2021.

   Liguori G, senior editor. *ACSM's Guidelines for Exercise Testing and Prescription*. 11th ed. Philadelphia (PA): Wolters Kluwer; 2021.

7. Because Bill is deconditioned with a moderate risk classification, a light-to-moderate range of 30%–40% is appropriate during the initial phase of aerobic training. This range can be beneficial in those who are deconditioned while also addressing the stated long-term goal of weight loss through a lower-intensity exercise program.

   Calculation:

   $HR_{max} = 220 - age$
   Target HR (lower end of range) =
   $\quad [(0.30) \times (HR_{max} - HR_{rest})] + HR_{rest}$
   Target HR (higher end of range) =
   $\quad [(0.40) \times (HR_{max} - HR_{rest})] + HR_{rest}$
   $HR_{max} = 220 - 62$
   Target HR (lower end of range) =
   $\quad [(0.30) \times (158 - 82)] + 82$
   Target HR (higher end of range) =
   $\quad [(0.40) \times (158 - 82)] + 82$

   The initial HR training range for Bill is 105–112 bpm.

   Resources: Hargens T, senior editor. *ACSM's Resources for the Personal Trainer*. 6th ed.

   Philadelphia (PA): Wolters Kluwer; 2021.

   Liguori G, senior editor. *ACSM's Guidelines for Exercise Testing and Prescription*. 11th ed. Philadelphia (PA): Wolters Kluwer; 2021.

MARY LOU CASE STUDY 2: ANSWERS

1. —A. Continue with current aerobic program of moderate-intensity running for $150-225$ min $\cdot$ wk^{-1}. Use resistance bands, machines, and body weight exercises in place of free weights and perform high repetition sets (12–15 repetitions) to moderate fatigue at 40%–60% of estimated 1-RM. Include at least 10 min 2–3 d $\cdot$ wk^{-1} of flexibility exercise

   Resources: Bushman BA, senior editor. *ACSM's Complete Guide to Fitness & Health*. 2nd ed. Champaign (IL):

   Human Kinetics; 2017.

   Liguori G, senior editor. *ACSM's Guidelines for Exercise Testing and Prescription*. 11th ed. Philadelphia (PA): Wolters Kluwer; 2021.

2. —B.

   Resources: Mottola MF, Davenport MH, Brun CR, Inglis SD, Charlesworth S, Sopper MM. $\dot{V}O_{2peak}$ prediction and exercise prescription for pregnant women. Med Sci Sports Exerc. 2006;38(8):1389–95.

Liguori G, senior editor. *ACSM's Guidelines for Exercise Testing and Prescription*. 11th ed. Philadelphia (PA): Wolters Kluwer; 2021.

3. —C. Decrease aerobic activity from moderate–vigorous to light activity only

   Resource: Bushman BA, senior editor. *ACSM's Complete Guide to Fitness & Health*. 2nd ed. Champaign (IL): Human Kinetics; 2017.

4. —D.

   Resource: Hargens T, senior editor. *ACSM's Resources for the Personal Trainer*. 6th ed. Philadelphia (PA): Wolters Kluwer; 2021.

5. —D. Increased fetal movement

   Resources: Hargens T, senior editor. *ACSM's Resources for the Personal Trainer*. 6th ed.

   Philadelphia (PA): Wolters Kluwer; 2021.

   Bushman BA, senior editor. *ACSM's Complete Guide to Fitness & Health*. 2nd ed. Champaign (IL):

   Human Kinetics; 2017.

6. Because Mary Lou is already a very active and healthy young woman and plans to continue her activity throughout her pregnancy, she will preserve much of her aerobic fitness (although it will decrease slightly) and muscle mass and will gain less fat mass. Mary Lou will notice an increase in her HR (due to increased gestational hormones during her first trimester and to maintain BP during second and third trimesters) and that her BP should remain relatively unchanged. Additionally, pregnant women experience a decrease in thermoregulatory control, so you will need to counsel Mary Lou on wearing appropriate attire, maintaining adequate hydration, and refraining from exercising in hot and humid environments. As Mary Lou progresses in her pregnancy, you should address modifications to her exercise prescription regarding her personal discomforts and abilities. You should also discuss the increased caloric need (approximately 300 kcal $\cdot$ d^{-1}) she will experience due to her pregnancy and determine the amount that will cover both this increased caloric need as well as cover the amount of kilocalories expended during her exercise sessions

   Resources: Hargens T, senior editor. *ACSM's Resources for the Personal Trainer*. 6th ed. Philadelphia (PA): Wolters Kluwer; 2021.

   Bushman BA, senior editor. *ACSM's Complete Guide to Fitness & Health*. 2nd ed. Champaign (IL): Human Kinetics; 2017.

7. Blood flow to the heart is reduced during exercise performed in the supine position due to the weight of the fetus lying compressing the inferior vena cava. In order to ensure that orthostatic hypotension and obstruction of venous return do not occur, exercises performed in the supine position are discouraged

   Resources: ACOG Committee on Obstetric Practice. ACOG Committee Opinion No. 650. Physical activity and exercise during pregnancy and the postpartum period. Obstet Gynecol. 2015;126:e135–e142.

   Hargens T, senior editor. *ACSM's Resources for the Personal Trainer*. 6th ed. Philadelphia (PA): Wolters Kluwer; 2021.

   Bushman BA, senior editor. *ACSM's Complete Guide to Fitness & Health*. 2nd ed. Champaign (IL): Human Kinetics; 2017.

CARL CASE STUDY 3: ANSWERS

1. —D. Training each muscle group for ≥1 set with 10–15 repetitions at a moderate intensity of 60%–70% of 1-RM per set, with a rest interval of 2–3 min between sets at an RPE of 5–6

   Resources: Bushman BA, senior editor. *ACSM's Complete Guide to Fitness & Health*. 2nd ed. Champaign (IL):

   Human Kinetics; 2017.

   Liguori G, senior editor. *ACSM's Guidelines for Exercise Testing and Prescription*. 11th ed. Philadelphia (PA): Wolters Kluwer; 2021.

   Carl is middle aged, deconditioned, and unaccustomed to resistance training. A gradual progression using ≥1 set of 10–15 repetitions of moderate intensity (*i.e.*, 60%–70% 1-RM) resistance is recommended.

2. —C. An initial exercise HR range and MET range of approximately 146–170 bpm and 7–7.8 METs, respectively (using the HRR and $\dot{V}O_2R$ methods)

   Resources: Hargens T, senior editor. *ACSM's Resources for the Personal Trainer*. 6th ed. Philadelphia (PA): Wolters Kluwer; 2021.

   Liguori G, senior editor. *ACSM's Guidelines for Exercise Testing and Prescription*. 11th ed. Philadelphia (PA): Wolters Kluwer; 2021.

   Carl has metabolic syndrome. The 40%–75% of $\dot{V}O_2R$ or HRR is recommended to help manage his dyslipidemia. This would equate to an intensity of 4.2–7 METs or an HR range of 112–146 bpm. Carl's directional preference is slight extension, so an upright posture will be most comfortable. Lastly, a progressively increasing exercise volume of ≥300 min · wk^{-1} will help him accomplish his weight loss and BP and blood lipid management goals.

3. —B. 40 min · session^{-1}; equivalent to 1,670 kcal · wk^{-1}

   Resources: Hargens T, senior editor. *ACSM's Resources for the Personal Trainer*.

   6th ed. Philadelphia (PA): Wolters Kluwer; 2021.

   Liguori G, senior editor. *ACSM's Guidelines for Exercise Testing and Prescription*. 11th ed. Philadelphia (PA): Wolters Kluwer; 2021.

   Carl must perform 200 MET-min of exercise per session. He must do that for 40 min if he wishes to achieve 200 MET-min. To convert METs to kcal · min^{-1}, use the following formula: kcal · min^{-1} = METs × 3.5 mL · kg^{-1} · min^{-1} × body weight (in kg) ÷ 1,000 × 5. Carl would expend approximately 8.35 kcal and 334 kcal per session.

   For more information about how to complete the math associated with this question, readers are referred to the 11th edition of the *ACSM's Guidelines for Exercise Testing and Prescription*, Box 5.3 on Page 152.

4. —D. Wall squats, body weight lunges, supine stability ball hamstring curls, standing cable chest press, cable scapular row in standing, machine shoulder press, latissimus dorsi pull-downs, opposite arm-leg raises (bird-dogs) in quadruped position, modified side bridges (side plank) with knees flexed, prone planks from the knees, accompanied by hip flexor and pectoral stretches

   Resources: Hargens T, senior editor. *ACSM's Resources for the Personal Trainer*. 6th ed. Philadelphia (PA): Wolters Kluwer; 2021.

   Haney W, Pabian P, Smith M, Patel C. Low back pain: movement considerations for exercise and training. Strength Cond J. 2013;35:99–106.

   Huynh L, Chimes GP. Get the lowdown on low back pain in athletes. ACSM's Health & Fitness Journal. 2014;18:15–22.

   Lee BC, McGill SM. Effect of long-term isometric training on core/torso stiffness. J Strength Cond Res. 2014;29:1515–26.

Liguori G, senior editor. *ACSM's Guidelines for Exercise Testing and Prescription*. 11th ed. Philadelphia (PA): Wolters Kluwer; 2021.

All of the other answers include workouts, which overemphasize activation of anterior chain muscles; use a preponderance of single-joint, isolation exercises; require extensive trunk flexion; or are too advanced for Carl's fitness level, training experience, and history of back pain and trunk flexion intolerance. Answer D includes exercises that promote muscle balance and adequate activation of posterior chain muscles, employ primarily multijoint exercises, elongate his overactive or shorter muscles, and avoid postures and motions, which cause him discomfort.

5. —D. Between 5.8 and 7.4 METs; no, basketball exceeds his current prescribed intensity range

    Resources: Hargens T, senior editor. *ACSM's Resources for the Personal Trainer*. 6th ed. Philadelphia (PA): Wolters Kluwer; 2021.

    Liguori G, senior editor. *ACSM's Guidelines for Exercise Testing and Prescription*. 11th ed. Philadelphia (PA): Wolters Kluwer; 2021.

    Carl would be engaging in "vigorous" activity for someone of his age, health, and fitness level and be above 80% of his $\dot{V}O_2R$ and HRR.

6. The Compendium of Physical Activities is an alphabetized directory of physical activities that are indexed by activity type, MET level, and kilocalorie expenditure rate. Activities can be selected within a client's desired or prescribed intensity levels to help the client accomplish their exercise volume goals for health improvement, weight loss, or rehabilitation

    Resource: Ainsworth BE, Haskell WL, Hermann, et al. 2011 Compendium of Physical Activities: a second update of codes and MET values. Med Sci Sports Exerc. 2011;43(8):1575–81.

7. It is apparent from Carl's fitness assessments and medical history that he is somewhat intolerant of trunk flexion, experiences relief from performing gentle extension exercises, and is doing his exercises in general with his spine in a neutral to slightly extended position. Exercise program design for persons with chronic low back pain should resemble those of apparently healthy individuals without low back pain. Exercise positions and postures (trunk flexion in Carl's case) which cause pain should be avoided, and exercises should be modified to accommodate client's exercise movement directional preferences. Carl will probably find it more comfortable to perform many of his exercises in a standing position or, if he must sit, with either a back support or chest pad

    Resources: Haney W, Pabian P, Smith M, Patel C. Low back pain: movement considerations for exercise and training. Strength Cond J. 2013;35:99–106.

    Hislop H, Avers D, Brown M. Daniels and Worthingham's Muscle Testing: Techniques of Manual Examination and Performance Testing. 9th ed. St. Louis (MO): Elsevier Saunders; 2014.

    Huynh L, Chimes GP. Get the lowdown on low back pain in athletes. ACSM's Health Fitness J. 2014;18:15–22.

    Lee BC, McGill SM. Effect of long-term isometric training on core/torso stiffness. J Strength Cond Res. 2014;29:1515–26.

    Long A, Donelson R, Fung T. Does it matter which exercise? A randomized control trial of exercise for low back pain. Spine (Philadelphia PA 1976). 2004;29:2593–602.

    Long A, May S, Fung T. Specific directional exercises for patients with low back pain: a case series. Physiother Can. 2008;60:307–17.

    McGill SM, Karpowicz A. Exercises for spine stabilization: motion/motor patters, stability progressions, and clinical technique. Arch Phys Med Rehabil. 2009;90(1):118–26.

(Continued)

CARL CASE STUDY 3: ANSWERS (Continued)

Nau E, Hanney WJ, Kolber MJ. Spinal conditioning for athletes with lumbar spondylolysis and spondylolisthesis. Strength Cond J. 2008;30:43–52.

Liguori G, senior editor. *ACSM's Guidelines for Exercise Testing and Prescription*. 11th ed. Philadelphia (PA): Wolters Kluwer; 2021.

Surkitt LD, Ford JJ, Hahne AJ, Pizzari T, McMeeken JM. Efficacy of directional preference management for low back pain: a systematic review. Phys Ther. 2012;92:652–65.

BEATRICE CASE STUDY 4: ANSWERS

1. —C. Class II obesity

    Resource: Liguori G, senior editor. *ACSM's Guidelines for Exercise Testing and Prescription*. 11th ed. Philadelphia (PA): Wolters Kluwer; 2021.

    Beatrice is classified as "Class II Obesity" (35.0–39.9). BMI is calculated by using the following formula:

    Weight in kg/(Height in m^2). Beatrice's BMI is 37.1 $kg \cdot m^{-2}$.

2. —B. 68 lb

    Resources: Hargens T, senior editor. *ACSM's Resources for the Personal Trainer*. 6th ed.

    Philadelphia (PA): Wolters Kluwer; 2021.

    Liguori G, senior editor. *ACSM's Guidelines for Exercise Testing and Prescription*. 11th ed. Philadelphia (PA): Wolters Kluwer; 2021.

    "Normal weight" is categorized by a BMI of 18.5–24.9. Because Beatrice wants to lose the minimal amount of weight, 24.9 will be her goal BMI.

    Use the formula for BMI with Beatrice's goal BMI and her current height to find what her new weight will be.

    $$24.9 = kg/(1.57^2)$$

    $$kg = 61.2 \text{ or } 134.6 \text{ lb}$$

    Subtract her goal weight from her current weight.

    $$203 \text{ lb} - 134.6 \text{ lb} = 68.4 \text{ lb}$$

3. —A. 0.4 lb

    Resource: Liguori G, senior editor. *ACSM's Guidelines for Exercise Testing and Prescription*. 11th ed. Philadelphia (PA): Wolters Kluwer; 2021.

    Beatrice is reducing 1400 $kcal \cdot wk^{-1}$ at this rate. There are 3,500 kcal in 1 lb. She will lose approximately 0.4 lb each week.

4. —C. 500–1,000 kcal

    Resource: Liguori G, senior editor. *ACSM's Guidelines for Exercise Testing and Prescription*. 11th ed. Philadelphia (PA): Wolters Kluwer; 2021.

    ACSM recommends weight loss of 1–2 $lb \cdot wk^{-1}$. This would mean a caloric deficit of 3,500–7,000 kcal each week or 500–1,000 kcal each day.

5. —A. Extrinsic rewards; intrinsic rewards

    Resource: Hargens T, senior editor. *ACSM's Resources for the Personal Trainer*. 6th ed. Philadelphia (PA): Wolters Kluwer; 2021.

    Extrinsic motivation is a motivation that helps to achieve a certain goal or reward. Extrinsic rewards are positive benefits that are often received through other people. Intrinsic rewards are rewards that are considered personal benefits because the goal achievement left the person feeling satisfied. Beatrice expressed several times that she feels motivated/encouraged when she sees results in her weight. This is an example of an extrinsic reward. Being able to keep up with her grandson would be an example of an intrinsic reward.

6. Beatrice is contemplating change but still lacks self-esteem. You can use every motivational tool in the book to help Beatrice. It is important to use active listening with Beatrice and to encourage her strengths. Reflect what she tells you and express that your concerns are the same as hers and provide nonthreatening feedback. Be sure that all praise and encouragement are genuine.

Although it is important to point out the long-term benefits of exercise, including the possible reduction in all of her risk factors, Beatrice is motivated most when she sees change. It is ideal to work with her on strategic planning. Work together to find several short-term goals that will help to motivate her as she slowly progresses toward her long-term goals. Set goals that are specific, measurable, achievable, realistic, and time constrained (SMART).

Use motivational interviewing skills. Approach her nutritional habits in a way that is nonconfrontational. Ask her if she is willing to discuss general nutrition information and appropriate portion control. Focus as much as possible on intrinsic motivators. If she is still unwilling to discuss nutritional habits, point out small achievements such as increases in time on a machine or overall increase in energy.

Resources: Hargens T, senior editor. *ACSM's Resources for the Personal Trainer.* 6th ed. Philadelphia (PA): Wolters Kluwer; 2021.

Liguori G, senior editor. *ACSM's Guidelines for Exercise Testing and Prescription.* 11th

ed. Philadelphia (PA): Wolters Kluwer; 2021.

7. Give specific and realistic guidelines. Explain that American Heart Association and ACSM have recommended that she engage in at least 150 min each week of moderate-intensity exercise. She will improve her cardiovascular and respiratory function, reduce her coronary artery disease risk factors, decrease morbidity and risk of early mortality, and improve quality of life.

When she appears to have improved confidence, encourage her to engage in any appropriate group fitness classes or neighborhood walking programs. Offer other ways that Beatrice can increase her overall physical activity. Use examples such as parking farther away, taking stairs whenever possible, taking short walks during commercial breaks, etc. Until she becomes fit enough to tolerate 30 min of nonstop aerobic activity, encourage her to engage in 10-min bouts of exercise that reach a moderate level of intensity. Without an HR monitor, you can describe moderate intensity as a level that makes her feel slightly short of breath or makes talking difficult. Find out what types of activities appeal to Beatrice and provide examples of how she can incorporate physical activity into her daily life.

Resources: Hargens T, senior editor. *ACSM's Resources for the Personal Trainer.* 6th ed. Philadelphia (PA): Wolters Kluwer; 2021.

Liguori G, senior editor. *ACSM's Guidelines for Exercise Testing and Prescription.* 11th ed. Philadelphia (PA): Wolters Kluwer; 2021.

HENRY CASE STUDY 5: ANSWERS

1. —C. 31.8 kg · m^{-2}

   Resource: Hargens T, senior editor. *ACSM's Resources for the Personal Trainer*. 6th ed. Philadelphia (PA): Wolters Kluwer; 2021.

2. —D. Class I obesity

   Resource: Hargens T, senior editor. *ACSM's Resources for the Personal Trainer*. 6th ed. Philadelphia (PA): Wolters Kluwer; 2021.

   A body mass index 30.0 and 34.9 is categorized as class I obesity.

3. —B. Preparation

   Resource: Hargens T, senior editor. *ACSM's Resources for the Personal Trainer*. 6th ed. Philadelphia (PA): Wolters Kluwer; 2021.

   Henry has decided to make the change to be more physically active. He is seeking help to formulate a plan.

4. —C. Emphasize self-liberation by helping Henry make a firm commitment to a goal and a start date

   Resource: Hargens T, senior editor. *ACSM's Resources for the Personal Trainer*. 6th ed. Philadelphia (PA): Wolters Kluwer; 2021.

   Commitment usually occurs at the beginning of the action stage. If Henry can set a firm time and date and stick to it, he will begin the action phase of adding exercise back into his life.

5. —A. 460 protein, 1,600 carbohydrate, 540 fat

   One gram of carbohydrate has approximately 4 kcal, 1 g of fat has approximately 9 kcal, and 1 g of protein has approximately 4 kcal.

   Resource: Swain D, senior editor. *ACSM'S Resource Manual for Guidelines for Exercise Testing and Prescription*, 7th ed. Philadelphia (PA): Wolters Kluwer; 2014.

6. —B. Mesosystem

   The mesosystem in the socioecological model includes environment, health agencies, community, competing sedentary activities, technology, mass media, and access to information. The proximity of a park to Henry's home would be a factor at the mesosystem level.

   Resource: Swain D, senior editor. *ACSM'S Resource Manual for Guidelines for Exercise Testing and Prescription*, 7th ed. Philadelphia (PA): Wolters Kluwer; 2014.

7. —A. 2,386 kcal

   If Henry wants to lose 1 lb a week and he will burn 2,000 extra kilocalories (kcal) each week with exercise, he will need to create an additional 1,500 kcal deficit with his diet per week. In order to do that, he needs to decrease his caloric intake by approximately 214 kcal · d^{-1}; this would equal 2,386 kcal each day.

   Resource: Liguori G, senior editor. *ACSM's Guidelines for Exercise Testing and Prescription*. 11th ed. Philadelphia (PA): Wolters Kluwer; 2021.

8. Answers might include family obligations, fatigue from work, and time management. Refer to his exam results and educate him about his six risk factors for disease. Ask him about how his health will affect his family and if he has support from his family and friends. Have him list ways he can overcome barriers such as working late, the boys' sports, and other family commitments. Make suggestions if he cannot think of anything. For example, he can walk or run while his boys are at practice. He can add in a short walk at lunch if he will not have time later for a longer exercise session

   Resource: Hargens T, senior editor. *ACSM's Resources for the Personal Trainer*. 6th ed. Philadelphia (PA): Wolters Kluwer; 2021.

9. Answers may include motivational interviewing and client-centered approach to questioning to determine SMART goals that Carl is ready to commit to. Agreeing with the client and not countering resistance, giving examples of specific SMART goals, and asking questions directed at determining, which specific goal is most important, confidence in accomplishing that goal on a scale of 1–10, etc. Be sure to clarify the scale of 1–10 and ask why they feel they are not a 1. If they are a 6 or less, the goal needs to be adjusted so they are closer to an 8

   Resource: Swain D, senior editor. *ACSM'S Resource Manual for Guidelines for Exercise Testing and Prescription*, 7th ed. Philadelphia (PA): Wolters Kluwer; 2014.

LEGAL & PROFESSIONAL RESPONSIBILITIES CASE STUDY 6: ANSWERS

1. —D. Physician consent form signed for your review

   Resource: Hargens T, senior editor. *ACSM's Resources for the Personal Trainer*. 6th ed. Philadelphia (PA): Wolters Kluwer; 2021.

   This client has two risk factors: no known disease and she is asymptomatic. She will be participating in moderate exercise. Therefore, a GXT with a physician present is not required. Getting medical clearance is not necessary unless she answers "yes" to any question under "General Health Questions" section on the Physical Activity Readiness Questionnaire + (PAR-Q+).

2. —C. Explain to her that the risks do not outweigh the benefits associated with this exercise technique

   Resource: Hargens T, senior editor. *ACSM's Resources for the Personal Trainer*. 6th ed. Philadelphia (PA): Wolters Kluwer; 2021.

   It is within the scope of practice for a personal trainer to correct bad form whether that patron is a client or not. It is also within the code of ethics to help prevent injury to participants.

3. —D. Use direct mail and host a fitness activity in the neighborhood park

   Resource: Hargens T, senior editor. *ACSM's Resources for the Personal Trainer*. 6th ed. Philadelphia (PA): Wolters Kluwer; 2021.

   Because the fitness facility is new in town, a direct mail to that specific neighborhood would be helpful. In combination with community involvement at the neighborhood park, the two approaches would target that specific market in multiple ways.

4. —C. Refer him to his physician or physical therapist

   Resource: Hargens T, senior editor. *ACSM's Resources for the Personal Trainer*. 6th ed. Philadelphia (PA): Wolters Kluwer; 2021.

   Pire N. ACSM's Career and Business Guide for the Fitness Professional. Philadelphia (PA): Wolters Kluwer; 2012.

   Attempting to treat an injury is beyond the scope of practice of a personal trainer, and the client should be referred to someone who is qualified to care for this injury.

5. —B. Write an incident report describing what happened and have her sign it

   Resource: Hargens T, senior editor. *ACSM's Resources for the Personal Trainer*. 6th ed. Philadelphia (PA): Wolters Kluwer; 2021.

   Even though the member does not appear to have any serious injury, the incident needs to be documented to protect the facility from further claims on the part of the member.

(Continued)

LEGAL & PROFESSIONAL RESPONSIBILITIES CASE STUDY 6: ANSWERS (Continued)

6. —B. Provide information to the client regarding participation options and risks

    Resource: Hargens T, senior editor. *ACSM's Resources for the Personal Trainer*. 6th ed. Philadelphia (PA): Wolters Kluwer; 2021.

    The purpose of the informed consent form is to ensure the client has full knowledge of tests to be performed, understands the relative risks, is informed of alternative procedures, is given the chance to ask questions, and gives consent voluntarily. The informed consent document does not protect the trainer from liability.

7. —C. More than 70% of fibers torn

    Resource: Hargens T, senior editor. *ACSM's Resources for the Personal Trainer*. 6th ed. Philadelphia (PA): Wolters Kluwer; 2021.

    Prentice W. Principles of Athletic Training (17th ed). New York NY: McGraw-Hill, 2021.

    Grade 2 hamstring strains are associated with partial tearing of muscle fibers. Typically, this value is no more than 70%. Loss of function and ecchymosis are associated with grade 3 strains. Soreness coming from muscle spasm as opposed to damaged tissue develops as a result of grade 1 strains.

8. Answers should include an ankle sprain of any degree, an injury to the peroneal tendons, or a fracture. She should stop working out, ice her injury, and stabilize with an elastic wrap. An incident report should be completed, and she should sign it. She should not participate in weight-bearing activities and not return to training without medical clearance

    Resource: Hargens T, senior editor. *ACSM's Resources for the Personal Trainer*. 6th ed. Philadelphia (PA): Wolters Kluwer; 2021.

    Prentice W. Principles of Athletic Training (17th ed). New York NY: McGraw-Hill, 2021.

9. Answers may include re-racking weights; checking bands for breaks; keeping the floor clear of debris and liquids; and checking stability balls, mats, and medicine balls for cleanliness and proper inflation. Machines should be in proper working order with no broken cables. Cardio equipment should be in proper working order with no broken pieces. Locker room floor should be dry and clear of clutter, and benches should be checked for stability. Locker rooms should be checked for members in distress. The group fitness floor should be dry, and equipment should be put away with the door locked so no one can enter without permission

    Resource: Hargens T, senior editor. *ACSM's Resources for the Personal Trainer*. 6th ed Philadelphia (PA): Wolters Kluwer; 2021.

PART 2

ACSM Certified Exercise Physiologist (ACSM-EP) Certification

Nicole Nelson, MSH, LMT, ACSM-EP
Associate Editor

DOMAIN NUMBER	I	II	III	IV
DOMAIN NAME	HEALTH AND FITNESS ASSESSMENT	EXERCISE PRESCRIPTION AND IMPLEMENTATION	EXERCISE COUNSELING AND BEHAVIOR MODIFICATION	RISK MANAGEMENT AND PROFESSIONAL RESPONSIBILITIES

ACSM-EP

OUTLINE OF THIS PART:

WHAT YOU NEED TO KNOW AND MULTIPLE CHOICE QUESTIONS DIVIDED BY SUBDOMAIN

DOMAIN I: HEALTH AND FITNESS ASSESSMENT

A. ADMINISTER AND INTERPRET PRE-PARTICIPATION HEALTH SCREENING PROCEDURES TO MAXIMIZE CLIENT SAFETY AND MINIMIZE RISK

Domain I Subdomain A: What you need to know

- The pre-participation screening algorithm and tools that provide accurate information about the client's health/medical history, current medical conditions, risk factors, sign/symptoms of disease, current physical activity habits, and medications.

- The key components included in informed consent and health/medical history.
- The limitations of informed consent and health/medical history.

Domain I Subdomain A: Multiple Choice Questions

1. The informed consent document _____.
   A) Is a legal document
   B) Provides immunity from prosecution
   C) Provides an explanation of the test to the client
   D) Legally protects the rights of the client

2. Which of the following is a *false* statement regarding an informed consent?
   A) The informed consent is not a legal document.
   B) The informed consent does not provide legal immunity to a facility or individual in the event of injury to an individual.
   C) Negligence, improper test administration, inadequate personnel qualifications, and insufficient safety procedures are all items that are expressly covered by the informed consent.
   D) The consent form does not relieve the facility or individual of the responsibility to do everything possible to ensure the safety of the individual.

3. What is the purpose of agreements, releases, and consent forms?
   A) To inform the client of participation risks as well as the rights of the client and the facility
   B) To inform the client what they can and cannot do in the facility
   C) To define the relationship between the facility operator and the ACSM-EP
   D) To detail the rights and responsibilities of the club owner to reject an application by a prospective client

4. In commercial settings, clients should be more extensively screened for potential health risks. The information solicited should include which of the following?
   A) Personal medical history
   B) Present medical status
   C) Medication
   D) All of the above

ACSM-EP

5. Identify the appropriate subjective self-evaluation tool used as a quick health screening before beginning any exercise program.
   A) Physical Activity Readiness Questionnaire + (PAR-Q+)
   B) Health Status Questionnaire (HSQ)
   C) Exercise electrocardiogram (E-ECG)
   D) RPE-Borg scale (RPE)

B. DETERMINE PARTICIPANT'S READINESS TO TAKE PART IN A HEALTH-RELATED PHYSICAL FITNESS ASSESSMENT AND EXERCISE PROGRAM

Domain I Subdomain B: What you need to know

- The pre-participation screening algorithm as delineated in the current edition of ACSM's Guidelines for Exercise Testing and Prescription.
- Cardiovascular risk factors or conditions that may require consultation with medical personnel prior to exercise testing or training (*e.g.,* inappropriate changes in resting heart rate and/or blood pressure; new onset discomfort in chest, neck, shoulder, or arm; changes in the pattern of discomfort during rest or exercise; fainting, dizzy spells, claudication).
- Pulmonary risk factors or conditions that may require consultation with medical personnel prior to exercise testing or training (*e.g.,* asthma, exercise-induced asthma/bronchospasm, extreme breathlessness at rest or during exercise, chronic bronchitis, emphysema).
- Metabolic risk factors or conditions that may require consultation with medical personnel prior to exercise testing or training (*e.g.,* obesity, metabolic syndrome, diabetes or glucose intolerance, hypoglycemia).
- Musculoskeletal risk factors or conditions that may require consultation with medical personnel prior to exercise testing or training (*e.g.,* acute or chronic pain, osteoarthritis, rheumatoid arthritis, osteoporosis, inflammation/pain, low back pain).
- ACSM pre-participation screening algorithm and the implications for medical clearance before participation in an exercise program.
- Risk factors that may be favorably modified by physical activity habits.
- Medical terminology (*e.g.,* total cholesterol (TC), high-density lipoprotein cholesterol (HDL-C), low-density lipoprotein cholesterol (LDL-C), triglycerides, impaired fasting glucose, impaired glucose tolerance, hypertension, atherosclerosis, myocardial infarction, dyspnea, tachycardia, claudication, syncope, ischemia).
- Recommended plasma cholesterol levels (*e.g.,* National Cholesterol Education Program/ATP Guidelines).
- Recommended blood pressure levels.
- Recommendations for medical clearance before initiating an exercise program.
- The components of a health-history questionnaire (*e.g.,* past and current medical history, family history of disease, orthopedic limitations, prescribed medications, activity patterns, nutritional habits, stress and anxiety levels, smoking, alcohol use).
- The administration of the pre-participation screening algorithm and recognition of major signs or symptoms suggestive of cardiovascular, or metabolic disease, and/or the presence of known cardiovascular, and metabolic disease status.
- The administration of the pre-participation screening algorithm to determine the need for medical clearance prior to initiating an exercise program and to select appropriate physical fitness assessment protocols.

Domain I Subdomain B: Multiple Choice Questions

1. Which of the following actions would be most appropriate if a client's pre-screening results indicated she has no known cardiovascular disease, has not been exercising in the previous year, and has been experiencing dyspnea at rest.
   A) Because she has no known disease, medical clearance is not necessary.
   B) Because she is currently experiencing symptoms, but does not have known disease, she should begin light- to moderate-intensity exercise immediately.
   C) Because she is currently experiencing symptoms, she should seek medical clearance prior to beginning exercise.
   D) Because she is experiencing dyspnea at rest, she should begin vigorous exercise immediately (without clearance) to increase her cardiorespiratory fitness.

2. Which of the following LDL cholesterol readings would be characterized as a risk factor for CVD?
    A) $<90 \text{ mg} \cdot \text{dL}^{-1}$
    B) $90-100 \text{ mg} \cdot \text{dL}^{-1}$
    C) $100-129 \text{ mg} \cdot \text{dL}^{-1}$
    D) $\geq130 \text{ mg} \cdot \text{dL}^{-1}$

3. Which of the following BP readings would be characterized as hypertension in an adult?
    A) SBP 100 and/or DBP 60 mm Hg
    B) SBP 110 and/or DBP 70 mm Hg
    C) SBP 140 and/or 90 mm Hg
    D) 118 and/or 78 mm Hg

4. Which of the following medications is designed to modify blood cholesterol levels?
    A) Nitrates
    B) β-blockers
    C) Antilipemics
    D) Aspirin

5. Which of the following represents more than 90% of the fat stored in the body and is composed of a glycerol molecule connected to three fatty acids?
    A) Phospholipids
    B) Cholesterol
    C) Triglycerides
    D) Free fatty acids

6. Which of the following BP readings represents the elevated blood pressure category in adults?
    A) 100/60 mm Hg
    B) 110/70 mm Hg
    C) 160/90 mm Hg
    D) 120/78 mm Hg

7. A source of intimal injury thought to initiate the process of atherogenesis is _____.
    A) Dyslipidemia
    B) Hypertension
    C) Turbulence of blood flow within the vessel
    D) All of the above

8. According to the ACSM, at what level is high-density lipoprotein (HDL) considered a risk factor in the development of cardiovascular disease (CVD)?
    A) $<200 \text{ mg} \cdot \text{dL}^{-1}$
    B) $<110 \text{ mg} \cdot \text{dL}^{-1}$
    C) $<60 \text{ mg} \cdot \text{dL}^{-1}$
    D) $<40 \text{ mg} \cdot \text{dL}^{-1}$

9. Which of the following describes pain and/or cramping in the lower leg due to inadequate blood flow to skeletal muscles?
    A) Dyspnea
    B) Syncope
    C) Claudication
    D) Angina

10. Which of the following results would be considered a positive cardiovascular disease (CVD) risk factor?
    A) Not participating in at least 30 min of moderate-intensity physical activity on at least $3 \text{ d} \cdot \text{wk}^{-1}$ for at least 3 months.
    B) HDL-C $>70 \text{ mg} \cdot \text{dL}^{-1}$
    C) Fasting blood glucose (FBG) = $80 \text{ mg} \cdot \text{dL}^{-1}$
    D) Body mass index (BMI) = $25 \text{ kg} \cdot \text{m}^{-2}$

11. Which of the following cardiovascular disease (CVD) risk factors may be favorably modified by physical activity?
    A) Obesity
    B) Hypertension
    C) Hypercholesterolemia
    D) All of the above

12. Which of the following would require consultation with medical personnel prior to exercise testing?
    A) Sedentary person, asymptomatic, BP = 140/90 mmHg
    B) A person who regularly exercises, but has recently experienced dyspnea at rest and with mild exertion
    C) A person who is inactive, no symptoms, no known disease
    D) A person who regularly exercises, has no symptoms, but has a history of cardiovascular disease.

13. Which term refers to an inadequate blood supply to an organ or part of the body?
    A) Ischemia
    B) Infarct
    C) Necrosis
    D) Oxidative stress

14. T/F based on the ACSM pre-participation algorithm, a participant with a history of heart valve disease, who does not currently exercise, and is currently asymptomatic, should seek medical clearance prior to exercise.
    A) True
    B) False

ACSM-EP

15. When using the ACSM pre-participation algorithm, what is considered meeting the criteria for exercise participation?
    A) Performing planned, structured physical activity (PA) at least 20 min at a light intensity on at least 2 d · wk⁻¹ for at least the last 2 months
    B) Performing planned, structured PA at least 30 min at a moderate intensity on at least 3 d · wk⁻¹ for at least the last 3 months
    C) Performing planned, structured PA at least 50 min at a vigorous intensity on at least 5 d · wk⁻¹ for at least the last 6 months
    D) Performing planned, structured PA for at least 60 min at a light intensity every day for at least 1 yr

C. DETERMINE AND ADMINISTER PHYSICAL FITNESS ASSESSMENTS FOR HEALTHY CLIENTS AND THOSE WITH CONTROLLED DISEASE

Domain I Subdomain C: What you need to know

- Physiological basis of the components of health-related physical fitness (cardiorespiratory fitness, muscular strength, muscular endurance, flexibility, body composition).
- Selecting the most appropriate testing protocols for each client based on preliminary screening data.
- Calibration techniques and proper use of fitness testing equipment.
- The purpose and procedures of fitness testing protocols for the components of health-related physical fitness.
- Test termination criteria and best practice procedures to be followed after stopping an exercise test.
- Fitness assessment sequencing.

- The effects of common medications and substances on exercise testing (*e.g.,* antianginals, antihypertensives, antiarrhythmics, bronchodilators, hypoglycemics, psychotropics, alcohol, diet pills, cold tablets, caffeine, nicotine).
- The physiologic and metabolic responses to exercise testing associated with chronic diseases and conditions (*e.g.,* heart disease, hypertension, diabetes mellitus, obesity, pulmonary disease).
- Analyzing information obtained from assessment of the components of health-related physical fitness.
- Modifying protocols and procedures for testing children, adolescents, older adults, and clients with special considerations.

Domain I Subdomain C: Multiple Choice Questions

1. Which of the following is *not* a purpose of physical fitness testing?
   A) To bring in extra income to pay off other major expenses of the testing company
   B) To educate participants about their present health and fitness status relative to health-related standards and age- and sex-matched norms
   C) To motivate participants by establishing reasonable and attainable health/fitness goals
   D) To allow evaluation of progress following an exercise program and long-term monitoring of participants

2. When performing a battery of tests in a single testing session, which of the following orders is most optimal for testing multiple health-related components of fitness?
   A) Resting heart rate (HR$_{rest}$), Queens College Step Test, ACSM push-up test
   B) Queens College Step Test, HR$_{rest}$, ACSM push-up test

   C) ACSM push-up test, Queens College Step Test, HR$_{rest}$
   D) HR$_{rest}$, Queens College Step Test, ACSM push-up test

3. _____ pertains to the ability to correctly identify patients who do not have a given condition.
   A) Sensitivity
   B) Specificity
   C) Positive percent value
   D) Negative predictive value

4. Which of the following would not require termination of a maximal or submaximal exercise test in a low-risk adult?
   A) Subject requests to stop
   B) Shortness of breath
   C) A slight decrease in diastolic pressure
   D) Failure of HR to increase with increased intensity

5. From rest to maximal exercise, the SBP should _____ progressively with an increasing workload.
   A) Increase
   B) Decrease
   C) Stay the same
   D) Decrease with isometric or increase with isotonic contractions

6. Fitness assessment is an important aspect of the training program because it provides information for which of the following?
   A) Developing the exercise prescription
   B) Evaluating proper nutritional choices
   C) Diagnosing musculoskeletal injury
   D) Developing appropriate billing categories

7. After completing an examination of your client's health screening documents and the prior physiological resting measurements that were recorded, you decide to proceed with a single session of fitness assessments. Identify the recommended order of administration.
   A) Body composition, flexibility, cardiorespiratory fitness, and muscular fitness
   B) Flexibility, body composition, muscular fitness, and cardiorespiratory fitness
   C) Flexibility, cardiorespiratory fitness, body composition, and muscular fitness
   D) Body composition, cardiorespiratory fitness, muscular fitness, and flexibility

8. Which of the following pathologies is associated with abnormally low systolic BP or a drop in systolic BP during a graded exercise test?
   A) Exercise-induced asthma (EIA)
   B) Cardiac dysfunction
   C) Deep vein thrombosis (DVT)
   D) Systemic vascular resistance (SVR)

9. Which of the following medications would result in a blunted HR response to graded exercise testing?
   A) Caffeine
   B) Nicotine
   C) β-blockers
   D) Adderall

10. Upon completion of a submaximal cardiorespiratory fitness assessment, how long should HR and BP be observed?
    A) <2 min
    B) 3 min
    C) 4 min
    D) at least 5 min

11. Which of the following would be considered a test of anaerobic power?
    A) Push-up test
    B) YMCA cycle test
    C) the Wingate test
    D) Balance error scoring system (BESS)

12. Which of the following best describes the rationale for performing a resting electrocardiogram (EKG)?
    A) To assess endothelial dysfunction
    B) To assess myocardial electrical conduction and oxygenation
    C) To determine systolic blood pressure
    D) To determine ejection fraction

13. Which of the following energy systems would contribute most to performance on vertical jump test?
    A) Aerobic system
    B) Oxidative phosphorylation
    C) Fast glycolysis
    D) Phosphagen system

14. Which of the following statements is true regarding exercise testing with children?
    A) Exercise testing for clinical purposes is generally not indicated for children unless there is a health concern.
    B) Compared to adults, children generally do not require any extra support during an exercise test.
    C) Compared to cycle ergometers, treadmills provide less risk for injury for exercise testing in children.
    D) In children, cycle ergometers tend to elicit a higher peak oxygen uptake compared to cycle ergometers.

D. CONDUCT AND INTEPRET CARDIORESPIRATORY FITNESS ASSESSMENTS

Domain I Subdomain D: What you need to know

- Common submaximal and maximal cardiorespiratory fitness assessment protocols.
- Blood pressure measurement techniques.
- Korotkoff sounds for determining systolic and diastolic blood pressure.
- The blood pressure response to exercise.
- Techniques of measuring heart rate and heart rate response to exercise.
- The rating of perceived exertion (RPE).

- Heart rate, blood pressure and RPE monitoring techniques before, during, and after cardiorespiratory fitness testing.
- The anatomy and physiology of the cardiovascular and pulmonary systems.
- Cardiorespiratory terminology (*e.g.,* angina pectoris, tachycardia, bradycardia, arrhythmia, hyperventilation).
- The pathophysiology of myocardial ischemia, myocardial infarction, stroke, hypertension, and hyperlipidemia.
- The effects of myocardial ischemia, myocardial infarction, hypertension, claudication, and dyspnea on cardiorespiratory responses during exercise.
- Oxygen consumption dynamics during exercise (*e.g.,* heart rate, stroke volume, cardiac output, ventilation, ventilatory threshold).

- Methods of calculating $\dot{V}O_{2max}$.
- Cardiorespiratory responses to acute graded exercise of conditioned and unconditioned clients.
- Analyzing and documenting cardiorespiratory fitness test results.
- Locating anatomic landmarks for palpation of peripheral pulses and blood pressure.
- Measuring heart rate, blood pressure, and RPE at rest and during exercise.
- Conducting submaximal exercise tests (*e.g.,* cycle ergometer, treadmill, field testing, step test).
- Determine cardiorespiratory fitness based on submaximal exercise test results.

Domain I Subdomain D: Multiple Choice Questions

1. Which of the following is accepted as the criterion measure of cardiorespiratory fitness?
   A) Field test performance
   B) Maximal volume of oxygen consumed per unit time ($\dot{V}O_{2max}$)
   C) Body fat percentage
   D) Maximal heart rate (HR_{max})

2. When estimating $\dot{V}O_{2max}$ using the YMCA cycle ergometer protocol, which of the following best describes the relationship between heart rate (HR) >110 bpm and 85% age-predicted HR_{max} or 70% heart rate reserve (HRR)?
   A) Logarithmic
   B) Inverse
   C) Curvilinear
   D) Linear

3. Which of the following variables is unique to the Rockport One-Mile Fitness Walking Test's regression equation to estimate $\dot{V}O_{2max}$?
   A) Age
   B) HR
   C) Gender
   D) Body mass

4. What is the suggested work rate for a deconditioned, female individual performing the Astrand-Rhyming cycle ergometer protocol?
   A) 150 or 300 kg · m · min^{-1} (25 or 50 W)
   B) 300 or 450 kg · m · min^{-1} (50 or 75 W)
   C) 450 or 600 kg · m · min^{-1} (75 or 100 W)
   D) 600 or 900 kg · m · min^{-1} (100 or 150 W)

5. The Queens College Step Test (also known as the McArdle Step Test) is performed for how long?
   A) 45 s
   B) 90 s
   C) 3 min
   D) 5 min

6. Which of the following is considered the "gold standard" to objectively measure cardiovascular exercise capacity?
   A) Maximal exercise test using indirect calorimetry
   B) Submaximal exercise test using hemodynamic responses
   C) Physician exam
   D) Walk/run field test

7. Which of the following graded exercise protocols is most widely used in the United States in a clinical setting?
   A) Bruce treadmill protocol
   B) Queens College Step Test
   C) Astrand-Rhyming cycle ergometer test
   D) All are used equally

8. HR, blood pressure (BP), and electrocardiogram (ECG) should be recorded regularly during the clinical exercise test and through at least _____ of recovery.
   A) 90 s
   B) 3 min
   C) 6 min
   D) 10 min

9. The normal HR response to incremental exercise is to increase workloads at an HR of _____ per 1 metabolic equivalent (MET).
   A) 10 bpm
   B) 5 bpm
   C) 20 bpm
   D) 15 bpm

10. Indirect calorimetry is a technique that analyzes volume of _____ to estimate energy production.
   A) Expired carbon monoxide
   B) Expired nitrogen
   C) Heat produced
   D) Expired oxygen

11. All of the following are among the ACSM guidelines to determine "maximal" effort during a maximally graded exercise test (GXT) except_____.
   A) Achievement of age-predicted HR_{max}
   B) A postexercise venous lactate concentration >8 mmol $\cdot L^{-1}$
   C) A rating of perceived exertion (RPE) at peak exercise >17 on the 6–20 scale or >7 on the 0–10 scale
   D) A peak respiratory exchange ratio (RER) ≥ 1.10

12. For every 1 MET increase in exercise intensity during submaximal exercise, SBP should increase _____.
   A) Approximately 10 mm Hg
   B) 15–20 mm Hg
   C) 25–30 mm Hg
   D) 30–35 mm Hg

13. Which of the following is true about the Bruce protocol?
   A) Speed and incline are increased every 3 min of the test.
   B) Stage one of the protocol involves the participant walking at 3 mph with a 10% grade.
   C) The Bruce protocol is performed on a cycle ergometer.
   D) The Bruce protocol is used to evaluate anaerobic power.

14. Which artery is considered the standard location for the auscultatory method of blood pressure measurement?
   A) Radial
   B) Brachial
   C) Femoral
   D) Tibial

15. Which of the following is a potential source of error in resting BP measurement?
   A) Auditory acuity
   B) Observer bias (*e.g.,* digit preference in reporting)
   C) Improper size of the cuff
   D) All of the above are correct

16. Which of the following are used as criteria to determine the achievement of $\dot{V}O_{2max}$ during a GXT?
   A) The client wishes to end the test.
   B) Borg rating of perceived exertion (RPE) 12–15.
   C) Achievement of 85% heart rate reserve (HRR).
   D) Respiratory exchange ratio (RER) ≥ 1.15.

17. Of the following GXT modes, which would be expected to yield the highest $\dot{V}O_2$ (assume the individual is equally experienced with each modality)?
   A) Treadmill.
   B) Cycle ergometer.
   C) Upper body ergometer.
   D) Each mode would yield the same $\dot{V}O_2$.

18. Which of the following ventilation ($\dot{V}_E$) ranges would likely be observed in a healthy individual during a maximal GXT?
   A) 5–10 L $\cdot min^{-1}$
   B) 10–25 L $\cdot min^{-1}$
   C) 45–65 L $\cdot min^{-1}$
   D) 70–125 L $\cdot min^{-1}$

19. At rest, tidal volume among healthy individuals tends to range between _____.
   A) 20–80 mL
   B) 100–200 mL
   C) 400–500 mL
   D) 1–2 L

20. _____ is not a contraindication of maximal exercise testing in the clinical setting.
   A) Acute myocarditis or pericarditis
   B) Ongoing unstable angina
   C) Recent stroke or transient ischemia attack
   D) Resting systolic blood pressure (SBP) between 125 and 140 mm Hg or diastolic blood pressure (DBP) between 60 and 75 mm Hg

E. CONDUCT ASSESSMENTS OF MUSCULAR STRENGTH, MUSCULAR ENDURANCE, AND FLEXIBILITY

Domain I Subdomain E: What you need to know

- Common muscular strength, muscular endurance, and flexibility assessment protocols.
- Relative strength, absolute strength, and repetition maximum (1-RM) estimation.
- The anatomy of bone, skeletal muscle, and connective tissues.
- The definition of the following terms: anterior, posterior, proximal, distal, inferior, superior, medial, lateral, supination, pronation, flexion, extension, adduction, abduction, hyperextension, rotation, circumduction, agonist, antagonist, and stabilizer.
- The planes and axes in which each movement action occurs.
- The interrelationships among center of gravity, base of support, balance, stability, posture, and spinal alignment.
- The location and function of muscles (*e.g.*, pectoralis major, trapezius, internal and external obliques, gastrocnemius).
- Joints and their associated movement.
- Conducting muscular strength, muscular endurance, and flexibility assessments (*e.g.*, 1-RM, hand grip dynamometer, push-ups).
- Estimating 1-RM using lower resistance (2–10 RM).

Domain I Subdomain E: Multiple Choice Questions

1. Which of the following is *not* a valid test for muscular strength?
   A) Grip strength test
   B) YMCA bench press test
   C) 3-repetition maximum (RM) bench press test
   D) 10-RM shoulder press test

2. A measure of muscular endurance is _____.
   A) 1-RM Bench press
   B) 3-RM Squat
   C) The YMCA bench press test
   D) The Wingate test

3. Which of the following would be considered the agonist of the bench press pattern?
   A) The biceps brachii
   B) Latissimus dorsi
   C) Pectoralis brevis
   D) Pectoralis major

4. The Romanian Deadlift (RDL) occurs primarily in which anatomical plane?
   A) Frontal plane
   B) Sagittal plane
   C) Transverse plane
   D) Coronal plane

5. The push-up test is an example of a(n) _____ muscular endurance test.
   A) Isoelectric
   B) Dynamic
   C) Isometric
   D) Isokinetic

6. A(n) _____ monitors the force a muscle generates at a constant speed.
   A) Isokinetic dynamometer
   B) Eccentric dynamometer

   C) Concentric sphygmomenometer
   D) Selectorized leg press

7. The joint action of the shoulder during the concentric phase of the bench press is _____.
   A) Flexion
   B) Extension
   C) Abduction
   D) Horizontal adduction

8. Which of the following is a benefit of muscular endurance testing?
   A) Provides information about strengths and weaknesses.
   B) Provides data for the development of the exercise prescription.
   C) Can highlight a participant's progress and provide positive feedback, which promotes exercise adherence.
   D) All of the above are benefits of muscular endurance testing.

9. A handgrip dynamometer is method of assessing _____ strength.
   A) Eccentric
   B) Isometric
   C) Isotonic
   D) Isokinetic

10. Which of the following would be a part of the procedures for conducting a 1-RM strength test?
    A) Provide adequate time for a dynamic warm-up.
    B) Ensure the participant is experienced with the strength pattern.
    C) Permit 3–5 min between attempts.

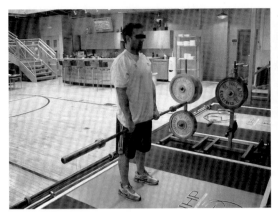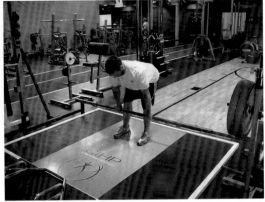

Figure 5.1 Romanian deadlift. Reprinted from *ACSM's Foundations of Strength Training and Conditioning,* second edition. 14.82.

D) All of the above should be included in 1-RM testing procedure.

11. Which of the following is NOT true about the performance of the push-up test?
    A) The male participant begins in the "up" or plank position.
    B) Females perform the push-up test with the knee as the pivot point.
    C) The test is terminated when the participant is unable to maintain proper technique within two repetitions.
    D) The participant should be familiarized of proper push-up technique.

12. During the eccentric phase of the Romanian Deadlift the hips are _____.
    See Figure 5.1.
    A) Extending
    B) Flexing
    C) Abducting
    D) Adducting

13. Which of the following terms is synonymous with cephalic?
    A) Inferior

B) Superior
C) Caudal
D) Lateral

14. Which of the following terms is used to describe an outward deviating knee?
    A) Genu varus
    B) Chondromalacia patella
    C) Genu valgus
    D) Patellar tendonitis

15. _____ muscles, such as the rectus femoris muscle, have fibers aligned at a small angle to a tendon running along the axis of a muscle.
    A) Pennate
    B) Parallel
    C) Circular
    D) Convergent

16. Which term is used to describe movements away from the midline of the body?
    A) Adduction
    B) Abduction
    C) Flexion
    D) Extension

F. CONDUCT ANTHROPOMETHRIC AND BODY COMPOSITION ASSESSMENTS

Domain I Subdomain F: What you need to know

- The advantages, disadvantages, and limitations of body composition techniques (*e.g.,* air displacement plethysmography (BOD POD®), dual-energy x-ray absorptiometry (DEXA), hydrostatic weighing, skinfolds, bioelectrical impedance).
- The standardized descriptions of circumference and skinfold sites.
- Procedures for determining BMI and taking skinfold and circumference measurements.

- The health implications of variation in body fat distribution patterns and the significance of BMI, waist circumference, and waist-to-hip ratio.
- Locating anatomic landmarks for skinfold (Fig. 5.2) and circumference measurements (for example of one measurement, see Fig. 5.3).
- Analyzing and documenting the results of anthropometric and body composition assessments.

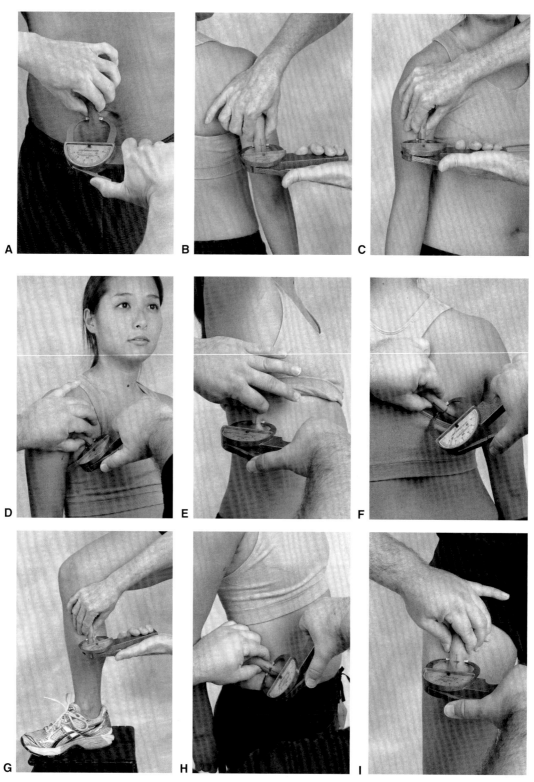

Figure 5.2 Anatomical sites for skinfold measurement. **A.** Abdominal: vertical fold, 2 cm to the right side of the umbilicus. **B.** Triceps: vertical fold on the posterior midline of the upper arm, halfway between the acromion and the olecranon processes, with the arm held freely to the side of the body. **C.** Biceps: vertical fold on the anterior aspect of the arm over the belly of the biceps muscle, 1 cm above the level used to mark the triceps site. **D.** Chest: diagonal fold, one-half the distance between the anterior axillary line and the nipple (men) or one third of the distance between the axillary line and the nipple (women). **E.** Midaxillary: vertical fold on the midaxillary line at the level of the xiphoid process of the sternum. **F.** Subscapular: diagonal fold (at a 45° angle), 1–2 cm below the inferior angle of the scapula. **G.** Medial calf: vertical fold at the maximum circumference of the calf on the midline of its medial border. **H.** Suprailium: diagonal fold in line with the natural angle of the iliac crest taken in the anterior axillary line immediately superior to the iliac crest. **I.** Thigh: vertical fold, on the anterior midline of the thigh, midway between the proximal border of the patella and the inguinal crease (hip). Reprinted from *ACSM's Resources for the Personal Trainer*, sixth edition. Figure 12.7.

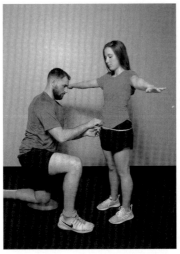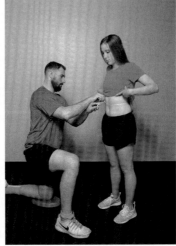

Figure 5.3 Anatomical sites for measurement of waist (narrowest part of the torso) and hip circumference (level of maximal hip circumference). Reprinted from *ACSM's Resources for the Personal Trainer*, sixth edition. Figure 12.6.

Domain I Subdomain F: Multiple Choice Questions

1. Underweight is classified as a body mass index (BMI) of _____.
   A) $<19.9 \text{ kg} \cdot \text{m}^{-2}$
   B) $<18.5 \text{ kg} \cdot \text{m}^{-2}$
   C) $<24.9 \text{ kg} \cdot \text{m}^{-2}$
   D) $<20.5 \text{ kg} \cdot \text{m}^{-2}$

2. When measuring regional body circumferences, an average of duplicate measures is used provided that those measurements do not differ by more than _____.
   A) 3 mm
   B) 10 mm
   C) 5 mm
   D) 12 mm

3. Which of the following represents the demarcation point of a *very high* health risk for young women when using waist-to-hip ratio (WHR)?
   A) >0.86
   B) >0.95
   C) >1.00
   D) >1.03

4. The _____ skinfold site is performed using a diagonal fold method.
   A) Thigh
   B) Medial calf
   C) Suprailiac
   D) Abdominal

5. Which of the following methods of body composition assessment measures body volume within the air?
   A) Bioelectrical impedance analysis (BIA)
   B) Air displacement plethysmography
   C) Dual energy x-ray absorptiometry (DEXA)
   D) Magnetic resonance imaging (MRI)

6. Hydrodensitometry is a body composition assessment technique that uses measures of body weight, volume, and residual lung volume _____.
   A) As the participant is partially submerged underwater
   B) As the participant is completely submerged underwater
   C) After the participant has consumed an isotope solution
   D) While resistance of small electrical currents are observed

7. Which of the following is NOT considered an assessment that provides an estimate of body composition?
   A) Body mass index (BMI) .
   B) Hydrodensitometry.
   C) Dual energy x-ray absorptiometry (DEXA)
   D) Skinfold assessment.

8. _____ obesity is associated with a higher risk of hypertension, metabolic syndrome, and Type 2 diabetes mellitus.
   A) Gynoid
   B) Android
   C) Distal
   D) Adrenergic

ACSM-EP

9. Which of the following is NOT correct regarding taking skinfold measurements?
   A) Take all measurements on the right side of the client's body.
   B) Take a minimum of two measurements at each site.
   C) Place the jaws of the caliper perpendicular to the fold, one inch above the fingers that are holding the skinfold.
   D) Take skinfold measures in rotational order to permit the skinfold site to regain its normal thickness.

10. For females, a waist circumference (WC) of more than _____ is associated with high health risk.
    A) 55 cm (21.6 in.)
    B) 66 cm (25.9 in.)
    C) 77 cm (30.3 in.)
    D) 88 cm (35 in.)

DOMAIN II: EXERCISE PRESCRIPTION AND IMPLEMENTATION

A. Determine safe and Effective exercise programs to achieve desired outcomes and goals, and Translate assessment results into appropriate exercise prescriptions

Domain II Subdomain A: What you need to know

- Strength-, aerobic-, and flexibility-based exercise.
- The benefits and precautions associated with exercise training in apparently healthy clients and those with controlled disease.
- Program development for specific client needs (*e.g.,* sport-specific training, performance, health, lifestyle, functional ability, balance, agility, aerobic, anaerobic).
- The six motor skill-related physical fitness components (agility, balance, coordination, reaction time, speed, and power).
- The physiologic changes associated with an acute bout of exercise.
- The physiologic adaptations following chronic exercise training.
- The FITT-VP principle for apparently healthy clients, clients with increased risk, and clients with controlled disease.
- The components and sequencing incorporated into an exercise session (*e.g.,* warm-up, stretching, conditioning or sports-related exercise, cooldown).
- The physiological principles related to warm-up and cooldown.

- The principles of reversibility, progressive overload, individual differences and specificity of training, and how they relate to exercise prescription.
- The role of aerobic and anaerobic energy systems in the performance of various physical activities.
- The basic biomechanical principles of human movement.
- The psychological and physiological signs and symptoms of overtraining.
- The signs and symptoms of common musculoskeletal injuries associated with exercise equipment (*e.g.,* sprain, strain, bursitis, tendonitis).
- The advantages and disadvantages of exercise equipment (*e.g.,* free weights, selectorized machines, aerobic equipment).
- Teaching and demonstrating exercises.
- Designing safe and effective training programs.
- Implementing the FITT-VP principle for apparently healthy clients, clients with increased risk, and clients with controlled disease.

Multiple Choice Practice Questions and Answers: Domain II Subdomain A

1. The purpose of the cooldown period following an exercise session includes all of the following *except* _____.
   A) Gradual recovery of HR
   B) Gradual recovery of BP
   C) Improvement in range of motion (ROM)
   D) Removal of metabolic end products

2. What does the acronym FITT-VP stand for?

   A) Fast, intense, time, type, volume, and progression
   B) Frequency, independent, time, type, volume, and persistence
   C) Frequency, intensity, time, type, volume, and progression
   D) Force, impulse, torque, time, volume, and progression

3. Muscular fitness refers to _____.
   A) Muscular endurance, muscular force, muscular strength
   B) Muscular endurance, muscular power, and muscular strength
   C) Muscular power, muscular force, and muscle soreness
   D) Muscular strength, anaerobic power, and muscular power

4. For higher-intensity activities, _____.
   A) The benefit outweighs any potential risk
   B) The risk of orthopedic and cardiovascular complications is increased
   C) The risk of orthopedic and cardiovascular complications is minimal
   D) There is no increased risk of orthopedic and cardiovascular complications

5. In the *2018 Physical Activity Guidelines for Americans*, it is recommended that adults need at least _____ min of moderate-intensity physical activity and should perform muscle strengthening exercises on _____ or more days per week.
   A) 90, 1
   B) 120, 2
   C) 150, 2
   D) 180, 1

6. If a client exercises too much without rest days or develops a minor injury and does not allow time for the injury to heal, what can occur?
   A) An overuse injury
   B) Shin splints
   C) Sleep deprivation
   D) Decreased physical conditioning

7. Which of the following activities would provide the greatest improvement in aerobic fitness for someone who is beginning an exercise program?
   A) Weight training
   B) Pilates
   C) Stretching
   D) Walking

8. Which of the following is a change seen as a result of regular aerobic exercise?
   A) Decreased HR at rest
   B) Increased stroke volume at rest
   C) No change for cardiac output at rest
   D) All of the above

9. Generally, low-fit or sedentary persons may benefit from _____.

A) Shorter duration, higher intensity, and higher frequency of exercise
B) Longer duration, higher intensity, and higher frequency of exercise
C) Shorter duration, lower intensity, and higher frequency of exercise
D) Shorter duration, higher intensity, and lower frequency of exercise

10. Which grouping lists the three training principles that you need to consider when prescribing exercise for individuals?
    A) Overload, intensity, progression
    B) Frequency, intensity, duration
    C) Specificity, overload, redundancy
    D) Overload, specificity, progression

11. Which of the following would be an example of a verbal external coaching cue that could be used while teaching the push-up?
    A) "Extend your elbows".
    B) "Squeeze your chest".
    C) "Push the floor away from you".
    D) "Tighten your abdominals".

12. Which of the following contribute to the increases in strength seen after a period of heavy resistance training?
    A) Decrease in muscle fiber diameter
    B) Increases in agonist motor unit recruitment
    C) Increases in neural inhibitory reflexes
    D) Decreases in tendon stiffness

13. Which of the following would be most appropriate to improve the performance of a throwing athlete (*e.g.,* shot put, hammer, javelin)?
    A) High-volume, low-intensity aerobic training
    B) Low-volume, low-intensity aerobic training
    C) Maximal resistance training with slow contraction velocities
    D) Submaximal resistance training with intermediate-high contraction velocities

14. Which of the following terms is characterized by prolonged performance decrements (>2 months), chronic injuries, and neuroendocrine disturbances associated with increases in training intensity or volume without adequate recovery.
    A) Functional overreaching
    B) Nonfunctional overreaching
    C) Overtraining syndrome
    D) Detraining syndrome

15. Which of the following is a purported benefit of a dynamic warm-up period?
    A) Increase in muscle temperature
    B) Gradually elevates oxygen consumption
    C) Increased psychological readiness for performance
    D) All of the above are correct

16. Given the same absolute exercise intensity and duration, who would be expected to have a higher excess post oxygen consumption (EPOC), the trained or untrained individual?
    A) Trained individual
    B) Untrained individual
    C) EPOC would be the same

17. Which of the following would be considered an advantage of using elastic bands when compared to free weights?
    A) Free weights rely on gravity to impose resistance, thus limiting the direction of the force vector (*i.e.,* direction of resistance) applied to the body.
    B) Bands are easily more easily transported compared to free weights.
    C) As the length of the band increases, more resistance is applied to the band, offering the potential for unique adaptations in variable ranges of motion.
    D) All of the above are correct.

18. Which of the following laws best describes how bone adapts to the loads under which it is placed?
    A) Wolff's law
    B) Boyle's law
    C) Poiseuille's law
    D) Newton's law

19. The functional unit of neuromuscular control involves the _____, which includes one motor neuron and all of the muscle fibers it innervates.
    A) Sarcomere
    B) Motor unit
    C) Sarcoplasmic reticulum
    D) Neuromuscular junction

20. The sequential recruitment of motor units from low threshold to high threshold based on force production demands best describes which principle?
    A) The all-or-none principle
    B) The size (or Henneman) principle
    C) The principle of specificity
    D) The principle of reversibility

21. During the final stage of a maximally graded exercise test, which value would be the highest?
    A) Cardiac Output ($\dot{Q}$)
    B) Minute Ventilation (V_E)
    C) Tidal Volume (TV)
    D) Absolute $\dot{V}O_2$

B. IMPLEMENT CARDIORESPIRATORY EXERCISE PRESCRIPTIONS FOR APPARENTLY HEALTHY CLIENTS AND THOSE WITH CONTROLLED DISEASE BASED ON CURRENT HEALTH STATUS, FITNESS GOALS, AND AVAILABILITY OF TIME

Domain II Subdomain B: What you need to know

- The recommended FITT-VP principle for the development of cardiorespiratory fitness.
- The benefits, risks, and contraindications of a wide variety of cardiovascular training exercises based on client experience, skill level, current fitness level and goals.
- The minimal threshold of physical activity required for health benefits and/or fitness development.
- Determining exercise intensity using HRR, $\dot{V}O_2R$, peak HR method, peak $\dot{V}O_2$ method, peak METs method, and the RPE scale.
- The accuracy of HRR, $\dot{V}O_2R$, peak HR method, peak $\dot{V}O_2$ method, peak METs method, and the RPE scale.
- Abnormal responses to exercise (*e.g.,* hemodynamic, cardiac, ventilatory).
- Metabolic calculations (*e.g.,* unit conversions, deriving energy cost of exercise, caloric expenditure).
- Calculating the caloric expenditure of an exercise session (kcal · session^{-1}).
- Methods for establishing and monitoring levels of exercise intensity, including heart rate, RPE, and METs.
- The applications of anaerobic training principles.
- The anatomy and physiology of the cardiovascular and pulmonary systems including the basic properties of cardiac muscle.
- The basic principles of gas exchange.

Domain II Subdomain B: Multiple Choice Questions

1. What is the frequency of combined aerobic exercise recommended for most adults?
   A) 5–7 d · wk^{-1}
   B) 4–6 d · wk^{-1}
   C) 3–5 d · wk^{-1}
   D) 1–3 d · wk^{-1}

2. Which of the following percentages of HRR would classify as "moderate" aerobic exercise intensity?
   A) 34%
   B) 52%
   C) 65%
   D) 91%

3. Which of the following methods is *NOT* recommended for estimating exercise intensity for exercise prescription?
   A) HRR
   B) Oxygen uptake reserve ($\dot{V}O_2R$)
   C) Ventilatory threshold (VT)
   D) Maximum heart rate percentage (%HR$_{max}$)

4. What is the minimum recommended target volume for energy expenditure (EE) to promote overall health and well-being in an Ex Rx?
   A) 500–1,000 MET-min · wk^{-1}
   B) 250–500 MET-min · wk^{-1}
   C) 150–250 MET-min · wk^{-1}
   D) 1,000–1,500 MET-min · wk^{-1}

5. The ACSM recommends a time of at least _____ min of moderate exercise or at least _____ min of vigorous exercise per week for aerobic exercise training.
   A) 150; 75
   B) 40; 40
   C) 30; 150
   D) 40; 200

6. If a 175-lb man jogged for 30-min treadmill at an intensity of 26 mL · kg^{-1} · min^{-1}, what would his approximate caloric expenditure be for the entire 30-min session?
   A) 10 kcal
   B) 80 kcal
   C) 310.5 kcal
   D) 3,900 kcal

7. A comprehensive exercise prescription should contain which of the following?
   A) Cardiorespiratory fitness, muscular strength, muscular endurance, flexibility, body composition, and neuromotor fitness
   B) Cardiorespiratory fitness, muscular power, muscular force, flexibility, body composition, and neuromotor fitness
   C) Cardiorespiratory fitness, muscular strength, muscular force, body composition, and neuromotor fitness
   D) Cardiorespiratory fitness, muscular power, muscular endurance, flexibility, and body composition

8. According to the most recent ACSM guidelines, in order to gain health benefits, it is recommended that moderate aerobic physical activity should be performed how many days per week?
   A) 2 d · wk^{-1}
   B) 7 d · wk^{-1}
   C) 5 d · wk^{-1}
   D) 3 d · wk^{-1}

9. For health benefits, it is recommended that vigorous aerobic physical activity should be performed how many days per week?
   A) 2 d · wk^{-1}
   B) 7 d · wk^{-1}
   C) 5 d · wk^{-1}
   D) 3 d · wk^{-1}

10. Moderate exercise is considered to be _____.
    A) 59%–79% HRR or $\dot{V}O_2R$
    B) 40%–59% HRR or $\dot{V}O_2R$
    C) 30%–45% HRR or $\dot{V}O_2R$
    D) 60%–89% HRR or $\dot{V}O_2R$

11. Vigorous exercise is considered to be _____.
    A) 59%–79% HRR or $\dot{V}O_2R$
    B) 40%–59% HRR or $\dot{V}O_2R$
    C) 30%–45% HRR or $\dot{V}O_2R$
    D) 60%–89% HRR or $\dot{V}O_2R$

12. The recommended exercise duration for moderate exercise is _____.
    A) 30–60 min · d^{-1}
    B) 20–50 min · d^{-1}
    C) 20–30 min · d^{-1}
    D) 30–40 min · d^{-1}

13. When using a pedometer, how many steps should most individuals achieve?
    A) 5,000 steps · d^{-1}
    B) 9,000 steps · d^{-1}
    C) 7,000 steps · d^{-1}
    D) 11,000 steps · d^{-1}

14. Which of the following is the correct MET value if a person's relative $\dot{V}O_2 = 34$ mL kg$^{-1} \cdot$ min^{-1}.
    A) 170 METs
    B) 6.8 METs
    C) 9.7 METs
    D) 15 METs

15. During aerobic exercise, which of the following responses would *not* be considered normal in individuals without CVD?
    A) Increased SBP
    B) Increased pulse pressure
    C) Increased mean arterial pressure
    D) Increased DBP

16. Which of the following variables is needed when using the Karvonen (HRR) formula to calculate target heart rate (THR)?
    A) HR$_{max}$
    B) Maximal SBP
    C) Rate pressure product (RPP)
    D) Maximal mean arterial pressure (MAP)

17. Your client is 24 years old. The exercise prescription calls for her to maintain an exercise intensity ranging between 55% and 70% HRmax. What is her target HR range for this workout?
    A) 97–123 bpm
    B) 108–137 bpm
    C) 110–140 bpm
    D) 121–154 bpm

18. When periodizing training for a marathon runner (26.2 mi) who is doing a long run each Sunday, which is appropriate? Each Sunday run should _____.
    A) Be the same distance at about 20–22 mi.
    B) Gradually increase in distance weekly with a slightly lower distance Sunday every fourth week or so.
    C) Gradually increase in distance every week by about 10%.
    D) Rapidly increase distance weekly then avoid all long runs the last 2 months.

19. Which of the following is true regarding the respiratory exchange ratio (RER)?
    A) At intensities exceeding the anaerobic threshold, the RER increases above 1.0.
    B) An RER of 0.7 would indicate the individual is using exclusively carbohydrate for energy.
    C) The RER can never exceed 1.
    D) An RER of 0.7 would indicate the individual is exercising at a vigorous intensity.

20. How many kilocalories did John expend if he performed 35 min of cycling at a relative $\dot{V}O_2$ of 35 mL $\cdot$ kg$^{-1} \cdot$ min^{-1}? His body mass is 75 kg.
    A) 250 kcal
    B) 300 kcal
    C) 410 kcal
    D) 460 kcal

21. Which of the following would be the most appropriate description of the Borg Rating of Perceived Exertion (RPE) = 13?
    A) Very light
    B) Somewhat hard
    C) Very hard
    D) Very, very hard

22. Assume your client's body mass = 165 lb, she is performing a step workout at a rate of 24 steps $\cdot$ min^{-1}. The step height is 8". What is her estimated relative $\dot{V}O_2$ during this step workout?
    A) 5 mL $\cdot$ kg$^{-1} \cdot$ min^{-1}
    B) 10 mL $\cdot$ kg$^{-1} \cdot$ min^{-1}
    C) 15 mL $\cdot$ kg$^{-1} \cdot$ min^{-1}
    D) 20 mL $\cdot$ kg$^{-1} \cdot$ min^{-1}

23. Your client's body mass = 180 lb. He is cycling at a relative $\dot{V}O_2 = 25$ mL $\cdot$ kg$^{-1} \cdot$ min^{-1}. How many minutes would he need to exercise at this intensity to expend 350 kcal?
    A) 25 min
    B) 34 min
    C) 45 min
    D) 60 min

C. IMPLEMENT EXERCISE PRESCRIPTIONS FOR FLEXIBILITY, MUSCULAR STRENGTH, MUSCULAR ENDURANCE, BALANCE, AGILITY, AND REACTION TIME FOR APPARENTLY HEALTHY CLIENTS AND THOSE WITH CONTROLLED DISEASE BASED ON CURRENT HEALTH STATUS, FITNESS GOALS AND AVAILABILITY OF TIME

Domain II Subdomain C: What you need to know

• The recommended FITT-VP principle for the development of muscular strength, muscular endurance, and flexibility.

• The minimal threshold of physical activity required for health benefits and/or fitness development.

- Safe and effective exercises designed to enhance muscular strength and/or endurance of muscle groups.
- Safe and effective stretches that enhance flexibility.
- Indications for water-based exercise (*e.g.,* arthritis, obesity).
- The types of resistance training programs (*e.g.,* total body, splitroutine) and modalities (*e.g.,* free weights, variable resistance equipment, pneumatic machines, bands).
- Acute (*e.g.,* load, volume, sets, repetitions, rest periods, order of exercises) and chronic training variables (*e.g.,* periodization).
- Types of muscle contractions (*e.g.,* eccentric, concentric, isometric).
- Joint movements (*e.g.,* flexion, extension, adduction, abduction) and the muscles responsible for them.
- Acute and delayed onset muscle soreness (DOMS).
- The anatomy and physiology of skeletal muscle fiber, the characteristics of fast- and slow-twitch muscle fibers, and the sliding filament theory of muscle contraction.
- The stretch reflex, proprioceptors, golgi tendon organ (GTO), muscle spindles, and how they relate to flexibility.
- Muscle-related terminology including atrophy, hyperplasia, hypertrophy.
- The Valsalva maneuver and its implications during exercise.

- The physiology underlying plyometric training and common plyometric exercises (*e.g.,* box jumps, leaps, bounds).
- The contraindications and potential risks associated with muscular conditioning activities (*e.g.,* straight-leg sit-ups, double leg raises, squats, hurdler's stretch, yoga plough, forceful back hyperextension, standing bent-over toe touch, behind neck press/lat pull-down).
- Spotting positions and techniques for injury prevention and exercise assistance.
- Periodization (*e.g.,* macro, micro, mesocycles) and associated theories.
- Safe and effective Olympic weight lifting exercises.
- Safe and effective core stability exercises (*e.g.,* planks, crunches, bridges, cable twists).
- Identifying and correcting improper technique in the use of resistive equipment (*e.g.,* stability balls, weights, bands, resistance bars, water exercise equipment).
- Teaching and demonstrating appropriate exercises for enhancing musculoskeletal flexibility.
- Teaching and demonstrating safe and effective muscular strength and endurance exercises (*e.g.,* free weights, weight machines, resistive bands, Swiss balls, body weight and all other major fitness equipment).
- Prescribing exercise using the calculated %1-RM.

Domain II Subdomain C: Multiple Choice Questions

1. What is the minimum recovery time recommended for a muscle group following a new or intense resistance training session?
   A) 12 h
   B) 24 h
   C) 48 h
   D) 72 h

2. A comprehensive exercise prescription should address which of the following?
   A) Cardiorespiratory (aerobic) fitness
   B) Body composition
   C) Neuromotor fitness
   D) All of the above

3. _____ involves holding the stretched position using the strength of the agonist muscle as is common in many forms of yoga.
   A) Passive static stretching
   B) Active static stretching

   C) Proprioceptive neuromuscular facilitation (PNF)
   D) Dynamic stretching

4. _____ is not recommended because of the significant chance of injury, severe muscle soreness, and serious complications such as exertional rhabdomyolysis that can ensue.
   A) Resistance training composed exclusively of supramaximal (>100% 1RM) eccentric actions
   B) The Valsalva maneuver
   C) Resistance training composed exclusively of static contractions for periods longer than 60 s
   D) The use of a weight belt during power lifting

ACSM-EP

5. Ideal resistance training volume for adults with the goal of general improvement of muscular fitness should be _____.
   A) 2–4 sets with 8–12 repetitions
   B) 1–2 sets with 8–12 repetitions
   C) 2–4 sets with 12–15 repetitions
   D) 3–5 sets with 8–12 repetitions

6. The ACSM recommends how many repetitions of each exercise to optimize improvement in muscular endurance?
   A) 5–6
   B) 6–10
   C) 11–14
   D) 15–25

7. What is the recommended repetition range for adults seeking the goal of general muscular fitness?
   A) 1–5
   B) 6–10
   C) 8–12
   D) 15–20

8. Which of the following muscle actions occurs when muscle tension increases but the length of the muscle does not change?
   A) Concentric isotonic
   B) Eccentric isotonic
   C) Isokinetic
   D) Isometric

9. Which of the following is an example of how to progressively overload the muscular system via resistance training?
   A) Increasing amount of resistance lifted
   B) Performing more sets per muscle group
   C) Increasing days per week the muscle groups are trained
   D) All of the above are examples of progressive overload

10. Which of the following will increase a person's postural stability?
    A) Lowering the center of gravity
    B) Raising the center of gravity
    C) Narrowing the width of stance
    D) Standing on an unstable surface such as an airex pad or a bosu

11. Which of the following methods of stretching involves a series of contract–relax cycles of the target muscle?
    A) Static
    B) Ballistic
    C) Proprioceptive neuromuscular facilitation (PNF)
    D) All of the above

D. IMPLEMENT EXERCISE PROGRESSION GUIDELINES FOR FLEXIBILITY, MUSCULAR STRENGTH, MUSCULAR ENDURANCE, BALANCE, AGILITY, AND REACTION TIME FOR APPARENTLY HEALTHY CLIENTS AND THOSE WITH CONTROLLED DISEASE BASED ON CURRENT HEALTH STATUS, FITNESS GOALS, AND AVAILABILITY OF TIME.

Domain II Subdomain D: What you need to know

- The basic principles of exercise progression.
- Adjusting the FITT-VP principle in response to individual changes in conditioning.
- The importance of performing periodic reevaluations to assess changes in fitness status.
- The training principles that promote improvements in muscular strength, muscular endurance, cardiorespiratory fitness, and flexibility.
- Recognizing the need for progression and communicating exercise prescription updates to clients.

Domain II Subdomain D: Multiple Choice Questions

1. Which of the following is a prudent rule of progression in exercise programming?
   A) 5%–10% rule
   B) 10%–15% rule
   C) 5–10 lb rule
   D) 10–15 lb rule

2. Among the FITT-VP principles, the letter P denotes
   A) Plan
   B) Progression
   C) Plyometric
   D) Prescription

3. Which of the following would be considered a method of introducing progression into an exercise program?
   A) Increase the load.
   B) Increase the number of repetitions performed.
   C) Modify the movement pattern.
   D) All of the above are correct.

4. Based on the 2 plus 2 rule, progression is warranted if the participant completes two additional repetitions above the desired number. This increase in performance must be repeated _____.
   A) At least one additional time within the next 2 months
   B) In two consecutive workouts
   C) In a 2-week period
   D) In a 2-month period

5. Which of the following would be the appropriate implementation of the 5%–10% progression rule for a participant that is currently using the following CV prescription?
   F: 3 d · wk^{-1}
   I: 65% HRR
   T. 30 min
   T: Running
   A) Increase the time to 40 min.
   B) Increase the intensity to 70% HRR.
   C) Increase the frequency to 5 d · wk^{-1}.
   D) All of the above.

6. Specific physiological adaptations to resistance training are determined by which of the following factors?
   A) Speed of movement
   B) Range of motion
   C) Rest between exercises
   D) All of the above.

E. IMPLEMENT A GENERAL WEIGHT MANAGEMENT PROGRAM AS INDICATED BY PERSONAL GOALS, AS NEEDED

Domain II Subdomain E: What you need to know

- Exercise prescriptions for achieving weight-related goals, including weight gain, weight loss, and weight maintenance.
- Energy balance and basic nutritional guidelines (*e.g.,* MyPlate, USDA Dietary Guidelines for Americans).
- Weight management terminology (*e.g.,* obesity, overweight, percent fat, BMI, lean body mass, anorexia nervosa, bulimia nervosa, binge eating, metabolic syndrome, body fat distribution, adipocyte, bariatrics, ergogenic aid, fat-free mass (FFM), resting metabolic rate (RMR) and thermogenesis).
- The relationship between body composition and health.
- The unique dietary needs of client populations (*e.g.,* women, children, older adults, pregnant women).
- Common nutritional ergogenic aids, their purported mechanisms of action, and associated risks and benefits (*e.g.,* protein/amino acids, vitamins, minerals, herbal products, creatine, steroids, caffeine).
- Methods for modifying body composition including diet, exercise, and behavior modification.
- Fuel sources for aerobic and anaerobic metabolism including carbohydrates, fats, and proteins.
- The effects of overall dietary composition on healthy weight management.
- The importance of maintaining normal hydration before, during and after exercise.
- The consequences of inappropriate weight loss methods (*e.g.,* saunas, dietary supplements, vibrating belts, body wraps, over-exercising, very low-calorie diets, electric stimulators, sweat suits, fad diets).
- The kilocalorie levels of carbohydrate, fat, protein, and alcohol.
- The relationship between kilocalorie expenditures and weight loss.
- Published position statements on obesity and the risks associated with it (*e.g.,* National Institutes of Health, American Dietetic Association, American College of Sports Medicine).
- The relationship between body fat distribution patterns and health.
- The physiology and pathophysiology of overweight and obese clients.
- The recommended FITT-VP principle for clients who are overweight or obese.
- Comorbidities and musculoskeletal conditions associated with overweight and obesity that may require medical clearance and/or modifications to exercise testing and prescription.
- Applying behavioral strategies (*e.g.,* exercise, diet, behavioral modification strategies) for weight management.
- Modifying exercises for clients limited by body size.
- Calculating the volume of exercise in terms of kcal · session^{-1}.

Domain II Subdomain E: Multiple Choice Questions

1. The kilocalorie yield of 1 g of carbohydrate isapproximately
   A) $2\,kcal \cdot g^{-1}$
   B) $4\,kcal \cdot g^{-1}$
   C) $7\,kcal \cdot g^{-1}$
   D) $9\,kcal \cdot g^{-1}$

2. As compared to being in a state of dehydration, which of the following is NOT associated with euhydration during exercise?
   A) Lower core temperature
   B) Lower heart rate
   C) Lower rating of perceived exertion (RPE)
   D) Lower stroke volume

3. The fastest method of producing ATP during exercise is through _____.
   A) Glycolysis
   B) Gluconeogenesis
   C) Aerobic metabolism
   D) The ATP-CP system

4. _____ energy production increases as exercise intensity exceeds the lactate threshold.
   A) Aerobic
   B) Anaerobic
   C) Oxidative phosphorylation
   D) Citric acid cycle

5. The stored form of sugar within skeletal muscle and the liver is _____.
   A) Pyruvate
   B) Fructose
   C) Glycogen
   D) Glucose

6. Aerobic production of ATP occurs in the _____ of the cell.
   A) Mitochondria
   B) Cytoplasm
   C) Ribosome
   D) Nucleus

7. Which of the following is a recommended weight management strategy?
   A) Very low-calorie diet
   B) Sweat suits
   C) Dietary supplements
   D) Combination of physical activity, behavior therapy, and proper nutrition

8. During pregnancy, an additional _____ $kcal \cdot d^{-1}$ is required to ensure sufficient nutrients are available for both mother and baby.
   A) 50
   B) 150
   C) 200
   D) 300

9. Based upon the 2015–2020 Dietary Guidelines for Americans, carbohydrate consumption for adults (including sedentary and recreational exercisers) should range between_____ of their daily macronutrient intake.
   A) 20% and 35%
   B) 30% and 45%
   C) 45% and 60%
   D) 45% and 65%

F. PRESCRIBE AND IMPLEMENT EXERCISE PROGRAMS FOR CLIENTS WITH CONTROLED CARDIOVASCULAR, PULMONARY, AND METABOLIC DISEASES AND OTHER CLINICAL POPULATIONS AND WORK CLOSELY WITH CLIENTS' HEALTHCARE PROVIDERS, AS NEEDED

Domain II Subdomain F: What you need to know

- ACSM pre-participation screening algorithm and the FITT-VP principle for clients with cardiovascular, pulmonary, and metabolic diseases and other clinical populations.
- Relative and absolute contraindications for initiating exercise sessions or exercise testing, and indications for terminating exercise sessions and exercise testing.
- Physiology and pathophysiology of diseases and conditions (*e.g.,* cardiac disease, arthritis, diabetes mellitus, dyslipidemia, hypertension, metabolic syndrome, musculoskeletal injuries, overweight and obesity, osteoporosis, peripheral artery disease, pulmonary disease).
- The effects of diet and exercise on blood glucose levels in diabetics.
- The recommended FITT-VP principle for the development of cardiorespiratory fitness, muscular fitness, and flexibility for clients with diseases and conditions (*e.g.,* cardiac disease, arthritis, diabetes mellitus, dyslipidemia, hypertension, metabolic syndrome, musculoskeletal injuries, overweight and obesity, osteoporosis, peripheral artery disease, pulmonary disease).

- Progressing exercise programs, according to the FITT-VP principle, in a safe and effective manner.
- Modifying the exercise prescription and/or exercise choice for clients with diseases and conditions (*e.g.,* cardiac disease, arthritis, diabetes mellitus, dyslipidemia, hypertension, metabolic syndrome, musculoskeletal injuries, overweight and obesity, osteoporosis, peripheral artery disease, pulmonary disease).
- Identifying improper exercise techniques and modifying exercise programs for clients with low back, neck, shoulder, elbow, wrist, hip, knee, and/or ankle pain.

Domain II Subdomain F: Multiple Choice Questions

1. The loss of elasticity (or "hardening") of the arteries is known as _____.
   A) Atherosclerosis
   B) Arteriosclerosis
   C) Atheroma
   D) Adventitia

2. Which type of exercise is considered most effective for reducing the risk of developing osteoporosis?
   A) Only chair exercises
   B) Aquatic exercise only
   C) Stationary cycling only
   D) All modes of weight-bearing exercise

3. Metabolic syndrome involves several metabolic risk factors. Which of the following health factors is NOT associated with the metabolic syndrome?
   A) Central adiposity
   B) Hypertension
   C) Hyperglycemia
   D) Asthma

4. Regular physical activity (PA) is believed to improve _____ among those with Type 2 diabetes mellitus (T2DM).
   A) Glycemic control
   B) Insulin sensitivity
   C) Blood pressure
   D) All of the above

5. Exercise frequency recommendations for individuals with diabetes mellitus (DM) include _____ $d \cdot wk^{-1}$.
   A) 2–3
   B) 3–4
   C) 4–5
   D) 3–7

6. For previously sedentary individuals that are considered very deconditioned, exercise bouts of _____ min may yield favorable adaptations.
   A) 10
   B) 30
   C) 50
   D) 60

7. A(n)_____ describes an event in which there is prolonged ischemia, resulting in myocardial tissue death.
   A) Palpitation
   B) Myocardial infarction
   C) Myocardial infection
   D) Embolism

8. In working with patients in a cardiac rehabilitation setting, which of the following is NOT a contraindication for the participation in exercise training?
   A) Unstable angina
   B) Acute systemic illness
   C) Recent embolism
   D) Stable heart failure

9. Exercise is not recommended during peak insulin action because_____ can result.
   A) Ketosis
   B) Hyperglycemia
   C) Hypoglycemia
   D) Hypertension

10. Which of the following are benefits of an acute bout of exercise in those with T2DM?
    A) Improved insulin sensitivity
    B) Improved glucose uptake
    C) Improved feelings of well-being
    D) All of the above

11. Which of the following is NOT a complication directly associated with diabetes mellitus.
    A) Coronary artery disease
    B) Peripheral neuropathy
    C) Osteoporosis
    D) Autonomic neuropathy

12. At what point should graded eccentric exercise be introduced for the improvement of tendinosis?
    A) When pain is at its peak
    B) When the pain subsides
    C) Eccentric exercise is contraindicated and should never be used in cases of tendinosis
    D) In the acute phase

G. PRESCRIBE AND IMPLEMENT EXERCISE PROGRAMS FOR HEALTHY SPECIAL POPULATIONS (E.G., OLDER ADULTS, CHILDREN, ADOLESCENTS, PREGNANT WOMEN)

Domain II Subdomain G: What you need to know

- Normal maturational changes across the life span and their effects (*e.g.,* skeletal muscle, bone, reaction time, coordination, posture, heat and cold tolerance, maximal oxygen consumption, strength, flexibility, body composition, resting and maximal heart rate, resting and maximal blood pressure).
- Techniques for the modification of cardiovascular, flexibility, and resistance exercises based on age, functional capacity, and physical condition.
- Techniques for the development of exercise prescriptions for children, adolescents and older adults with regard to strength, functional capacity, and motor skills.
- The unique adaptations to exercise training in children, adolescents, and older adults with regard to strength, functional capacity, and motor skills.
- The benefits and precautions associated with exercise training across the life span.
- The recommended FITT-VP principle for the development of cardiorespiratory fitness, muscular fitness, balance, and flexibility in apparently healthy children and adolescents.
- The effects of the aging process on the musculoskeletal and cardiovascular structures and functions during rest, exercise, and recovery.
- The recommended FITT-VP principle necessary for the development of cardiorespiratory fitness, muscular fitness, balance, and flexibility in apparently healthy older adults.
- Common orthopedic and cardiovascular exercise considerations for older adults.
- The relationship between regular physical activity and the successful performance of activities of daily living (ADLs) for older adults.
- The recommended FITT-VP principle necessary for the development of cardiorespiratory fitness, muscular fitness, balance, and flexibility in apparently healthy pregnant women.
- Teaching and demonstrating appropriate exercises for healthy populations with special considerations.
- Modifying exercises based on age, physical condition, and current health status.

Domain II Subdomain G: Multiple Choice Questions

1. Which of the following is *not* true regarding the psychological benefits of regular exercise in the older adults?
   A) Improved Self-concept
   B) Life satisfaction
   C) Stimulation of appetite
   D) Improved Self-efficacy

2. Which statement is true regarding ACSM physical activity guidelines for children?
   A) Children should participate in several bouts of physical activity lasting more than $120 \min \cdot d^{-1}$.
   B) Children should perform $\geq 60 \min \cdot d^{-1}$ of physical activity.
   C) Children should focus on just one or two modes of physical activity to develop exceptional skills in those areas.
   D) Children need to have several periods of 2 h or more of inactivity during the day in order to have adequate rest.

3. An exercise program for older adult persons generally should emphasize increased _____.
   A) Frequency
   B) Intensity

C) Duration
D) Intensity and frequency

4. Which of the following exercises should be avoided after the first trimester for a pregnant woman?
   A) Upright exercises such as walking on an outdoor track
   B) Sitting exercises such as semi-recumbent cycling
   C) Prone position exercises
   D) Supine position exercises

5. Which of the following are true regarding exercise recommendations during pregnancy?
   A) Maximal exercise testing should not be performed on women who are pregnant unless medically necessary.
   B) Exercise intensity can be monitored by using the Borg RPE scale (between 12 and 14).
   C) Exercises performed in the supine position should be modified or avoided after week 16 of pregnancy.
   D) All of the above are correct.

6. Which of the following measures at rest tend to be higher in children compared to adults?
   A) Heart rate (HR)
   B) Systolic blood pressure (SBP)
   C) Sweat rates
   D) Stroke volume (SV)

7. Which of the following statements is true regarding pregnant women that have been sedentary but have no contraindications?
   A) To rapidly improve health of mother and baby, exercise duration should begin with longer bouts (>30 min).
   B) Previously sedentary pregnant women should perform maximal exercise testing to establish their baseline fitness level.
   C) Intensity recommendations for previously sedentary pregnant women include 70%–85% HRR.
   D) Previously inactive women should progress from 15 $min \cdot d^{-1}$.

8. Based on ACSM recommendations, older adults should perform at least _____ days of moderate-intensity aerobic activity each week.

A) 2
B) 3
C) 4
D) 5

9. Which of the following is considered an exercise prescription recommendation for children and adolescents?
   A) Children and adolescents should perform 1–2 $d \cdot wk^{-1}$ of resistance exercise
   B) Children and adolescents should perform at least 85% 1-RM for strength prescription
   C) Children and adolescents should perform resistance exercise at least 3 $d \cdot wk^{-1}$.
   D) Children and adolescents should perform 3–5 $d \cdot wk^{-1}$ of aerobic activity.

10. Which of the following is NOT a relative contraindication for exercising during pregnancy?
   A) Severe anemia
   B) Poorly controlled hypertension
   C) Low back pain
   D) Modest increase in HR during exercise compared to nonpregnancy

H. MODIFY EXERCISE PRESCRIPTIONS BASED ON VARIOUS ENVIRONMENTAL CONDITIONS

Domain II Subdomain H: What you need to know

- The effects of various environmental conditions on the physiologic response to exercise (*e.g.,* altitude, variable ambient temperatures, humidity, environmental pollution).
- Special precautions and program modifications for exercise in various environmental conditions (*e.g.,* altitude, variable ambient temperatures, humidity, environmental pollution).

- The role of acclimatization when exercising in various environmental conditions (*e.g.,* altitude, variable ambient temperatures, humidity, environmental pollution).
- Appropriate fluid intake during exercise in various environmental conditions (*e.g.,* altitude, variable ambient temperatures, humidity, environmental pollution).

Domain II Subdomain H: Multiple Choice Questions

1. When participating in exercise at high altitudes, HR will _____ at the same RPE as compared to when exercising at sea level.
   A) Be lower
   B) Have no relation and cannot be monitored
   C) Be higher
   D) Remain the same

2. Maximal oxygen consumption is reduced in high altitudes as a result of _____.
   A) Lower percent of oxygen in the air
   B) Reduced partial pressure of oxygen (PO_2)
   C) Delayed onset of the lactate threshold
   D) Reduced maximal HR

3. Which of the following are established adaptations that occur as a result of chronic altitude exposure?
   A) Increased hemoglobin levels
   B) Increase in maximal HR
   C) Increase in PO_2
   D) Decrease in sweat rates

4. _____ refers to the physiologic adaptive changes that improve heat tolerance.
   A) Heat stress
   B) Heat acclimatization
   C) Heat compensation
   D) Heat loss

DOMAIN III: EXERCISE COUNSELING AND BEHAVIOR MODIFICATION

A. OPTIMIZE ADOPTION AND ADHERENCE OF EXERCISE AND OTHER HEALTHY BEHAVIORS BY APPLYING EFFECTIVE COMMUNICATION TECHNIQUES.

Domain III Subdomain A: What you need to know

- Verbal and nonverbal behaviors that communicate positive reinforcement and encouragement (*e.g.,* eye contact, targeted praise, empathy).
- Group leadership techniques for working with clients of all ages.
- Learning preferences (auditory, visual, kinesthetic) and how to apply teaching and training techniques to optimize training session.
- Applying active listening techniques.
- Using feedback to optimize a client's training sessions.
- Effective use of a variety of communication modes (*e.g.,* telephone, newsletters, email, social media).

Domain III Subdomain A: Multiple Choice Questions

1. Which of the following is NOT a positive communication technique to reinforce the adoption of healthy exercise behavior?
   A) Provide the client with targeted praise.
   B) Listen and encourage with verbal and nonverbal prompts.
   C) Convey interest and empathy.
   D) Tell the client what their behavior change barrier is and how to correct it.

2. Which of the following is a client-centered communication technique where the practitioner makes reflective statements to convey that he or she has heard and understood what the client is saying?
   A) Synergistic approach
   B) Communication bridging
   C) Active listening
   D) Preparation phase

3. Which of the following reflects motivational interviewing?
   A) Express empathy.

   B) Avoid arguing, demonstrate patience and flexibility.
   C) Instill confidence in the ability to adopt healthy behaviors such as exercise.
   D) Tell the client why they have been unsuccessful in their pursuit of weight loss goals.

4. Which of the following environmental variables might help create an inviting exercise environment for an individual that is apprehensive about beginning exercise?
   A) Playing loud, aggressive music
   B) Multiple mirrors on the walls
   C) Hostile artwork on the walls
   D) Professional attire worn by staff

5. Which of the following are strategies used to help prevent inactivity relapse?
   A) Expect lapses and have a plan to restart the desired behavior change
   B) Realistic goal setting
   C) Methods of self-monitoring
   D) All of the above are correct

B. OPTIMIZE ADOPTION AND ADHERENCE OF EXERCISE AND OTHER HEALTHY BEHAVIORS BY APPLYING EFFECTIVE BEHAVIORAL STRATEGIES AND MOTIVATIONAL TECHNIQUES

Domain III Subdomain B: What you need to know

- Behavior change models and theories (*e.g.,* transtheoretical model, social cognitive theory, social ecological model, health belief model, theory of planned behavior, self-determination theory, cognitive evaluation theory).
- The basic principles involved in motivational interviewing (MI).
- Intervention strategies and stress management techniques.
- Behavioral strategies to enhance exercise and health behavior change (*e.g.,* reinforcement, S.M.A.R.T. goal setting, social support).
- Behavior modification terminology (*e.g.,* self-esteem, self-efficacy, antecedents, cues to action, behavioral beliefs, behavioral intentions, reinforcing factors).
- Behavioral strategies (*e.g.,* exercise, diet, behavioral modification strategies) for weight management.

- The role that affect, mood, and emotion play in exercise adherence.
- Barriers to exercise adherence and compliance (*e.g.,* time management, injury, fear, lack of knowledge, weather).
- Techniques that facilitate intrinsic and extrinsic motivation (*e.g.,* goal setting, incentive programs, achievement recognition, social support).
- The role extrinsic and intrinsic motivation plays in the adoption and maintenance of behavior change.
- Health coaching principles and lifestyle management techniques related to behavior change.

- Strategies to increase nonstructured physical activity (*e.g.,* stair walking, parking farther away, biking to work).
- Explaining the purpose and value of understanding perceived exertion.
- Using imagery as a motivational tool.
- Evaluating behavioral readiness to optimize exercise adherence.
- Applying the theories related to behavior change to diverse populations.
- Developing intervention strategies to increase self-efficacy and self-confidence.
- Developing reward systems that support and maintain program adherence.
- Setting effective behavioral goals.

Domain III Subdomain B: Multiple Choice Questions

1. Feeling good about being able to perform an activity or skill, such as finally being able to run a mile or to increase the speed of walking a mile, is an example of an _____.
   A) Extrinsic reward
   B) Intrinsic reward
   C) External stimulus
   D) Internal stimulus

2. The health belief model assumes that people will engage in a behavior, such as exercise, when _____.
   A) There is a perceived threat of disease
   B) External motivation is provided
   C) Optimal environmental conditions are met
   D) Internal motivation outweighs external circumstances

3. To determine program effectiveness, psychological theories provide a conceptual framework for assessment and _____.
   A) Management of programs or interventions
   B) Application of cognitive-behavioral or motivational principles
   C) Measurement
   D) All of the above

4. Exercise adherence is increased when _____.
   A) There is social and health care provider support for the individual
   B) A regular schedule of exercise is established
   C) Muscle soreness and injury are minimal
   D) Individualized, attainable goals and objectives are identified
   E) All of the above

5. While assessing the behavioral changes associated with an exercise program, which of the following would be categorized under the cognitive process of the transtheoretical model?
   A) Stimulus control
   B) Reinforcement management
   C) Self-reevaluation
   D) Self-liberation

6. Which of the following assumes that a person will adopt appropriate health behaviors if they feel the consequences are severe and feel personally vulnerable?
   A) Learning theories
   B) Health belief model
   C) Transtheoretical model
   D) Stages of motivational readiness

C. PROVIDE EDUCATIONAL RESOURCES TO SUPPORT CLIENTS IN THE ADOPTION AND MAINTENANCE OF HEALTHY LIFESTYLE BEHAVIORS

Domain III Subdomain C: What you need to know

- The relationship between physical inactivity and common chronic diseases and conditions (*e.g.,* diabetes mellitus, obesity, stroke, dyslipidemia, arthritis, low back pain, hypertension).

- The dynamic interrelationship between fitness level, body composition, stress, and overall health.
- Modifications necessary to promote healthy lifestyle behaviors for diverse populations.

- Stress management techniques and relaxation techniques (*e.g.,* progressive relaxation, guided imagery, massage therapy).
- Activities of daily living (ADLs) and how they relate to overall health.
- Specific, age-appropriate leadership techniques and educational methods to increase client engagement.

- Community-based exercise programs that provide social support and structured activities (*e.g.,* walking clubs, intramural sports, golf leagues, cycling clubs).
- Accessing and disseminating scientifically based, relevant fitness-, nutrition-, and wellness-related resources and information.
- Educating clients about benefits and risks of exercise and the risks of sedentary behavior.

Domain III Subdomain C: Multiple Choice Questions

1. The degenerative loss of muscle mass and, thus, strength due to reduced physical activity and aging is known as _____.
   A) Rheumatoid arthritis
   B) Sarcopenia
   C) Hypertension
   D) Osteoporosis

2. Considering the following list of activities, which are considered activities of daily living (ADLs)?
   A) Walking (transferring)
   B) Singing
   C) Lifting extremely heavy items
   D) Reading and writing

3. Which of the following would be considered a stress reduction technique?
   A) Diaphragmatic breathing

   B) Meditation
   C) Progressive relaxation technique
   D) All of the above

4. Which of the following is true regarding physical activity in those with nonspecific low back pain (LBP)?
   A) Bed rest is recommended until the pain subsides.
   B) Individuals with nonspecific LBP should sit in a chair for the majority of the day in order to reduce spinal compression.
   C) Nonspecific LBP is extremely rare and not worth worrying about.
   D) Individuals with nonspecific LBP should remain active and continue ordinary activity within pain limits.

D. PROVIDE SUPPORT WITHIN THE SCOPE OF PRACTICE OF AN ACSM CERTIFIED EXERCISE PHYSIOLOGIST AND REFER TO OTHER HEALTH PROFESSIONALS AS INDICATED

Domain III Subdomain D: What you need to know

- The side effects of common over the counter and prescription.
- Drugs that may impact a client's ability to exercise.
- Signs and symptoms of mental health states (*e.g.,* anxiety, depression, eating disorders) that may necessitate referral to a medical or mental health professional.
- Symptoms and causal factors of test anxiety (*i.e.,* performance, appraisal threat during

exercise testing) and how they may affect physiological responses to testing.
- Client needs and learning styles that may impact exercise sessions and exercise testing procedures.
- Conflict resolution techniques that facilitate communication among exercise cohorts.
- Communicating the need for medical, nutritional, or mental health intervention.

Domain III Subdomain D: Multiple Choice Questions

1. Following an acute musculoskeletal injury, the appropriate action calls for stabilization of the area and incorporating the RICES treatment method. RICES is the acronym for which of the following?
   A) Recovery, ibuprofen, compression, education, stabilization
   B) Rest and ice, care for injury, support

   C) Rest, ice, compression, elevation, and stabilization
   D) Rotate, ice, care, evaluate, support

2. _____ can reduce HR response to exercise by as much as 30 bpm.
   A) Analgesics
   B) Antilipemics

C) Antibiotics

D) β-blockers

3. Due to its mechanism of action, which of the following medications is associated with dehydration, which could result in an increased risk for developing heat illness?
A) Calcium channel blockers
B) Diuretics
C) β-blockers
D) NSAIDS

4. Which of the following should the ACSM-EP consider when performing fitness and body composition testing on those with lower baseline fitness levels or who are classified as overweight or obese?
A) The results of fitness tests can elicit feelings of distress.
B) Elevated body fat percentage results can reduce enthusiasm to begin an exercise program.
C) Viewing the results of fitness tests may be most intimidating for those that are new to exercise or that have lower baseline fitness.
D) All of the above should be considered.

DOMAIN IV: RISK MANAGEMENT AND PROFESSIONAL RESPONSIBILITIES

A. DEVELOP AND DISSEMINATE RISK MANAGEMENT GUIDELINES FOR A HEALTH/FITNESS FACILITY TO REDUCE MEMBER, EMPLOYEE, AND BUSINESS RISK

Domain IV Subdomain A: What you need to know

- Employee criminal background checks, child abuse clearances, and drug and alcohol screenings.
- Employment verification requirements mandated by state and federal laws.
- Safe handling and disposal of body fluids and employee safety (OSHA guidelines).
- Insurance coverage common to the health/fitness industry including general liability, professional liability, workers' compensation, property, and business interruption
- Sexual harassment policies and procedures
- Interviewing techniques
- Precautions taken in an exercise setting to ensure client safety
- Pre-participation screening algorithm, medical release, and waiver of liability for normal and at-risk clients
- Emergency action plan (EAP); response systems and procedures

- The legal implications of documented safety procedures, the use of incident report documents, and ongoing safety training documentation
- Maintaining employee records/documents (CPR/AED certification, certifications for maintaining job position).
- The components of the ACSM Code of Ethics and the ACSM Certified Exercise Physiologist scope of practice.
- Developing and/or modifying a policies and procedures manual.
- Enforcing confidentiality policies.
- Maintaining a safe exercise environment (*e.g.,* equipment operation and regular maintenance schedules, safety and scheduled maintenance of exercise areas, overall facility maintenance, proper sanitation, proper signage).
- Clearly communicating human resource risk management policies and procedures.
- Training employees to identify and limit/reduce high risk.

Domain IV Subdomain A: Multiple Choice Questions

1. Whose legal responsibility is it to supervise the clinical exercise laboratory and interpret all clinical exercise testing results in a diagnostic setting?
A) The test administrator
B) The clinical exercise physiologist
C) The on-call physician assistant
D) The supervising physician

2. An important safety consideration for exercise equipment in a fitness center includes _____.
A) Flexibility of equipment to allow for different body sizes
B) Affordability of equipment to allow for changing out equipment periodically
C) Mobility of equipment to allow for easy rearrangement
D) None of the above

3. Which of the following personnel is responsible for overall facility management and is often responsible for assisting the development of programs?
   A) Administrative assistant
   B) Front desk staff
   C) Facility operator or program director
   D) Certified personal trainer

4. Which of the following statements is NOT true regarding sexual harassment?
   A) To avoid any suggestion of impropriety, it is suggested the ACSM-EP ask permission prior to touching a client.
   B) Sexual harassment would include any kind of intimidation or coercion of a sexual nature.
   C) Only males can be guilty of sexual harassment.
   D) Sexual harassment is a form of sex discrimination.

5. The Health Insurance Portability and Accountability Act (HIPPA) requires _____.
   A) the ACSM-EP to wear protective equipment to prevent exposure to blood-borne pathogens
   B) the ACSM-EP to purchase limited liability insurance
   C) the ACSM-EP to keep all information gathered about a client's health status confidential
   D) the ACSM-EP to attend a sexual harassment sensitivity class

6. Which of the following federal laws regarding hiring of employees prohibits discrimination on the basis of race, color, gender, religion, and national origin?
   A) The Drug-Free Workplace Act
   B) The Americans with Disabilities Act
   C) The Civil Rights Act
   D) HIPPA

B. ENSURE THAT EMERGENCY POLICIES AND PROCEDURES ARE IN PLACE

Domain IV Subdomain B: What you need to know

- Emergency procedures (*i.e.,* telephone procedures, written emergency action plan and procedures, personnel responsibilities) in a health fitness setting.
- The initial management and first-aid procedures for exercise-related injuries (*e.g.,* bleeding, strains/sprains, fractures, shortness of breath, palpitations, hypoglycemia, allergic reactions, fainting/syncope).
- The responsibilities, limitations, and legal implications for the Certified Exercise Physiologist of carrying out emergency procedures.
- Safety plans, emergency procedures, and first-aid techniques needed during fitness evaluations, exercise testing, and exercise training.
- Potential musculoskeletal injuries (*e.g.,* contusions, sprains, strains, fractures), cardiovascular/pulmonary complications (*e.g.,* chest pain, palpitations/arrhythmias, tachycardia, bradycardia, hypotension/hypertension, hyperventilation), and metabolic abnormalities (*e.g.,* fainting/syncope, hypoglycemia/hyperglycemia, hypothermia/hyperthermia).
- Appropriate documentation of emergencies.
- Applying first-aid procedures for exercise-related injuries (*e.g.,* bleeding, strains/sprains, fractures, shortness of breath, palpitations, hypoglycemia, allergic reactions, fainting/syncope).
- Applying basic life support, first aid, cardiopulmonary resuscitation, and automated external defibrillator techniques.
- Developing and/or modifying an evacuation plan.
- Demonstrating emergency procedures during exercise testing and/or training.

Domain IV Subdomain B: Multiple Choice Questions

1. Which of the following is a possible medical emergency that a client can experience during an exercise session?
   A) Hypoglycemia
   B) Hypotension
   C) Hyperglycemia
   D) All of the above

2. Implementation of emergency procedures must include the fitness center's _____.
   A) Management
   B) Staff
   C) Clients
   D) Management and staff

3. The top priority of any facility should be the health and safety of its membership.
    A) True
    B) False

4. Which of the following policies is (are) thought to help ensure client safety within an exercise facility?
    A) Performance of pre-participation screening of members

    B) Designing exercise programs which consider the participants exercise history, medical history, and current fitness level
    C) Training staff to respond effectively to emergency situations
    D) All of the above

ACSM-EP

DOMAIN I

Doman I Subdomain A: Multiple Choice Answers

1. —C. Provides an explanation of the test to the client

   Explanation: Informed consent is not a legal document. It does not provide legal immunity to a facility or individual in the event of injury to a client nor does it legally protect the rights of the client. It simply provides evidence that the client was made aware of the purposes, procedures, and risks associated with the test or exercise program. The consent form does not relieve the facility or individual of the responsibility to do everything possible to ensure the safety of the client. Negligence, improper test administration, inadequate personnel qualifications, and insufficient safety procedures all are items that are not expressly covered by informed consent. Because of the limitations associated with informed consent documents, legal counsel should be sought during the development of the document.

2. —C. Negligence, improper test administration, inadequate personnel qualifications, and insufficient safety procedures are all items that are expressly covered by the informed consent

   Explanation: Negligence, improper test administration, inadequate personnel qualifications, and insufficient safety procedures are all items that are expressly *not* covered by the informed consent. The informed consent is also not a legal document; it does not provide legal immunity to a facility or individual in the event of injury to a person, and it does not relieve the facility or individual of the responsibility to do everything possible to ensure the safety of an individual.

3. —A. To inform the client of participation risks as well as the rights of the client and the facility

   Explanation: Agreements, releases, and consents are documents that clearly describe what the client is participating in, the risks involved, and the rights of the client and the facility. If signed by the client, they are accepting some of the responsibility and risk by participating in this program. All fitness facilities are strongly encouraged to have program or service agreements and informed consents drafted by a lawyer for their protection.

4. —D. All of the above

   Explanation: Different types of health screenings are used for various purposes. In commercial settings, clients should be screened more extensively for potential health risks. At minimum, a personal medical history should be taken. In addition, present medical status should be examined and questions asked regarding the use of medications (both prescription and over the counter).

5. —A. Physical Activity Readiness Questionnaire + (PAR-Q+)

   Explanation: The PAR-Q+ is a screening tool for self-directed exercise programming. The HSQ is a screening tool with similarities to the PAR-Q+, but it takes longer to complete versus the quick completion of the PAR-Q+. The RPE-Borg scale is used to measure or to RPE during exercise or during an exercise test. The E-ECG would involve continuous electrical heart monitoring during exercise stress test used in a clinical setting when deemed appropriate by a physician.

Doman I Subdomain B: Multiple Choice Answers

1. —C. Because she is currently experiencing symptoms, she should seek medical clearance prior to beginning exercise

   Explanation: Based on the ACSM screening algorithm, symptomatic participants who do not currently exercise should seek medical clearance regardless of disease status.

2. —D. ≥ 130 mg $\cdot$ dL^{-1}

   Explanation: An LDL-C mg $\cdot$ dL^{-1} is considered a risk factor for CVD. According to the ATP III, an LDL-C ranging between 100 and 129 mg $\cdot$ dL^{-1} is considered near or above optimal, while an LDL-C <100 mg $\cdot$ dL^{-1} is considered optimal.

3. —C. SBP 140 and/or DBP 90 mm Hg

   Explanation: To be classified as hypertensive, the SBP must equal or exceed 130 mm Hg or the DBP must equal or exceed 80 mm Hg as measured on two separate occasions, preferably days apart. An elevation of either the systolic or diastolic pressure is classified as hypertension.

4. —C. Antilipemics

   Explanation: Nitrates and nitroglycerine are antianginals (used to reduce chest pain associated with angina pectoris). β-blockers are antihypertensives (used to reduce BP by inhibiting the action of adrenergic neurotransmitters at the β-receptor, thereby promoting peripheral vasodilation). β-blockers also are designed to reduce BP by inhibiting the action of adrenergic neurotransmitters at the β-receptors, thereby decreasing. Antilipemics control blood lipids, especially cholesterol and low-density lipoprotein (LDL). Aspirin is used to control for blood platelet stickiness.

5. —C. Triglycerides

   Explanation: Dietary fats include triglycerides, sterols (*e.g.,* cholesterol), and phospholipids. Triglycerides represent more than 90% of the fat stored in the body. A *triglyceride* is a glycerol molecule connected to three fatty acid molecules. The fatty acids are identified by the amount of "saturation" or the number of single or double bonds that link the carbon atoms. Saturated fatty acids only have single bonds. Monounsaturated fatty acids have one double bond, and polyunsaturated fatty acids have two or more double bonds.

6. —D. 120/78 mm Hg

   The elevated category is SBP 120–129 mm Hg and DBP <80 mm Hg. To be classified as hypertensive, the SBP must equal or exceed 130 mm Hg, or the diastolic pressure must equal or exceed 80 mm Hg as measured on two separate occasions, preferably days apart. An elevation of either the systolic or diastolic pressure is classified as hypertension.

7. —D. All of the above

   Initial causes of coronary artery disease (CAD) are thought to be an irritation of, or an injury to, the tunica intima (the innermost of the three layers in the wall) of the blood vessel. Sources of this initial injury are thought to be caused by dyslipidemia (elevated total blood cholesterol), hypertension (chronic high BP, either an elevation of SBP or DBP measured on two different days), immune responses, smoking, tumultuous and nonlaminar blood flow in the lumen of the coronary artery (turbulence), vasoconstrictor substances (chemicals that cause the smooth muscle cells in the walls of the vessel to contract, resulting in a reduction in the diameter of the lumen), and viral infections.

8. —D. <40 mg $\cdot$ dL^{-1}

   Risk factors that contribute to the development of CAD include age (men, >45 yr; women, >55 yr), a family history of myocardial infarction or sudden death (male first-degree relatives <55 yr and female first-degree relatives <65 yr), cigarette smoking, hypertension (BP >130/80 mm Hg measured on two separate occasions), hypercholesterolemia (total cholesterol >200 mg $\cdot$ dL^{-1} or 5.2 mmol $\cdot$ L^{-1}, or HDL <40 mg $\cdot$ dL^{-1} or 1.04 mmol $\cdot$ L^{-1}), and Type 1 and 2 diabetes mellitus.

9. —C. Claudication

   Explanation: Claudication describes the ischemic pain/cramping experienced as a result of impaired blood flow. Claudication can be experienced in individuals with peripheral vascular disease during exertion (*e.g.,* during walking). Pain tends to ease with rest. Dyspnea describes shortness of breath, syncope describes a temporary loss of consciousness, which is commonly related to insufficient blood flow to the brain, and angina describes discomfort in the chest as a result of reduced blood flow to the heart.

ACSM-EP

10. —A. Not participating in at least 30 min of moderate-intensity physical activity on at least 3 d · wk^{-1} for at least 3 months

    Explanation: Physical inactivity is a CVD risk factor. HDL-C >80 mg · dL^{-1} is considered cardioprotective, thus a negative risk factor (cut point ≥60 mg · dL^{-1}). Of note, HDL-C <40 mg · dL^{-1} is associated with CVD risk. FBG is normal, the cut point for diabetes ≥126 mg · dL^{-1}. BMI of 25 kg · m^{-2} would be categorized as overweight, not obese (cut point ≥30 kg · m^{-2}).

11. —D. All of the above

    Explanation: It is well documented that increases in physical activity (with a goal of >150 min · wk^{-1}) can reduce elevated BP, reduce elevated cholesterol, and assist in weight loss.

12. —B. A person who regularly exercises but has recently experienced dyspnea (shortness of breath or difficulty breathing) at rest and with mild exertion

    Explanation: Regardless of physical activity participation, a person experiencing dyspnea at rest is a sign of CV disease and discontinues exercise and seeks medical clearance.

    Based on the ACSM algorithm, each of the other conditions would not require medical clearance prior to testing or exercise.

13. —A. Ischemia is characterized by a restriction in blood supply to tissues, resulting in a reduction of oxygen, which is required for cellular metabolism. The term infarct refers to necrosis (*i.e.,* tissue death), which is related to the loss of local blood supply. Oxidative stress is characterized by the stress on the body resultant of free radical exposure

14. —A. True

    Explanation: Based on the ACSM algorithm, those who do not exercise and have known CV disease (in this case heart valve disease) and are asymptomatic should obtain medical clearance prior to exercise of any intensity.

15. —B. Performing planned, structured PA at least 30 min at a moderate intensity on at least 3 d · wk^{-1} for at least the last 3 months

Doman I Subdomain C: Multiple Choice Answers

1. —A. To bring in extra income to pay off other major expenses of the testing company

   Explanation: The purpose of physical fitness testing is not and should not be for any reason other than to benefit the participant. Even research studies involving physical fitness testing should offer beneficial data for the study's participants. Educating, motivating, and evaluating the progress of participants are all effective purposes of physical fitness testing.

2. —D. HR$_{rest}$, Queens College Step Test, ACSM push-up test

   Explanation: To get the most accurate and appropriate information, the following order of testing is recommended: resting measurements (*e.g.,* HR, BP, blood analysis), body composition, cardiorespiratory fitness (*e.g.,* Queens College Step Test), muscular fitness (*e.g.,* ACSM push-up test), and flexibility. Often, several methods of body composition assessment are sensitive to hydration status, and some tests of cardiorespiratory and muscular fitness may affect hydration. Therefore, it is inappropriate to administer those specific tests before the body composition assessment. Assessing cardiorespiratory fitness often uses measures of HR. Some tests of muscular fitness and flexibility affect HR. Hence, they are inappropriate to administer before cardiorespiratory fitness testing since the elevated HR from those assessments may have a negative impact on the cardiorespiratory fitness testing results.

3. —B. Specificity

   Explanation: As indicated in Box 4.6 in regard to ischemic heart disease (IHD), specificity is the percentage of patients without IHD who have a negative test for IHD. So, specificity represents the true negative cases among the test sample.

   Resource: Liguori G, senior editor. ACSM's Guidelines for Exercise Testing and Prescription. 11th ed. Philadelphia (PA): Wolters Kluwer; 2021.

4. —C. A slight decrease in diastolic pressure

   Explanation: During dynamic exercise, DBP may not change much or even decrease slightly because it represents the pressure in heart during diastole (rest).

5. —A. Increase

   Explanation: SBP is an indicator of the amount of blood pumped out of the heart in 1 min in a healthy vascular system and normally increases as workload increases because the peripheral and central stimuli that control this specific process also normally increase with an increase in workload. Thus, SBP should increase with an increase in workload. Failure of the SBP to increase as workload increases indicates an abnormal response to increasing workload. Additionally, an abnormally elevated SBP response to aerobic exercise indicates an unhealthy vascular system.

6. —A. Developing the exercise prescription

   Explanation: The purpose of the fitness assessment is to develop a proper exercise prescription (the data collected through appropriate fitness assessments assist the health fitness specialist in developing safe, effective programs of exercise based on the individual client's current fitness status), to evaluate the rate of progress (baseline and follow-up testing indicate progression toward fitness goals), and to motivate (fitness assessments provide information needed to develop reasonable, attainable goals). Progress toward or attainment of a goal is a strong motivator for continued participation in an exercise program.

7. —D. Body composition, cardiorespiratory fitness, muscular fitness, and flexibility

   Explanation: To get the most accurate and appropriate information, the following order of testing is recommended: resting measurements (*e.g.,* HR, BP, blood analysis), body composition, cardiorespiratory fitness, muscular fitness, and flexibility. Often, several methods of body composition assessment are sensitive to hydration status, and some tests of cardiorespiratory and muscular fitness may affect hydration. Therefore, it is inappropriate to administer those specific tests before the body composition assessment. Assessing cardiorespiratory fitness often uses measures of HR. Some tests of muscular fitness and flexibility affect HR. Hence, they are inappropriate to administer before cardiorespiratory fitness testing because the elevated HR from those assessments may have a negative impact on the cardiorespiratory fitness testing results.

8. —B. Cardiac dysfunction

   Explanation: The "normal" response to graded exercise is an increase in sympathetic outflow (accompanied by increases in boosts in contractility and heart rate), which results in increases in cardiac output. Increases in cardiac output results in an increase in systolic BP. If systolic BP does not increase with increases in workload, this suggests a failure of the heart to pump blood with normal efficiency. In most cases, the primary effects of EIA, DVT, and SVR would not result in attenuated systolic BP during exercise.

9. —C. β-blockers

   Explanation: β-blockers tend to attenuate the work of the heart, resulting in reduced exercise HR and BP. Caffeine, nicotine, and Adderall are stimulants and would likely result in increased HR responses.

10. —C. At least 5 min

    Explanation: All physiological observations, including HR, BP, signs, and symptoms, should be monitored for at least 5 min following a submaximal exercise test. If abnormal responses occur, a longer posttest monitoring period is recommended.

11. —C. The Wingate test

    Explanation: The Wingate is a 30-s test of anaerobic power. Specifically peak anaerobic power, mean anaerobic power, total work, and fatigue index are often measured. The push-up test is a muscular endurance test, the YMCA is a submaximal cardiorespiratory fitness test, and the BESS is a test of static postural stability.

12. —B. To assess myocardial electrical conduction and oxygenation

    Explanation: The EKG is a graphical representation of the electrical conduction of the heart. The electrical signals that occur during conduction are detected by electrodes placed on the skin. The EKG also provides an accurate measure of HR. Endothelial function is characterized by a reduction of vasodilators resulting in impaired vasodilation. Endothelial dysfunction is generally measured with the use of ultrasound, Doppler imaging or flow-mediated MRI. Systolic blood pressure is the pressure exerted on vessel walls during systole and is generally assessed using a sphygmomenometer.

ACSM-EP

Ejection fraction is the percentage of blood that is pumped out of the ventricles with each contraction and is measured with the use of imaging techniques including an echocardiogram.

13. —D. Phosphagen system

Explanation: Due to the short duration of the vertical jump test, the phosphagen system is thought to be the primary energy contributor. The phosphagen system is thought to be the predominant provider of energy for tasks under 15 s.

14. —A. Exercise testing for clinical purposes is generally not indicated for children unless there is a health concern

Doman I Subdomain D: Multiple Choice Answers

1. —B. Maximal volume of oxygen consumed per unit time ($\dot{V}O_{2max}$)

Explanation: $\dot{V}O_{2max}$ is the best (only) direct measure of cardiorespiratory fitness. $\dot{V}O_{2max}$ is less subject to overestimations and is a far more stable and valid indicator of cardiorespiratory fitness. This is in large part due to the close relation $\dot{V}O_{2max}$ has to the functional capacity of the heart (stroke volume, HR, arteriovenous O_2 difference).

2. —D. Linear

Explanation: As work rate on a submaximal test increases, HR will respond in a linear manner once it surpasses 110 bpm. HR increases and reaches a steady state at each exercise work rate and will rise incrementally with each stage of exercise. This response will continue at each stage as long as the physiological limits of that individual are not reached.

3. —C. Gender

Explanation: Males have approximately 15% higher relative $\dot{V}O_{2max}$ than females across different ages and physical activity levels. The Rockport One-Mile Fitness Walking Test formula is $\dot{V}O_{2max}$ (mL · kg^{-1} min^{-1}) = 132.853 − (0.1692 × body mass in kg) − (0.3877 × age in years) + (6.315 × gender) − (3.2649 × time in min) − (0.1565 × HR), where gender = 0 for female, 1 for male. The Rockport regression equation adjusts for the physiological advantage males have over females.

4. —B. 300 or 450 kg · m · min^{-1} (50 or 75 W)

Explanation: The Astrand-Rhyming protocol provides varying work rates depending on gender and fitness level. For untrained female individuals, the minimum recommendation protocol is 50 revolutions per minute (RPM) with a load of 1 kg (on a Monark cycle ergometer with 6 m flywheel circumference). 1 kg 6 m 50 RPM = 300 kg · m · min^{-1}. The range of up to 450 kg · m · min^{-1} allows for some physical fitness variation within the population.

5. —C. 3 min

Explanation: The Queens College Step Test lasts 3 min in order to provide steady-state HR as a result of aerobic exercise. Then, to estimate $\dot{V}O_{2max}$, early recovery HR is measured for 15 s (multiplied by 4). Exercise <3 min runs the risk of not establishing steady-state HR, and exercise >5 min is redundant, as HR has plateaued and continued exercise introduces the potential of local muscular fatigue.

6. —A. Maximal exercise test using indirect calorimetry

Explanation: Indirect calorimetry is a technique used to measure energy expenditure. Indirect calorimetry measures a person's expired oxygen and CO_2. Because oxygen consumption and energy expenditure are directly related, the volume of oxygen consumed ($\dot{V}O_2$) can be used to estimate the amount of energy expended. Maximal exercise testing, usually conducted as a graded exercise or exercise tolerance test, provides the truest measure of exercise capacity (*e.g.,* peak oxygen uptake [$\dot{V}O_{2peak}$]) for each individual. All other forms of testing/examination rely on estimations, which, although beneficial, often over- or undercompensate and can therefore be misleading.

7. —A. Bruce treadmill protocol

Explanation: Treadmill protocols remain the most popular form of clinical exercise testing in the United States. Cycle ergometry has become increasingly popular in Europe; however, it has been shown that cycle ergometry can underestimate peak exercise capacity by 5%–20%. The Bruce protocol continues to be the most commonly used protocol for exercise testing due to its familiarity among physicians, amount of research supporting the protocol, and ability to be modified to meet the needs of low-functional capacity clients.

8. —C. 6 min

Explanation: Following completion of peak exercise during a clinical exercise test, the test administrator should continue to monitor the vital signs of the client regularly (*e.g.*, every 1–2 min) through at least 6 min of recovery. This timeframe is used to help determine the rate of return of vital signs as well as to ensure the health and safety of the client following exhaustive work. This is particularly true in cases where low-functional capacity exists or the risk of a sudden cardiac event is elevated.

9. —A. 10 bpm

Explanation: Research has suggested that for every MET increase, the subsequent HR response should be approximately 10 bpm. This rise is sufficient to challenge the heart to appropriately respond to the increased metabolic demand.

10. —D. Expired oxygen

Because there is a direct relationship between oxygen consumption and energy production, $\dot{V}O_2$ can be used as means to estimate caloric expenditure.

11. —A. Achievement of age-predicted HR_{max}

Explanation: ACSM considers "failure of HR to increase with increases in workload" as the criterion used to confirm that a maximal effort has been elicited.

12. —A. Approximately 10 mm Hg

Explanation: During dynamic exercise, SBP will increase in a direct proportion to exercise intensity. The increase in SBP is due to the increase in which helps to facilitate increase in blood flow to the exercising muscles. The increase in SBP is expected to rise 5–10 mm Hg/MET of effort; by definition, 1 MET being roughly equivalent to the energy expended during rest.

13. —A. Speed and incline are increased every 3 min of the test

Explanation: The Bruce protocol involves increases in speed and inclination every 3 min. The test is performed on a treadmill and is used to evaluate cardiac function. Stage 1 of the Bruce protocol is performed at 1.7 mph and a 10% grade.

14. —B. Brachial

Explanation: The brachial artery is the standard location for BP measurement. Systolic and diastolic pressures can vary in different parts of the arterial tree, thus the brachial artery is generally recommended for purposes of standardization.

15. —D. All of the above are correct

Explanation: Cuff size must be suited to the diameter of the arm. Use of too small of a cuff will result in an overestimation of pressure, while too large of a cuff will underestimate pressure. Observer error is an established source of error, whether it involves differences in auditory acuity or the observer having a digit preference (*e.g.*, reporting readings ending in 2 or 0).

16. —D. Respiratory exchange ratio (RER) ≥ 1.15

Explanation: For a GXT to be considered maximal, several criteria may be used, RER ≥ 1.15. RER is the ratio of oxygen consumed and carbon dioxide produced ($\dot{V}CO_2/\dot{V}O_2$). Naturally, the client may end the test at any time, however, this is not a criteria indicating $\dot{V}O_{2max}$ achievement. Other criteria suggestive of $\dot{V}O_{2max}$ achievement include Borg RPE ≥ 17 (on a 6–20 scale), HR within 10 bpm of HR_{max}, and a plateau in $\dot{V}O_2$ despite an increase in workload.

17. —A. Treadmill

Explanation: Treadmill protocols would likely elicit $\dot{V}O_{2max}$ values higher than cycle or upper body ergometer protocols because of the increased amount of muscle mass used during ambulation. Upper body and cycle ergometry use less muscle mass, thus aerobic metabolism and oxygen consumption would likely be lower compared to weight bearing, total body activities such as running.

18. —D. 70–125 $L \cdot min^{-1}$

Explanation: During exhaustive exercise minute ventilation tends to range from 70 to 125 $L \cdot min^{-1}$. Ventilation (the total volume of air exhaled per minute) at rest tends to range between 5 and 10 $L \cdot min^{-1}$. Ventilation increases in a linear fashion with increasing submaximal workloads. Ventilation increases exponentially at intensities that exceed the ventilatory threshold in order to remove excess CO_2 produced during higher-intensity exercise.

19. —C. 400–500 mL

Tidal volume (TV) is the volume of air inspired or expired in one normal breath. Tidal volume in the healthy adult male is approximately 500 mL and approximately 400 mL in healthy adult females.

20. —D. Resting systolic blood pressure (SBP) between 125 and 140 mm Hg or diastolic blood pressure (DBP) between 60 and 75 mm Hg

Explanation: A contraindication is any situation in which the risk associated with undergoing the exercise test is likely to exceed the information to be gained from it. Box 4.1: Contraindications to Symptom-Limited Maximal Exercise Testing outlines the contraindications of clinical exercise testing. Resting SBP above 200 mm Hg or DBP above 110 mm Hg are the appropriate contraindications.

Resource: Liguori G, senior editor. ACSM's Guidelines for Exercise Testing and Prescription. 11th ed. Philadelphia (PA): Wolters Kluwer; 2021.

Doman I Subdomain E: Multiple Choice Answers

1. —B. YMCA bench press test

Explanation: The YMCA bench press test is a valid test for upper body muscular endurance because the test is conducted with a set resistance, and the goal is to successfully complete as many repetitions as possible.

2. —C. The YMCA bench press test

Explanation: Two common assessments for upper body muscular endurance include the YMCA bench press and the push-up test. The YMCA bench press test involves gender-specific loading of the bench press pattern. Males use 80 lb and females use 35 lb. The load is lifted in cadence with a metronome paced at 60 bpm. Generally, 1 or 3 RM tests are considered muscular strength tests. The Wingate test is considered an anaerobic power test.

3. —D. Pectoralis major

Explanation: Agonists, or prime movers, are considered to be the muscles that are most responsible for accomplishing a given movement. In the case of the bench press, the pectoralis major muscles are the main muscles responsible for pushing the bar away from you.

4. —B. Sagittal plane

Explanation: The Sagittal plane divides the body into right and left slices. Sagittal plane exercises typically include flexion and extension patterns. The RDL involves hip flexion and extension. Other examples of sagittal plane patterns include bicep curls and the split squat.

5. —B. Dynamic

Explanation: The push-up test is considered a dynamic muscular endurance test involving both concentric and eccentric phases of contraction. The term isometric generally denotes muscular contraction where there is no change in muscle length. Isokinetic testing is performed on specialized equipment with a constant speed of angular motion.

6. —A. Isokinetic dynamometer

Explanation: The term isokinetics typically refers to a type of muscular contraction that accompanies a constant rate of limb movement. Isokinetic dynamometers are special devices that measure force through a joint range of motion at a predetermined, constant speed.

7. —D. Horizontal adduction

Explanation: It is important to note that adduction and horizontal adduction occur in different anatomical planes. Adduction involves bones moving closer to the midline in the frontal plane. For example, adduction occurs during the jumping jack when you bring your arms back to your sides. Horizontal adduction is adduction within the horizontal plane, as seen when performing the lifting phase of the bench press.

8. —D. All of the above are benefits of muscular endurance testing

Explanation: Muscular endurance testing serves many purposes, including exposing weakness of specific muscles, which left unnoticed, could result in injury. In addition, use of muscular endurance assessment results should be used to formulate the resistance training prescription. Retesting and comparing results to baseline muscular endurance values can also quantify progress of the program.

9. —B. Isometric

Explanation: Isometric contraction occurs when muscular force is developed but the length of the muscle is constant. Use of the handgrip dynamometer involves the participant holding the device as they squeeze with maximum isometric effort for at least 5 s. The purpose of using the hand dynamometer is to measure the maximum isometric strength of the hand and forearm muscles.

10. —D. All of the above should be included in 1-RM testing procedure

Explanation: 1 RM testing should only be conducted if the participant is experienced with the pattern. Prior to attempting 1 RM, the participant should perform an adequate dynamic warm-up. Sufficient rest (3–5 min) should be permitted between attempts to minimize the effects of fatigue on performance.

11. —A. The participant begins in the "up" or plank position

Explanation: The push-up test for males begins with the participant in the "down" position.

12. —B. Flexing

Explanation: Joint actions are all referenced from anatomical position (standing tall, with feet pointing forward). Flexion refers to a movement that decreases the angle between two body parts. The eccentric phase (lowering the load to the floor) of the RDL involves hip flexion. In which case, the angle between the torso and femur decreases.

13. —B. Superior

Explanation: Superior is synonymous with cephalic. Inferior is synonymous with caudal.

14. —A. Genu varus

Explanation: Genu (knee) varus describes an outward deviation of the knee (*i.e.*, bow-legged appearance). Genu valgus describes an inward deviation of the knee joint. Chondromalacia patella describes the softening and breakdown of the cartilage on the underside of the kneecap. Patellar tendonitis (*i.e.*, jumper's knee) describes inflammation of the patellar tendon.

15. —A. Pennate

Explanation: Skeletal muscle is often characterized by its architecture or fiber arrangement. In a pennate muscle, the tendon runs through the length of the muscle with the fibers attaching diagonally. The rectus femoris is actually considered a bipennate muscle, as the fibers lie on both sides of the tendon. Parallel muscles run parallel to one another (*e.g.*, biceps brachii and rectus abdominis). Circular muscles are characterized by a ring-like architecture that surrounds a bodily opening (*e.g.*, orbicularis oris controls the opening of the mouth). Convergent muscles are triangular in shape and have a common point of attachment from which the muscle fibers reach outward, which enables the muscle to cover a large surface area (*e.g.*, pectoralis major).

16. —B. Abduction

Abduction describes movement patterns in which a body part moves away from the midline. Adduction describes movement toward the midline. Flexion involves a decrease in joint angle (*e.g.*, bicep curl involves elbow flexion), while extension involves increasing joint angle (*e.g.*, tricep curl involves elbow extension).

Doman I Subdomain F: Multiple Choice Answers

1. —B. <18.5 kg · m^{-2}

Explanation: BMI, a calculation of body weight in kilograms divided by height in squared meters, is generally used to establish a relationship between the height of an individual and the amount of mass on that frame. BMI norms have been established by the ACSM and the Expert Panel on the Identification, Evaluation, and Treatment of Overweight and Obesity in Adults.

"Normal" BMI is defined as a number between 18.5 and 24.9 kg · m^{-2}. Therefore, a BMI below 18.5 kg · m^{-2} would classify as "underweight," meaning that there is too little mass on the body given its height.

2. —C. 5 mm

Explanation: When recording regional body circumferences, it is recommended that two measurements be recorded (in rotational order) and then averaged together. This helps ensure reliability and accuracy of the measurement. Acceptable error is ±5 mm between measurements. In the event that the two measurements exceed 5 mm in difference, the administrator should remeasure to ensure accurate results.

3. —A. >0.86

Explanation: Due to the different distribution of fat between males and females, risk stratification using WHR is different between men and women. Males tend to carry more visceral fat around the abdomen and subsequently have higher WHR than females. A *very high* risk value is set at >0.95 for young men and >1.03 for men between the ages of 60 and 69 yrs. Women carry excess adipose tissue around the hips and buttocks; therefore, the risk of cardiovascular and other diseases is higher at lower ratios compared to males.

4. —C. Suprailiac

Explanation: The suprailiac skinfold site should be a diagonal fold in line with the natural angle of the iliac crest taken in the anterior axillary line immediately superior to the iliac crest.

5. —B. Air displacement plethysmography

Explanation: Air displacement plethysmography measures body volume using changes in air pressure within a sealed chamber. The volume of air displaced is calculated indirectly by subtracting the volume of air remaining in the chamber when the subject is inside from the volume of air in the chamber when it is empty.

6. —B. As the participant is completely submerged underwater

Explanation: Hydrodensitometry (aka "underwater weighing") is a technique that estimates body composition using measures of body weight, body volume, and residual lung volume as the subject is completely submerged underwater. This is an inherent limitation to this method as many subjects find it difficult to submerge entirely underwater during testing.

7. —A. BMI

Explanation: BMI is a ratio of body mass and height ($kg \cdot m^{-2}$). Although BMI is considered a valid measure for CV and metabolic risk classification, it does not differentiate between fat mass and fat-free mass.

8. —B. Android

Explanation: Distribution of body fat is a valuable indicator of CV and metabolic disease risk. Android (or central) adiposity is associated with higher risk for many CV and metabolic diseases.

9. —C. Place the jaws of the caliper horizontal to the fold, one inch above the fingers

Explanation: The jaws of the caliper should be perpendicular to the fold. The jaws of the caliper should be positioned one centimeter below the fingers that are holding the skinfold.

10. —D. 88 cm (35 in.)

Explanation: Females with a WC >88 cm have been shown to have an increase risk for the development of Type 2 diabetes, hypertension, and CV disease. Because WC reflects the level of abdominal adiposity, it is useful in determining health risk. It is worth noting, when used in concert with BMI, WC measures may provide a more precise approximate of CV and metabolic disease risk.

DOMAIN II

Doman II Subdomain A: Multiple Choice Answers

1. —C. Improvement in range of motion (ROM)

Improvements in ROM are a benefit of the stretching phase of an exercise session. Although oftentimes included as part of the cooldown, the stretching phase is distinct and should follow the cooldown phase. This is to promote improved flexibility and ROM in the muscles, as they will still be warm from the increased blood flow during the exercise session.

2. —C. Frequency, intensity, time, type, volume, and progression

Explanation: Frequency (how often), intensity (how hard), time (duration or how long), type (mode or what kind), total volume (amount), and progression (advancement) or the FITT-VP principle of exercise prescription provides recommendations on exercise pattern to be consistent with the ACSM recommendations made in its companion evidence-based position stand (Garber CE, Blissmer B, Deschenes MR, et al. 2011).

3. —B. Muscular endurance, muscular power, and muscular strength

Explanation: The ACSM uses the phrase "muscular fitness" to refer collectively to muscular strength, endurance, and power.

4. —B. The risk of orthopedic and cardiovascular complications is increased

Explanation: The risk of orthopedic and, perhaps, cardiovascular complications can be increased with high-intensity activity. Factors to consider when determining exercise intensity include the individual's level of fitness, presence of medications that may influence exercise performance, risk of cardiovascular or orthopedic injury, and individual preference for exercise and individual program objectives.

5. —C. 150, 2

Explanation: The *2018 Physical Activity Guidelines for Americans* recommends that adults need at least 150 min of moderate-intensity physical activity and should perform muscle-strengthening exercises on 2 or more days each week.

6. —A. An overuse injury

Explanation: An overuse injury describes an injury that results from repetitive stress to tissues over time. The risk of overuse injuries increases if a person increases exercise volume and intensity beyond the tolerance of the tissues (bones, myofascia, ligaments, or tendons).

7. —D. Walking

Explanation: Large muscle group activity performed in rhythmic fashion over prolonged periods facilitates the greatest improvements in aerobic fitness. Walking, running, cycling, swimming, stair climbing, aerobic dance, rowing, and cross-country skiing are examples of these types of activities. Weight training should not be considered an appropriate activity for enhancing aerobic fitness but should be part of in a comprehensive exercise program to improve muscular strength and muscular endurance. The mode of activity should be selected based on the principle of specificity—that is, with attention to the desired outcomes—and to maintain the participation and enjoyment of the individual.

8. —D. All of the above

Explanation: The effects of regular (chronic) exercise can be classified or grouped into those that occur at rest, during moderate (or submaximal) exercise, and during maximal effort work. For example, you can measure an untrained individual's HR_{rest}, train the person for several weeks or months, and then measure HR_{rest} again to see what change has occurred. HR_{rest} declines with regular exercise probably because of a combination of decreased sympathetic tone, increased parasympathetic tone, and decreased intrinsic firing rate of the sinoatrial node. Stroke volume increases at rest as a result of increased time for ventricular filling and an increased myocardial contractility. Little or no change occurs in cardiac output at rest because the decline in HR is compensated for by the increase in stroke volume.

9. —C. Shorter duration, lower intensity, and higher frequency of exercise

Explanation: The number of times per day or per week that a person exercises is interrelated with both the intensity and the duration of activity. Generally, those with poor levels of fitness may benefit from multiple short-duration, low-intensity exercise sessions per day. Individual goals, preferences, limitations, and time constraints also will determine frequency and the relationship between duration, frequency, and intensity.

10. —D. Overload, specificity, progression

Explanation: The three training principles are overload, specificity, and progression. Though redundancy should be considered when writing exercise prescriptions, it is not recognized by the ACSM as a training principle. Although redundancy, frequency, intensity, and duration are important factors to consider with exercise programming, they are not considered training principles. *Overload* is pushing the body beyond what it is used to, *specificity* is being careful to choose exercises that closely relate to the outcome goal, and *progression* has to do with developing a systematic method of improving.

11. —C. "Push the floor away from you."

Explanation: There are two primary verbal coaching cues exercise practitioners can provide while teaching movement patterns:

internal and external. External cues direct a client's focus toward the effect the movement will have on the surrounding environment (*i.e.,* external focus of attention). Internal cues direct a client's focus toward their body while the movement is performed (*i.e.,* internal focus of attention). Answers A, B, and D direct the individual's attention toward agonists or joints that are most involved in the performance of the push-up. Answer C directs the client's attention toward the environment (pushing the floor away) while the push-up is performed.

12. —B. Increases in agonist motor unit recruitment

    Explanation: Strength increases after chronic resistance training as a result of several physiological mechanisms. Heavy strength training augments agonist motor recruitment (along with improved motor unit synchronization), thus leading to increases in force development. In addition, protective inhibitory reflexes that limit strength expression in untrained individuals are reduced. Other known adaptations that contribute to strength improvement include increases in muscle fiber diameter and increased tendon stiffness.

13. —D. Submaximal resistance training with intermediate–high lifting velocities

    Explanation: Power is the product of force and velocity; therefore, both variables should be addressed in a program aimed at optimizing power production. The force–velocity curve indicates that the greater the amount of force generated, the slower the muscle shortening, thus reducing movement velocity. Therefore, to optimize power training outcomes, intermediate–high velocity movements using submaximal loads are recommended.

14. —C. Overtraining syndrome

    Explanation: Functional overreaching includes the deliberate increase in training intensity or volume, which results in a transient decline in performance, soon followed by recovery and improvements in performance. Nonfunctional overreaching involves the increase in intensity or volume with more prolonged decreases in performance; where several weeks of recovery are needed for performance to return to baseline levels.

Overtraining syndrome is considered more severe than nonfunctional overreaching and results in chronic performance decline along with more severe symptoms.

15. —D. All of the above are correct

    A dynamic warm-up has many physiological and psychological benefits, which can improve the quality of a workout. As a dynamic warm-up increases muscle and core temperature, this is thought to aid in oxygen release from hemoglobin (Bohr effect), reduce risk of myofascial strains, and increase enzymatic activity. In addition, the dynamic warm-up may contribute to improved mental preparedness for upcoming performance.

16. —B. The untrained individual

    Explanation: Given the same workout, the trained person will recover much faster, thus all factors that contribute to EPOC (increased body temperature and HR, resynthesis of anaerobic fuels) would return to resting levels at a faster rate.

17. —D. All of the above are correct

    Though research is still needed to fully elucidate the benefits of band training, the use of elastic band training does offer some advantages over free weight training. Using bands enables users to easily change the direction of resistance by repositioning the anchor point. As bands increase in length, more force is needed to complete a movement, thus the resistance at end ROM will be greater. Conversely, because free weights use gravity (a constant) for resistance, external resistance does not change during the ROM. In addition, bands are cheaper than free weights and much easier to transport, increasing the possibility of participation in resistance training at home or while traveling.

18. —A. Wolff's law

    Explanation: Wolff's law describes how bone in a healthy individual will adapt to stress. If bone is stressed, the bone will remodel itself to provide the strength needed for loading. Boyle's law describes how the pressure of a gas will increase as the volume of the container decreases. Poiseuille's law describes the relationship between velocity of blood flow, fluid viscosity, and vessel radius.

Newton's laws relate to motion and describe the relationship between a body and the forces acting upon it.

19. —B. Motor unit

Explanation: The motor unit is one motor neuron and all of the muscle fibers that the neuron innervates. The motor unit is considered the functional unit in the recruitment of muscle. The sarcomere is the structural unit of a myofibril, consisting of actin and myosin filaments. The sarcoplasmic reticulum is an organelle within muscle cells; its main purpose is to store calcium. The neuromuscular junction is a synaptic connection between the terminal end of a motor nerve and a muscle.

20. —B. The size (or Henneman) principle

The size principle states that motor units are recruited progressively from low threshold to high threshold. Increase in muscle force production is one factor that will elicit the increases in motor unit recruitment. The all-or-none principle states that if recruitment threshold is met, every fiber within the motor unit is activated. The principle of specificity, or the SAID principle, describes the adaptations that result from training are specific to the demands of the activity. The principle of reversibility describes how training adaptations can fade if the training stimulus is insufficient.

21. —B. Minute ventilation

Explanation: During maximal exercise, V_E can rise as high as 150 L $\cdot$ min^{-1}. For most recreationally trained individuals, TV can reach up to 3 L $\cdot$ breath^{-1}. Cardiac output during maximal exercise can range from 25 to 30 L $\cdot$ min^{-1}, while absolute $\dot{V}O_{2max}$ values can range from 2.0 to 5 L $\cdot$ min^{-1} in recreationally trained individuals.

Doman II Subdomain B: Multiple Choice Answers

1. —C. 3–5 d $\cdot$ wk^{-1}

Explanation: It is recommended that individuals perform a minimum of 5 d $\cdot$ wk^{-1}, or vigorous-intensity aerobic exercise done at least 3 d $\cdot$ wk^{-1}, or a weekly combination of 3–5 d $\cdot$ wk^{-1} of moderate- and vigorous-intensity exercise to promote and maintain health and fitness benefits. Aerobic exercise performed <3 d $\cdot$ wk^{-1} does not provide the body with enough stimulus to maximize improvements in cardiorespiratory fitness. Benefits from aerobic exercise performed in excess of 5 d $\cdot$ wk^{-1} have been suggested to plateau as well as increase the risk of musculoskeletal injury and burnout.

2. —B. 52%

Explanation: Moderate-intensity aerobic exercise is considered to fall in the range of 40%–59% of an individual's HRR (HR$_{max}$ – – HR$_{rest}$). Vigorous exercise includes an HRR range of 60%–89%.

3. —D. Maximum heart rate percentage (%HR$_{max}$)

Explanation: It is not recommended to use HR-dependent methods when prescribing exercise intensities because of the over-/underestimation that can occur. Additionally, HR can vary depending on the method used to establish HR (*e.g.,* palpation, HR monitor). Measures such as VO2R and the ventilatory threshold are generally preferred as these measures tend to be less subject to variation and provide a truer indication of fitness.

4. —A. 500–1,000 MET-min $\cdot$ wk^{-1}

Explanation: This volume of EE is considered adequate for most adults. An exercise volume between 500 and 1,000 MET-min $\cdot$ wk^{-1} is roughly equivalent to (a) 1,000 kcal $\cdot$ wk^{-1} of moderate-intensity physical activity (or about 150 min $\cdot$ wk^{-1}); (b) an exercise intensity of 3–5.9 METs (for individuals weighing ~68–91 kg [~150–200 lb]); and (c) 10 MET-h $\cdot$ wk^{-1}. These have all been associated with improved physical health and well-being as well as significantly lower rates of CVD and premature mortality.

5. —A. 150; 75

Explanation: The ACSM provides evidence-based recommendations (Table 5.1) of at least 150 min $\cdot$ wk^{-1} of moderate exercise, or at least 75 min $\cdot$ wk^{-1} of vigorous exercise, or a combination of moderate and vigorous exercise daily to attain the recommended targeted volumes of exercise.

Resource: Liguori G, senior editor. ACSM's Guidelines for Exercise Testing and Prescription. 11th ed. Philadelphia (PA): Wolters Kluwer; 2021.

6. —C. 310.5 kcal

Explanation: Caloric expenditure = Absolute O_2 consumed × Caloric equivalent

The steps are as follows:
- Convert 175 lb to 79.55 kg (divide by 2.2).
- Convert relative O_2 of 26 mL · kg^{-1} min^{-1} to absolute O_2 of 2.07 L · min^{-1}. For this converstion, multiply the relative $\dot{V}O_2$ by body mass in kg, then divide by 1,000.
- With an absolute O_2 consumption of 2.07 L · min^{-1}, you can then multiply by 5 kcal · min^{-1} (caloric equivalent) and then by 30 min of exercise, which will give you 310 kcal total for the exercise session.

7. —A. Cardiorespiratory fitness, muscular strength, muscular endurance, flexibility, body composition, and neuromotor fitness

Explanation: A comprehensive exercise prescription should address cardiorespiratory (aerobic) fitness, muscular strength and endurance, flexibility, body composition, and neuromotor fitness.

8. —C. 5 d · wk^{-1}

Explanation: Moderate-intensity aerobic exercise done at least 5 d · wk^{-1}, or vigorous-intensity aerobic exercise done at least 3 d · wk^{-1}, or a weekly combination of 3–5 d · wk^{-1} of moderate- and vigorous-intensity exercise is recommended for most adults to achieve and maintain health/fitness benefits.

9. —D. 3 d · wk^{-1}

Explanation: Moderate-intensity aerobic exercise done at least 5 d · wk^{-1}, or vigorous-intensity aerobic exercise done at least 3 d · wk^{-1} or a weekly combination of 3–5 d · wk^{-1} of moderate- and vigorous-intensity exercise is recommended for most adults to achieve and maintain health/fitness benefits.

10. —B. 40%–59% HRR or $\dot{V}O_2R$

Explanation: Moderate (e.g., 40%–59% HRR or $\dot{V}O_2R$) to vigorous (e.g., 60%–89% HRR or $\dot{V}O_2R$) intensity aerobic exercise is recommended for most adults, and light (e.g., 30%–39% HRR or $\dot{V}O_2R$) to moderate intensity aerobic exercise can be beneficial in individuals who are deconditioned.

11. —D. 60%–89% HRR or $\dot{V}O_2R$

Explanation: Moderate (e.g., 40%–59% HRR or $\dot{V}O_2R$) to vigorous (e.g., 60%–89% HRR or $\dot{V}O_2R$) intensity aerobic exercise is recommended for most adults, and light

(e.g., 30%–39% HRR or $\dot{V}O_2R$) to moderate intensity aerobic exercise can be beneficial in individuals who are deconditioned.

12. —A. 30–60 min · d^{-1}

Explanation: Most adults are recommended to accumulate 30–60 min · d^{-1} (≥150 min · wk^{-1}) of moderate-intensity exercise, 20–60 min · d^{-1} (≥75 min · wk^{-1}) of vigorous-intensity exercise, or a combination of moderate- and vigorous-intensity exercise per day to attain the volumes of exercise recommended (Garber CE, Blissmer B, Deschenes MR, et al. 2011; U.S. Department of Health and Human Services. 2008 Physical Activity Guidelines for Americans [Internet] 2008).

13. —C. 7,000 steps · d^{-1}

Explanation: The goal of 10,000 steps · d^{-1} is often cited, but achieving a pedometer step count of at least 5,400–7,900 steps · d^{-1} can meet recommended exercise targets, with the higher end of the range showing more consistent benefit (Garber CE, Blissmer B, Deschenes MR, et al. 2011; Tudor-Locke C, Hatano Y, Pangrazi RP, Kang M. 2008). For this reason and the imprecision of step counting devices, a daily target of at least 7,000 steps is recommended for most people.

14. —C. 9.7 METs

Explanation: To convert relative $\dot{V}O_2$ to METs, simply divide the $\dot{V}O_2$ value by 3.5.

34/3.5 = 9.7

15. —D. Increased DBP

Explanation: Because of exercise-induced vasodilation, DBP remains unchanged, or even slightly decreases, during aerobic exercise in healthy individuals. In those with known CVD, aerobic exercise may illicit increases in DBP at the beginning of exercise. This is the result of impaired vasodilation in working skeletal muscle, which leads to increases in total peripheral resistance.

16. —A. HR$_{max}$

Explanation: The Karvonen formula for calculating % HRR = [(HR$_{max}$–HR$_{rest}$)] × %intensity] + resting HR. The Karvonen formula and calculation of a % HRR do not involve SBP, MAP, or RPP.

17. —B. 108–137 bpm

Explanation: You begin by subtracting her age of 24 yr from 220, which is her estimated HR$_{max}$. In this case, the estimated HR$_{max}$ is

196 bpm. To get the low end of THR, multiply 196 by the recommended intensity of 55% (0.55). $196 \times 0.55 = 108$ bpm.

To calculate the high end of the THR, multiply 196 by 70%. $196 \times 0.70 = 137$ bpm. Answer A is incorrect because it subtracted her age from 200 instead of 220. Answer C is incorrect because it used 200 with no age adjustment, and answer D is incorrect because it used 220 with no age adjustment, which results in too high of a value.

18. —B. Gradually increase in distance weekly with a slight lower distance Sunday every fourth week or so

Explanation: The runner could become overtrained if they just built up to a longer distance each week without a down week built in periodically, even if done gradually. Doing the same distance weekly will not allow the runner to reach the race distance, therefore never allowing them to prepare for the actual race mileage. Periodization must be done gradually. If increased too rapidly, the runner may become injured or overtrained.

19. —A. At intensities exceeding the anaerobic threshold, the RER increases above 1.0.

Explanation: The RER is a measure typically obtained using methods of indirect calorimetry, where expired gases are analyzed for CO_2 and O_2 concentrations. The RER is a useful indicator of nutrient metabolism at rest and during steady-state exercise. Importantly, the RER does not necessarily reflect cellular energy metabolism during nonsteady-state exercise due to additional non-metabolic CO_2 production and elimination. When exercising at intensities above the anaerobic threshold, the RER can exceed 1 as a result of acid buffering, which artificially inflates (above cellular metabolism) CO_2 in expired air. An RER of 0.7 would indicate the individual is at rest and relying on lipids for energy.

20. —D. 460 kcal

Explanation: To best approach this problem, first convert relative (rel) $\dot{V}O_2$ to absolute (abs) $\dot{V}O_2$.

$Abs\dot{V}O_2 = 35 \text{ mL} \cdot \text{kg}^{-1} \text{ min}^{-1} \times 75 \text{ kg} \times 1 \text{ L} \cdot 1000 \text{ mL}^{-1}$
$Abs\dot{V}O_2 = 2.63 \text{ L} \cdot \text{min}^{-1}$

Once in absolute terms, convert $\dot{V}O_2$ to kcal by using the kcal equivalent of 5 kcal $\cdot \text{L}^{-1}$.
$\text{kcal} \cdot \text{min}^{-1} = 2.63 \text{ L} \cdot \text{min}^{-1} \times 5 \text{ kcal} \cdot \text{L}^{-1}$
$\text{kcal} \cdot \text{min}^{-1} = 13.15$

John performed this activity for 35 min.

Total kcal = $13.15 \text{ kcal} \cdot \text{min}^{-1} \times 35 \text{ min}$
Total kcal = 460 kcal

21. —B. Somewhat hard

Explanation: The Borg scale uses a subjective rating of intensity on a numerical scale of 6–20. An RPE of 13 corresponds to approximately 70% HR_{max}.

22. —D. 20 mL $\cdot \text{kg}^{-1} \cdot \text{min}^{-1}$

Explanation: To begin, you would use the metabolic equation for step exercise:

$\dot{V}O_2 = 0.2$ (step rate) $+ 1.33 \times 1.8$ (step height (m))(step rate) $+ 3.5$

Next, you will need to convert the step height from inches to meters.

$= 8'' \times 0.0254 = .203$
$\dot{V}O_2 = 0.2 (24) + 1.33 \times 1.8(.203)(24) + 3.5$
$\dot{V}O_2 = 20 \text{ mL} \cdot \text{kg}^{-1} \cdot \text{min}^{-1}$

23. —B. 34 min

Explanation: For this type of problem, you will need to determine how many kilocalories per minute are expended. Once you know how many kilocalories are expended in 1 min and you know how many total kilocalories are expended, you can solve for time.

Step 1: You will need to convert the person's body mass from pounds to kilograms.

$180/2.2 = 81.8 \text{ kg}$
Step 2: Convert relative $\dot{V}O_2$ to absolute $\dot{V}O_2$.
$(81.8 \times 25)/1000 = 2.045 \text{ L} \cdot \text{min}^{-1}$

Step 3: Using absolute $\dot{V}O_2$ and the expenditure estimate of 5 kcal for every 1 L of oxygen consumed, calculate how many kilocalories would be expended at this intensity in 1 min.

$= 2.045 \text{ L} \cdot \text{min}^{-1} \times 5 \text{ kcal} \cdot \text{L}^{-1}$
$= 10.225 \text{ kcal} \cdot \text{min}^{-1}$

Step 4: If 10.225 kcal are expended in 1 min and the goal is to expend 350 kcal, divide 350 by 10.225 to get the number of total minutes.

$= 350/10.225$
$= 34 \text{ min}$

ACSM-EP

Doman II Subdomain C: Multiple Choice Answers

1. —C. 48 h

   Explanation: Exercising muscle requires time to recover/repair between bouts. Several factors, such as exercise intensity, goals, individual training status, and total exercise volume can influence the amount of time needed for recovery; however, in most cases, 48 h is recommended. It is important to note that split routines and other variations of resistance training can allow for individuals to continue to work within that 48 h window as long as care is given to not engage the previously exercised muscle group(s) during succeeding bouts.

2. —D. All of the above

   Explanation: In addition to cardiorespiratory fitness, body composition, and neuromotor fitness, the ideal exercise training program should also address muscular strength, muscular endurance, and flexibility in most adults who are seeking to maintain or improve their all-around fitness.

3. —B. Active static stretching

   Explanation: Static stretching does not involve movement once the desired ROM is achieved and the stretch is held for a period of time (*i.e.,* 10–30 s). The primary difference between active and passive static stretching is the source of assistance. In passive static stretching, the muscle/tendon group being stretched is held by a partner or device such as an elastic band.

4. —A. Resistance training composed exclusively of eccentric contractions conducted at very high intensities

   Explanation: The 2009 ACSM position statement on progression models in resistance training recommends the use of concentric, eccentric, and isometric actions. Of note, very high intensity (>100% 1RM) eccentric actions can result in extensive damage to muscle fibers. As such, the risk of severe health complications such as exertional rhabdomyolysis is significantly increased.

5. —A. 2–4 sets with 8–12 repetitions

   Explanation: Unless the participant is advanced in training status and has specific training goals (*e.g.,* increase power or strength), most adults should train each muscle group for a total of 2–4 sets with 8–12 repetitions per set as described in the Resistance Training section in Chapter 5 of *ACSM's Guidelines For Exercise Testing and Prescription*, 11th edition.

6. —D. 15–25

   Explanation: Per *ACSM's Guidelines For Exercise Testing and Prescription* (GETP), 11th edition, "To improve muscular endurance rather than strength and mass, a higher number of repetitions, perhaps 15–25 or more, should be performed per set along with shorter rest intervals and fewer sets (*i.e.,* 1 or 2 sets per muscle group). This regimen necessitates a lower intensity of resistance, typically of no more than 50% 1 RM."

7. —C. 8–12

   Explanation: Eight to 12 repetitions represent a relatively low intensity of 67%–80% of 1 RM. This low intensity allows the development of muscular endurance and reduces the risk of musculoskeletal related injuries.

8. —D. Isometric

   Explanation: Isometric muscle action, also known as static muscle action, occurs when muscle tension increases with no overt muscular or limb movement; the length of the muscle does not change. These actions occur when with an attempt to push or pull against an immovable object. Measures of static strength are specific to both the muscle group and joint angle being tested; therefore, these tests' usefulness to generalize overall muscular strength is limited.

9. —D. All of the above are examples of progressive overload

   Explanation: By definition, progressive overload is a principle of training that states that the stress on the musculoskeletal system needs to progressively increase in order to keep producing greater force. This could be achieved by increasing the intensity (resistance), the number of rep or sets, and/or the number of exercise session per week.

10. —A. Lowering the center of gravity

    Explanation: Lowering the center of gravity (*i.e.,* center of body mass) will increase a person's postural stability. Stability would also be increased by increasing the width of stance or by standing on a stable surface.

11. —C. PNF

    Explanation: PNF encompasses a few techniques aimed at improving ROM. Generally, the techniques involve the use of isometric contractions of the target or antagonist muscle followed by relaxation and either active or passive static stretching of the target muscle.

Doman II Subdomain D: Multiple Choice Answers

1. —A. 5%–10% rule

    Explanation: Generally, progression should be relative to the participant's current fitness level and movement capacity, thus using absolute values may not provide sufficient stimulus for adaptation, or it may prove to be too much of an increase for the participant. Using a relative percentage helps customize the increase in stress to the individual. ACSM recommends increases of 5%–10% weekly.

2. —B. Progression

    Explanation: The principle of progression refers to the need to increase the demands on the body over time in order to elicit adaptation. The notable principles of progression include overload, specificity, and variation. Progression should be introduced gradually and systematically and should not outpace the participant's functional movement capacity.

3. —D. All of the above are correct

    Explanation: Each of the approaches would alter or increase the exercise stimulus, thus each would be considered a means of progression.

4. —B. In two consecutive workouts

    Explanation: The 2 plus 2 rule is a conservative approach to progression, which requires the participant to repeat their performance in the subsequent workout. This helps ensure that the initial increase in performance was not the result of having a singular great day, rather the effect was the result of actual strength adaptations.

5. —B. Increase the intensity to 70% HRR

    Currently, the participant is performing $3 \cdot d \cdot wk^{-1}$ for 30 min at 65%. Prudent progressive planning could involve changing any of the FITT variables by 5%–10%. In this case, an increase up to 40 min (answer A) would be a 25% increase. This is a sizable and abrupt increase in volume and may exceed the participant's current myofascial tissue tolerance. If the tissues are not prepared for this exercise volume, injury could result. Increasing to $5 \cdot d \cdot wk^{-1}$ (answer C) would result in an additional 60 min of weekly running time; once again exceeding the 5%–10% rule. The increase to 70% HRR is an increase of 5% and falls within the 5%–10% margin. In all likelihood, when making increases to intensity, it may be prudent to shorten the duration of the workout by a few minutes in order for the participant to adapt to the increase in intensity.

6. —D. All of the above

    Based on the principle of specificity, all training adaptations are specific to the stimulus applied. Therefore, modification of a particular training stimulus, such as speed of movement, ROM, or rest, would elicit a unique response.

Doman II Subdomain E: Multiple Choice Answers

1. —B. 4 kcal/g

    Explanation: Carbohydrate provides roughly $kcal \cdot g^{-1}$, while fat provides $9 \text{ kcal} \cdot g^{-1}$. Protein provides approximately $4 \text{ kcal} \cdot g^{-1}$.

2. —D. Lower stroke volume

    Explanation: Euhydration describes the normal state of body water content. Dehydration describes a state of decreased body water content. When in a dehydrated state during exercise, plasma volume tends to be reduced, which is associated with reductions in plasma volume. When normally hydrated during exercise, core temperature, heart rate, and RPE tend to remain at lower levels as compared to being in a dehydrated state.

3. —D. the ATP-CP system

    Explanation: The ATP-CP system involves one simple reaction, thus it is the speediest energy pathway. In contrast, glycolysis, gluconeogenesis, and aerobic pathways involve several reactions, which require a bit more time to produce ATP.

ACSM-EP

4. —B. Anaerobic

Explanation: Once the lactate threshold is exceeded, there is an increased reliance on anaerobic pathways for ATP production. Generally, when exercising at intensities below the lactate threshold, the participant achieves a steady state of energy production, which relies primarily on aerobic metabolism. The citric acid cycle and oxidative phosphorylation (*i.e.*, the electron transport chain) are the primary contributors of ATP in aerobic metabolism.

5. —C. Glycogen

Explanation: Glucose is packaged and stored as glycogen in the liver and skeletal muscle. Pyruvate is a product of glycolysis, while fructose is a type of simple sugar (*i.e.*, monosaccharide) that is found in fruits and some vegetables.

6. —A. Mitochondria

Explanation: The aerobic energy pathway produces ATP in the mitochondria in a process called oxidative phosphorylation.

7. —D. Combination of physical activity, behavior therapy, and proper nutrition

Explanation: Interventions that include diet, PA, and behavior changes, including goal setting, stimulus control, and problem-solving strategies, tend to be the most effective for weight loss and weight maintenance.

Very low-calorie diets can restrict specific nutrient, vitamin, and mineral consumption and can lead to dehydration or fatigue. Sweat suits can induce dehydration and any weight loss is related to body water, where body composition remains unchanged. Dietary supplements aimed at weight reduction could result in side effects including sleeplessness, nausea, dizziness, and racing heart. In addition, the FDA does not regulate dietary supplements, thus actual purity and contents are uncertain.

8. —D. 300

Explanation: During pregnancy, there are increased nutrient and energy demands to support fetal growth. In addition to an increase in energy intake, authorities recommend increased intake of folic acid and iron, which can be provided in a prenatal vitamin.

9. —D. 45–65

Explanation: Based on the 2015–2020 Dietary Guidelines for Americans, most adults should consume a diet that includes between 45% and 65% carbohydrate.

Doman II Subdomain F: Multiple Choice Answers

1. —B. Arteriosclerosis

Explanation: Arteriosclerosis, also called hardening of the arteries, is a loss of arterial elasticity and is associated with aging. Atherosclerosis is a form of arteriosclerosis characterized by an accumulation of obstructive lesions within the arterial wall. The adventitia is the outermost layer of the artery wall that provides the media and intima with oxygen and other nutrients.

2. —D. All modes of weight-bearing exercise

Explanation: Regularly participating in weight-bearing exercises such as walking or running is important to keep bone mineral density high in order to decrease risk of developing osteoporosis. Water exercise is not considered weight-bearing because of the buoyancy effect of the water. Intensity, whether it is high or low, is not relevant in this case. What matters is if the exercise involves supporting the weight.

3. —D. Asthma

Explanation: To date, an association between asthma and the metabolic syndrome has not been established. Metabolic syndrome involves several metabolic risk factors including hyperglycemia, hypertension, dyslipidemia, and central adiposity.

4. —D. All of the above

Explanation: Regular PA has been shown effective for lowering blood pressure. In addition, among those with type 2 DM, insulin action and glycemic control has been shown to improve with both cardiovascular and resistance exercise.

5. —D. 3–7

Explanation: $3-7 \text{ d} \cdot \text{wk}^{-1}$ is recommended for those with DM. As a part of the $3-7 \text{ d} \cdot \text{wk}^{-1}$, resistance training is recommended, provided the absence of contraindications such as retinopathy.

6. —A. 10

Explanation: Ten minute bouts of exercise is recommended for individuals that are very deconditioned. Clients that have been sedentary and are deconditioned have lower functional capacity, thus, shorter bouts of lower-intensity exercise are best tolerated.

7. —B. Myocardial infarction

Explanation: A myocardial infarction (MI) occurs after a period of myocardial ischemia to heart tissue resulting in tissue death or necrosis. Importantly, the ACSM-EP must be aware of the client's ischemic threshold and take steps, such as monitoring rate pressure product (HR × SBP), RPE, and symptoms (*e.g.*, angina, dyspnea, claudication), to ensure exercise intensity not exceed this level.

8. —D. Stable heart failure

Explanation: In patients with stable heart failure, exercise is encouraged and is thought to improve functional capacity and exercise tolerance and reduce the risk of experiencing other CV complications. Acute systemic illness, recent embolism, and unstable angina are absolute contraindications to exercise.

9. —C. Hypoglycemia

Explanation: Hypoglycemic events are a concern among individual's that take insulin or antihyperglycemic agents, particularly during or following exercise. Awareness of the impact of specific exercise intensities and duration has on blood glucose, routine monitoring of blood glucose prior, during, and after exercise and adequate carbohydrate intake are essential steps to avoid hypoglycemia. It may also be the case that insulin dosages be reduced when preparing for exercise.

10. —D. All of the above

Explanation: Physical activity is associated with improvements in insulin sensitivity, glucose uptake and use, as well as overall feelings of well-being in those with T2DM.

11. —C. Osteoporosis

Explanation: There are several chronic diabetes-related complications including peripheral neuropathy, autonomic neuropathy, and coronary artery disease. These conditions are the result of chronic impaired glucose control and elevated BP. Osteoarthritis is a skeletal condition characterized by compromised bone mineral density and an increased risk for fracture.

12. —B. When the pain subsides

Explanation: Tendinosis involves degenerative changes to a tendon without inflammation and is often the result of mechanically overloading the tissue via abrupt increases in exercise volume or improper biomechanics. Until pain subsides, pain-provoking activity should be reduced to decrease the loading of the damaged tendon. Once symptoms have improved, appropriately graded eccentric exercise has been shown to be a safe and effective method for strengthening the muscle-tendon unit (MTU).

Doman II Subdomain G: Multiple Choice Answers

1. —C. Stimulation of appetite

Explanation: Older people who exercise regularly report greater life satisfaction (older people who exercise regularly have a more positive attitude toward their work and generally are in better health than sedentary persons), greater happiness (strong correlations have been reported between the activity level of older adults and self-reported happiness), higher self-efficacy (older persons taking part in exercise programs commonly report that they can do everyday tasks more easily than before they began exercising), improved self-concept and self-esteem (older adults improve their score on self-concept questionnaires following participation in an exercise program), and reduced psychological stress (exercise is effective in reducing psychological stress without unwanted side effects).

2. —B. Children should perform ≥ 60 min of physical activity each day

Explanation: Children should attempt to accumulate ≥60 min of physical activity daily, this may be continuous or discontinuous activity. Children should not focus on just one or two modes. Exposing them to a wide variety of physical activities is suggested to enhance adherence. Finally, children should not have prolonged periods during the day that are sedentary because this may promote negative health consequences.

ACSM-EP

3. —A. Frequency

Explanation: Increased frequency of exercise is generally recommended for older adults to optimize cardiovascular as well as balance and flexibility adaptations. The recommended duration of exercise depends on the intensity of the activity because higher-intensity activity should be conducted over a shorter period of time.

4. —D. Supine position exercises

Explanation: Exercises in the supine (lying on your back) position could cause mild obstruction of venous return, which decreases, and may cause BP to drop dangerously low. Exercise in the prone position may be uncomfortable if not contraindicated. Walking is a good exercise for most pregnant women with no other special conditions. Sitting exercises such as riding an upright stationary bicycle (*i.e.,* leg ergometer) may be fine to do at an adequate comfort level, but caution should occur with semi-recumbent cycling to ensure that the knees are not hitting the torso of the pregnant woman.

5. —D. All of the above are correct

Explanation: The risk of maximal exercise testing pregnancy does not outweigh the benefit. If a maximal test is warranted, the test should be performed with physician supervision. Because pregnancy can alter HR response to exercise, intensity should be monitored using methods other than HR, including RPE. After the first trimester, supine exercises should be modified or avoided because of the risk of reduced venous return as a result of the growing fetus.

6. —A. Heart rate

Explanation: SBP and SV all tend to be lower in children compared to adults. Despite having a higher number of sweat glands per unit of skin area, children tend to have lower sweat rates when exposed to hot conditions. The HR of children at rest ranges between 100 and 110 bpm.

7. —D. Previously inactive women should progress from 15 min/day

Explanation: Exercise should begin with short bouts (10–15 min) and gradually increase to at least 30 min/day of accumulated physical activity. Maximal exercise testing should not be performed during pregnancy unless deemed medically necessary. Because HR response to exercise tends to be altered during pregnancy, RPE or the "talk test" are preferred methods of monitoring intensity. Intensity should be adjusted based on the individual's current fitness level. Prudent recommendations include beginning with low intensity and gradually increase to moderate (RPE 12–14 on a 6–20 scale) as tolerated.

8. —D. 5

Explanation: Aerobic frequency recommendations suggest older adults perform at least $5 \text{ d} \cdot \text{wk}^{-1}$ of moderate-intensity aerobic exercise or $3 \text{ d} \cdot \text{wk}^{-1}$ of vigorous-intensity aerobic exercise.

9. —C. Children and adolescents should perform resistance exercise at least $3 \text{ d} \cdot \text{wk}^{-1}$

Explanation: Resistance training can include structured (*e.g.,* lifting weights, use of resistance bands) or unstructured (*e.g.,* climbing trees, use of playground equipment) muscle strengthening activities. Younger participants, with appropriate supervision, adequate experience, and proper mechanics can safely participate in heavier resistance training, but most evidence supports the use of body weight or 8–15 submaximal repetitions performed to the point of moderate fatigue. Children and adolescents should also perform daily aerobic activity.

10. —D. Modest increase in HR during exercise compared to nonpregnancy

Explanation: Stroke volume and heart rate tend to be higher during an acute bout of exercise during pregnancy in order to support sufficient blood flow to both mother and baby.

Doman II Subdomain H: Multiple Choice Answers

1. —C. Be higher

Explanation: When engaging in physical activity or exercise at high altitude, HR will be higher than at sea level for the same perceived exertion because of the decreased supply of oxygen available. If one was to compete in endurance-oriented events at

high altitude, it would be wise to properly acclimate to the "competition or event" altitude prior to the actual competitive event. Also note that dehydration is often an issue at high altitude, so it is important to adequately hydrate before, during, and after training or competing.

2. —B. Reduced partial pressure of oxygen (PO_2)

Explanation: As altitude increases, barometric pressure reduces resulting in lower PO_2, meaning there is less oxygen available to the body resulting in less O_2 uptake by skeletal muscle. On Earth, regardless of location or altitude, air comprises 21% oxygen. Maximal HR remains the same at altitude, though HR will be higher at rest and any submaximal intensity when compared to sea level. The lactate threshold, or point where lactate begins to accumulate in the blood, may occur at reduced intensities (earlier on) due to the reduced PO_2 at altitude.

3. —A. Increased hemoglobin levels

Explanation: Long-term exposure to altitude induces several positive physiological adaptations that can improve performance at elevation. These adaptations do include increased hemoglobin and hematocrit levels.

As such, the potential to deliver and extract oxygen improves. Maximal HR remains the same at altitude. Sweat rates may change, but this is generally the result of heat acclimatization (in which case, sweat rates tend to increase), not necessarily altitude exposure. PO_2 is an environmental factor, which is not impacted by exposure.

4. —B. Heat acclimatization

Explanation: Heat acclimatization refers to the adaptations that can improve heat tolerance. Acclimatization is the result of earlier onset and more efficient thermoregulatory responses. These responses include increased sweat rates over a larger surface area and early onset of sweating. Salt concentrations in sweat are reduced resulting in greater electrolyte availability to the body. In addition, distribution of cardiac output improves, which aids circulatory cooling, while continuing to meet metabolic demands.

DOMAIN III

Doman III Subdomain A: Multiple Choice Answers

1. —D. Tell the client what their behavior change barrier is and how to correct it

Explanation: Effective communication uses a client-centered approach. This involves asking the client open-ended questions related to their goals and any perceived barriers to performing regular physical activity, which provides the client the opportunity to reflect on and recognize what is important to them.

2. —C. Active listening

Explanation: Active listening is a process where the practitioner works to understand the underlying meaning of what the client is by making statements that aim to bridge the gap between what the client is saying and the meaning behind the statements. Reflective statements help demonstrate understanding of the client's viewpoint and can help develop client rapport and empathy.

3. —D. Tell the client why they have been unsuccessful in their pursuit of weight loss goals

Explanation: Motivational interviewing involves client self-discovery and consideration of the factors that lead to positive health behavior. Successful motivational interviewing is directed by the client.

4. —D. Professional attire worn by staff

Explanation: The exercise environment can create unintended barriers to apprehensive new exercisers. These barriers include use of mirrors, aggressive colors and artwork, and revealing instructor clothing.

5. —D. All of the above are correct

Explanation: Relapse prevention incorporates many techniques in order to prevent an individual from returning to an inactive lifestyle after establishing exercise as a habit. Relapse prevention considers the recognition that lapses do occur and exercise resumption plans may be needed. Additionally, setting of realistic goals and continued assessment of progress will reinforce exercise adherence.

Doman III Subdomain B: Multiple Choice Answers

1. —B. Intrinsic reward

Explanation: Reinforcement is the positive or negative consequence for performing or not performing a behavior. Positive conse-

quences are rewards that motivate behavior. This can include both intrinsic and extrinsic rewards. Intrinsic rewards are the benefits gained because of the rewarding nature of the activity. Extrinsic or external rewards are the positive outcomes received from others, which may include encouragement and praise or material reinforcements such as T-shirts and money.

2. —A. There is a perceived threat of disease

Explanation: The health belief model assumes that people will engage in a behavior (*e.g.*, exercise) when there exist a perceived threat of disease and a belief of susceptibility to disease, and the threat of disease is severe. This model also incorporates cues to action as critical to adopting and maintaining behavior. The concept of self-efficacy (confidence) is also added to this model. Motivation and environmental considerations are not a part of the health belief model.

3. —B. Application of cognitive-behavioral or motivational principles

Explanation: Psychological theories are the foundations for effective use of strategies and techniques of effective counseling and motivational skill building for exercise adoption and maintenance. Theories provide a conceptual framework for development rather than management, of programs or interventions. Psychological theories facilitate evaluation of program effectiveness, not just measurement of outcomes. Within the field of behavioral change, a theory is a set of assumptions that accounts for the relationships between certain variables and the behavior of interest.

4. —E. All of the above

Explanation: Different factors affect exercise adherence. Some are situational in nature such as social support and time commitment, whereas others are personal (individualized). In order for a trainee to "stick" to an exercise routine, many of these factors must be met.

5. —C. Self-reevaluation

Explanation: Key components of the transtheoretical model are the processes of behavioral change. These processes include five cognitive processes (consciousness raising, dramatic relief, environmental reevaluation, self-reevaluation, and social liberation) and five behavioral processes (counterconditioning, helping relationships, reinforcement management, self-liberation, and stimulus control).

6. —B. Health belief model

Explanation: The health belief model is a theoretical framework to help explain and predict interventions to increase physical activity. The model originated in the 1950s based on work by Rosenstock. Learning theories assume that an overall complex behavior arises from many small simple behaviors. By reinforcing partial behaviors and modifying cues in the environment, it is possible to shape the desired behavior.

Doman III Subdomain C: Multiple Choice Answers

1. —B. Sarcopenia

Explanation: Similar to osteoporosis (loss of bone mass due to aging and reduced physical activity), sarcopenia is associated with a reduced ability to perform ADL and increases the risk of musculoskeletal injury. Muscular strength and endurance may improve or maintain bone mass and muscle mass, thus reducing the risk of osteoporosis and sarcopenia.

2. —A. Walking (transferring)

Explanation: Out of the list of possible choices, walking is the only choice that is considered an ADL. The six ADLs are eating, bathing, dressing, toileting, transferring (walking), and continence. Although it is great to be able to lift a medium to moderately heavy weights, sing, read, and write, these tasks are not necessary for ADL.

3. —D. All of the above

Stress reduction is critical for the maintenance of physical health, the attenuation of anxiety and to enhance a feeling of well-being. Well-recognized stress reduction techniques include practicing breathing patterns that involve slow, deep breathing versus shallow and rapid breathing. Meditation is considered a practice of mind–body medicine that helps the participant focus their attention and promote relaxation. Progressive Relaxation Technique involves the participant systematically tensing, then relaxing muscle groups. The tensing following by relaxation is thought to bring attention to any unnecessary tension in the body.

4. —D. Individuals with nonspecific LBP should remain active and continue ordinary activity within pain limits

   Explanation: Nonspecific LBP is described as LBP with no known physiological cause such as cancer, stenosis, fracture, etc. Nonspecific LBP accounts for 85% of all LBP cases. Movement that does not provoke pain should be encouraged in those with nonspecific LBP in order to reduce the risk of disability.

Doman III Subdomain D: Multiple Choice Answers

1. —C. Rest, ice, compression, elevation, and stabilization

   Explanation: Basic principles of acute care for musculoskeletal injuries include the objectives for care of exercise-related injuries, which are to decrease pain, reduce swelling, and prevent further injury. These objectives can be met in most cases by following "RICES" guidelines. RICES stands for rest, ice, compression, elevation, and stabilization. Rest will prevent further injury and ensure that the healing process will begin. Ice is used to reduce swelling, bleeding, inflammation, and pain. Compression also helps to reduce swelling and bleeding. Compression is achieved by the use of elastic wraps or tape. Elevation helps to decrease the blood flow and excessive pressure to the injured area. Stabilization (or splinting) is thought to protect the injury from further damage, helps attenuate pain, and potentially lessens neural inhibition.

2. —D. β-blockers

   Explanation: β-blockers work by blocking the acceleratory effects of epinephrine on the heart. This results in a blunted HR response to exercise.

3. —B. Diuretics

   Explanation: Diuretics are a type of antihypertensive medication. Diuretics increase urine output by the kidney, which can cause dehydration as well as electrolyte abnormalities.

4. —D. All of the above should be considered

   Explanation: The ACSM-EP should be mindful that the results of fitness and body composition tests can increase the participants stress and undermine participation in regular physical activity. As such, it is essential that the ACSM-EP provide encouragement and explain that baseline results are a starting point for positive behavior change and improved health and wellness.

DOMAIN IV

Doman IV Subdomain A: Multiple Choice Answers

1. —D. The supervising physician

   Explanation: In a diagnostic clinical setting, exercise testing should be conducted under the auspices of a physician. However, recent trends have moved many exercise testing laboratories away from the physician and toward allied health paraprofessionals (*e.g.,* clinical exercise physiologists, physician assistants). This has been done in large part as a cost-cutting move as well as to free-up time for physicians. The use of these paraprofessionals to administer exercise testing can be done legally as long as the supervising physician is "in the immediate vicinity . . . and available for emergencies." However, it is important to note that the safety of the client is still the priority of the supervising physician.

2. —A. Flexibility of equipment to allow for different body sizes

   Explanation: Creating a safe environment in which to exercise is a primary responsibility of any fitness facility. In developing and operating facilities and equipment for use by exercisers, the managers and staff are obligated to meet a standard of care for exerciser safety. The equipment to be used includes not only testing, cardiovascular, strength, and flexibility pieces but also rehabilitation, pool, locker room, and emergency equipment. You must evaluate several criteria when selecting equipment. These criteria include correct anatomic positioning, ability to adjust to different body sizes, quality of design and materials, durability, repair records, and then price.

ACSM-EP

3. —C. Facility operator or program director

Explanation: The facility operator or program director is tasked with designing programs and monitoring the implementation of programs. In addition, they purchase equipment and supplies for the facility, as well as monitor the safety of the facility.

4. —C. Only males can be guilty of sexual harassment

Explanation: Though more sexual harassment claims are brought against men, both sexes may be guilty of sexual harassment.

5. —C. the ACSM-EP to keep all information gathered about a client's health status confidential

Explanation: HIPAA was established by the U.S. Dept of Health and Human Services to protect the privacy of health information. HIPAA requires that all information gathered about a client's health status be kept confidential in the fitness facility.

6. —C. The Civil Rights Act

Explanation: The ACSM-EP must understand the laws that govern the hiring of employees. One such statute is the Civil Rights Act of 1964, which prohibits any discrimination based upon color, race, gender, religion, or national origin.

Doman IV Subdomain B: Multiple Choice Answers

1. —D. All of the above

Explanation: Possible medical emergencies during exercise include, but are not limited to, heat exhaustion or heat stroke, fainting, hypoglycemia, hyperglycemia, simple or compound fractures, bronchospasm, hypotension or shock, seizures, bleeding, and other cardiac symptoms.

2. —D. Management and staff

Explanation: When an emergency or injury occurs, safe and effective management of the situation will assure the best care for the individual. Implementing emergency procedures is an important part of the training of the staff. In-services, safety plans, and emergency procedures should be a part of the staff training. In addition, all exercise staff should be CPR certified and knowledgeable of first aid. Therefore, the fitness center management and staff all are included in the implementation of an emergency plan.

3. —A. True

Explanation: There are several policies and procedures that relate to the business and financial operations of a fitness center; however, the most important priority is to protect the health and safety of the members. This can be accomplished by conducting pre-participation screening, fitness testing, orientations, equipment maintenance, and emergency procedures.

4. —D. All of the above

Explanation: There are several measures that facilities can use to ensure membership safety. Prepaticipation screening, designing appropriate exercise programs, and development of emergency policy are just a few. Other health facility policies include conducting emergency response training for the staff, requiring certification of fitness staff, maintaining a clean environment, performance of regular maintenance of all exercise equipment, and providing supervision of member activities.

ACSM-EP

There are five case studies: Mike, Mr. McCain, Sarah, Mrs. Kelly, and Jimmy Strawn in this section.

CASE STUDY 1: MIKE
Author: Will Peveler, PhD

You are working as a personal trainer at a university recreation facility. You have been assigned a new client, Mike. He has been relatively active but has never worked with a trainer or been on a structured program. He is a prior college football player but has been inactive since graduation (6 years prior). He plays softball a couple times a week and has been walking 3 times a week for 30 min for the past 3 months at a moderate intensity. He is a software programmer and sits at a desk all day during his working hours. Although he feels fatigued, his overall goal is to become healthier and get in better shape.

Mike completes an informed consent and health status questionnaire. Mike is a 40-year-old Caucasian, with a body mass of 95.24 kg and a height of 181 cm. His blood pressure (BP) is 112/78 mm Hg, total cholesterol is 221 mg $\cdot$ dL^{-1} (high-density lipoprotein [HDL] and low-density lipoprotein [LDL] are unknown), and fasting blood glucose is unknown. Both his father and his paternal grandfather have known cardiovascular disease. There are no known cardiovascular or metabolic diseases on his mother's side.

- Once you have determined that Mike is clear to participate using the most recent American College of Sports Medicine (ACSM) guidelines, conduct a fitness assessment in order to establish baseline data.
- Cardiovascular measures—Resting heart rate (HR$_{rest}$) was found to be 77 bpm and BP was found to be 118/78 mm Hg.
- Body composition—After using skinfold calipers, a three-site formula was used to determine body composition: Chest = 14 mm, abdomen = 28 mm, and thigh = 19 mm.
- Cardiovascular endurance—The 1.5-mi walk/run test was chosen because it allows Mike to pace himself. He completed the distance in 14 min and 0 s.
- Muscular endurance—The push-up was conducted as per ACSM guidelines. Mike successfully completed 30 push-ups.
- Muscular strength—Bench press one repetition maximum (1-RM) and leg press 1-RM were chosen to determine Mike's muscular strength, per ACSM guidelines. Mike was able to bench press 225 lb and leg press 455 lb.

Mike: Case Study 1 Questions

1. Is medical clearance recommended prior to Mike's participation in moderate exercise?
   A) Yes
   B) No

2. Is medical clearance recommended prior to Mike's participation in vigorous exercise?
   A) Yes
   B) No

(Continued)

ACSM-EP

CASE STUDY 1: MIKE (Continued)

3. In addition to the given question's variables, if Mike mentioned to you that he was also recently experiencing shortness of breath at rest, would you automatically refer him to a physician for medical clearance?

4. You have decided to assess Mike's cardiorespiratory endurance and have selected the 1.5-mi run test. Discuss the steps involved in conducting the 1.5-mi run test for Mike.

5. Assuming Mike completed the 1.5-mi walk/run test in 14 min, please calculate Mike's estimated maximal volume of oxygen consumed per unit time ($\dot{V}O_{2max}$) using the below equation:

   $\dot{V}O_{2max}$(ml kg^{-1} · min^{-1}) = 3.5 + 483/1.5 mi time (min)
   A) 34.5 mL · kg^{-1} · min^{-1}
   B) 52.8 mL · kg^{-1} · min^{-1}
   C) 29.5 mL · kg^{-1} · min^{-1}
   D) 38.0 mL · kg^{-1} · min^{-1}

6. Using the table ("Cardiorespiratory Fitness Classifications ($\dot{V}O_{2max}$) by Age and Sex") from the most recent edition of the guidelines, Mike's $\dot{V}O_{2max}$ would place him in which of the following categories?
   A) Superior
   B) Good
   C) Fair
   D) Poor

7. Mike expressed a desire to have his muscular strength assessed on the bench press exercise and you determined that using the 1-RM test would be a good choice. Identify the necessary steps that are needed to successfully conduct this specific test on Mike.

8. The push-up result for Mike would place him in which of the following fitness categories?
   A) Excellent
   B) Very good
   C) Good
   D) Fair

9. The bench press 1-RM result for Mike would place him in which of the following fitness categories?
   A) Superior
   B) Excellent
   C) Fair
   D) Poor

10. The leg press 1-RM result for Mike would place him in which of the following fitness categories?
    A) Well above average
    B) Above average
    C) Average
    D) Below average

11. What is Mike's body mass index (BMI)? Note: BMI = weight (kg) divided by height (m^2).
    A) 14.43 kg · m^{-2}
    B) 39.71 kg · m^{-2}
    C) 29.07 kg · m^{-2}
    D) 52.62 kg · m^{-2}

12. Using Mike's BMI from the previous question, what is his BMI classification?
    A) Underweight
    B) Normal
    C) Overweight
    D) Obese

13. ACSM provides moderate-intensity exercise guidelines using heart rate reserve (HRR), $\dot{V}O_2R$, and Borg rating of perceived exertion (RPE). The Borg RPE scale is 6–20. List the exercise intensity parameters for each measure.

CASE STUDY 2: MR. McCAIN
Author: Shawn Drake, PT, PhD
Author's Certifications: ACSM-CEP, EIM3

Mr. McCain is a 36-year-old, African American male, who works as a construction worker. He is not participating in any exercise program because he is tired after working in the hot sun all day. At work, he is getting more than 30 min of physical activity 5 d · wk^{-1} and has done so for the past year. His father died of a heart attack at the age of 40 years. Now that he is approaching the age of 40 years, he wants to take steps to improve his health.

Mr. McCain is interested in a cross-fit program that he has heard about at work. He states that he would like to start that program but wants to make sure he is fit enough to begin the high-intensity program. Mr. McCain takes a β-blocker for hypertension. He is a nonsmoker and otherwise healthy.

On today's visit, his HR$_{rest}$ was 65 bpm and his resting BP was 140/84 mm Hg. Mr. McCain mentioned that he forgot to take his β-blocker today. He weighs 202 lb and is 72 in. tall, and his body fat is 22%. His fasting blood lipid profile results were as follows; HDL-cholesterol (HDL-C) = 46 mg · dL^{-1}; LDL = 140 mg · dL^{-1}; triglycerides = 220 mg · dL^{-1}. Fasting blood glucose result was 80 mg · dL^{-1}.

Mr. McCain completed a max Bruce treadmill exercise test in 11 min and 55 s (estimated $\dot{V}O_{2max}$ = 45.5 mL · kg^{-1} · min^{-1}). His maximal heart rate (HR$_{max}$) reached 185 bpm, and his BP was 186/98 mm Hg. Other health-related physical fitness parameters included 21 push-ups.

Mr. McCain: Case Study 2 Questions

1. Does Mr. McCain need medical clearance to participate in moderate-intensity exercise?
   A) Yes
   B) No

2. Identify Mr. McCain's cardiovascular risk factors.
   none

3. What is Mr. McCain's BP classification?
   A) Normal
   B) Elevated
   C) Stage I hypertension
   D) Stage II hypertension

4. Based on his $\dot{V}O_{2max}$, Mr. McCain would fall within which of the following fitness categories?
   A) Superior
   B) Excellent
   C) Good
   D) Fair

5. Design an exercise program for Mr. McCain using the frequency, intensity, time, and type (FITT) framework based on his current health/fitness status.

6. What is Mr. McCain's target $\dot{V}O_2R$ if prescribing at 60% intensity level?
   A) 29.4 mL · kg^{-1} · min^{-1}
   B) 31.9 mL · kg^{-1} · min^{-1}
   C) 28.7 mL · kg^{-1} · min^{-1}
   D) 34.3 mL · kg^{-1} · min^{-1}

7. You have suggested that Mr. McCain maintain his HR between 55% and 65% HRR during his elliptical workout. What would his specific HR range be for this prescribed intensity?
   A) 110–125 bpm
   B) 125–131 bpm
   C) 131–143 bpm
   D) 143–155 bpm

8. How many kilocalories (kcal) would Mr. McCain burn if he exercised at 60% $\dot{V}O_2R$ for 30 min?
   A) 90 kcal
   B) 396 kcal
   C) 454 kcal
   D) 560 kcal

ACSM-EP

CASE STUDY 3: SARAH
Author: Nicole Nelson MSH, LMT
Author's Certifications: ACSM-EP

Sarah is a 21-year-old female collegiate tennis player. She is currently preparing for her upcoming season and would like to begin training with you in order to improve her aerobic capacity and speed on the court. Her typical daily practice consists of 2 hours of on-court drills. She also performs 20 min of sprint interval training 2 d · wk^{-1}. She has never participated in any formal resistance training. She was diagnosed with type 1 DM at the age of 6 years. Currently, she is not experiencing cardiovascular, metabolic, or renal signs or symptoms. She relies on an insulin pump to manage her blood glucose and understands the importance of regularly monitoring her blood glucose prior to and after exercise.

Sarah's parents have no known disease.
Resting HR = 54 bpm
Resting BP = 118/65 mm Hg
Fasting blood glucose = 70 mL · dL^{-1}
LDL-C = 110 mg · dL^{-1}
HDL-C = 70 mg · dL^{-1}
Body fat % (Lange three-site) = 18%
Push-ups = 15
Right side plank = 60 s
Left side plank = 50 s
Biering–Sorensen Test (trunk extension endurance): 110 s
Leg press weight ration: weight pushed in pounds/body weight in pounds = 1.76
Bruce protocol $\dot{V}O_{2max}$ test = 45 mL · kg^{-1} · min^{-1}

Sarah: Case Study 3 Questions

1. Based on Sarah's medical history and assessment results, should she seek medical clearance before continuing to participate in vigorous intensity exercise?

2. Based on Sarah's medical history and assessment results, should she seek medical clearance if she continues to participate in moderate-intensity exercise?

3. List Sarah's cardiovascular disease (CVD) risk factors.

4. In addition to the assessments listed within Sarah's history, what other active or resting assessments might you consider conducting?

5. You decided to perform a graded exercise test (GXT) to determine Sarah's $\dot{V}O_{2max}$. Sarah is familiar with treadmill running so you chose the Bruce protocol. Describe the BP and HR responses that would cause you to terminate the test early (prior to reaching fatigue).

6. Describe the procedures involved in conducting the push-up test for Sarah.

7. You perform a glenohumeral internal rotation (also considered medial rotation) ROM test on Sarah; right = 55°; left = 75°. What are your impressions of the results?

8. You decided to perform the three-site Lange skinfold test for Sarah's body composition assessment. Describe the specific locations for the tricep, suprailiac, and thigh measurements.

9. Describe the limitations of using skinfold testing to assess body fat percentage.

CASE STUDY 4: MRS. KELLY
Author: Melissa Conway-Hartman Med, LAT, ATC
Author's Certifications: ACSM-EP, EIM2

Mrs. Kelly is a 55-year-old female who has come to your fitness center looking for help with her workout. Her goals include becoming more active, losing a few pounds, and increasing strength and endurance for enhanced ability to carry out activities of daily living. She walks her dog around the block for approximately 15 min · d^{-1}. She has worked out in the past in a fitness center and is familiar with cardiovascular equipment and prefers the treadmill. She is not as familiar with resistance training but is comfortable if she has someone to instruct her. She does not like to work out with her husband because he intimidates her. She has also expressed her dislike of coming to the gym during busy hours because she feels as though people are watching her.

As you are interviewing her, she tells you she takes medication for high BP and her doctor wants her to work out to improve her cardiovascular health. She has problems periodically with her right knee. Her doctor diagnosed her with a tear in her medial meniscus. She is also in physical therapy for a sore left shoulder and has a history of adhesive capsulitis. She also reveals that she has struggled to keep her weight down over the last 5 years; she currently weighs 210 lb and is 5 ft 6 in. tall. Her results from her latest physical include the following:

Total cholesterol—	202 mg · dL^{-1}
Triglycerides—	155 mg · dL^{-1}
HDL-C—	40 mg · dL^{-1}
LDL-cholesterol (LDL-C)—	131 mg · dL^{-1}
Fasting glucose—	105 mg · dL^{-1}
BP—	122/78 mm Hg

Mrs. Kelly expresses to you that she knows she needs to make changes and feels ready to succeed this time but is still afraid to fail due to her intermittent success in the past. Fear of having severe cardiovascular issues is a big motivator for her this time around. She does not currently work outside of the home, spends much of her time caring for her sick nephew and mother, and frequently travels to visit family on the West coast.

Assume you have addressed her medical issues with proper medical clearance forms and assessments.

Mrs. Kelly: Case Study 4 Questions

1. What is Mrs. Kelly's BMI?
   A) 23 kg · m^{-2}
   B) 30 kg · m^{-2}
   C) 34 kg · m^{-2}
   D) 40 kg · m^{-2}

2. Based on the initial information given, which of the following would be an appropriate *initial* goal you would suggest for Mrs. Kelly?
   A) Decrease caloric intake.
   B) Increase total volume of cardiovascular exercise as tolerated until she meets the ACSM recommended amount of a minimum of 150 min of moderate-to-vigorous intensity activity each week.
   C) Incorporate abdominal exercises into her program.
   D) Because she does not like to work out with her husband, suggest she get a friend to work out with.

3. According to the stages of change model or the transtheoretical model (TTM) of behavior change, which stage is Mrs. Kelly in?
   A) Precontemplation
   B) Action
   C) Maintenance
   D) Preparation

4. Given Mrs. Kelly's fear of developing severe cardiovascular issues, what behavior model would you use to help progress her behavior change?
   A) TTM
   B) Health belief model
   C) Social ecological model
   D) Self-efficacy model

5. Given that Mrs. Kelly has been unable to maintain her exercise plan, what strategy would you use to find out how you can best help her adhere to her program this time and facilitate behavior change?

(Continued)

ACSM-EP

CASE STUDY 4: MRS. KELLY (Continued)

A) Goal setting
B) Client-centered approach
C) Decisional balance sheet
D) Creating an exercise plan for her

6. You noticed that Mrs. Kelly has some self-efficacy issues due to her injuries. What is one way you can increase her self-efficacy so she will feel comfortable with her resistance training exercises?
   A) Include Mrs. Kelly in a small group resistance training session with women of similar age and interests.
   B) Educate her on the benefits of resistance training.
   C) Help her identify her barriers.
   D) Ask what made her successful in the past.

7. As Mrs. Kelly begins to have success in her program and enters the maintenance stage of the TTM, what strategies can you use to help her maintain her program?
   A) Enlist social support (*e.g.*, working out with a friend).
   B) Inform her of the benefits of being active.

C) Help her replace her bad habits with good ones.
D) Help her see that the pros outweigh the cons.

8. The model or approach that combines behavioral skill training, cognitive intervention, and lifestyle coaching is which of the following?
   A) Relapse prevention
   B) The social cognitive model
   C) The TTM
   D) The socioecological model

9. List a few cognitive and behavioral strategies you may help Mrs. Kelly with overcoming barriers with injuries, travel, and relapse prevention.

10. Looking at Mrs. Kelly's past exercise and medical history, list specific health metrics that increase her cardiometabolic risk. What is her BMI? How would you help her develop a goal to address her cardiometabolic profile?

CASE STUDY 5: JIMMY STRAWN
Author: Matthew W. Parrot, PhD

Jimmy Strawn graduated with his Bachelor of Science in Exercise Physiology and attained the ACSM-EP certification soon after. After researching his job options, Jimmy decided to start his own personal training studio and borrowed $100,000 with his parents cosigning the loan. In 2010, Westport Fitness Training became a reality. This small training studio was developed in the heart of an up-and-coming part of the city that appeared to mirror Jimmy's target market demographic. Jimmy started the facility with himself and one other employee along with 3,000 sq ft of commercial space filled with brand new fitness equipment. Shortly after the grand opening, another large commercial facility in the area closed its doors. As a result, Westport Fitness Training grew quickly from two employees to four, plus five contract personal trainers within the first 12 months. Business was booming.

The influx of customers meant long hours for Jimmy and his staff. The trainers were busy with clients, and Jimmy could barely keep up with the increasing administrative demands and new business opportunities. Consequently, no preventive maintenance was performed on the exercise equipment in the first 5 years of operation. The fact that the equipment was purchased brand new gave Jimmy the false impression that it would last for years without regular attention.

One summer day in July 2015, a Westport Fitness Training client was working with Jimmy's top contract personal trainer when the unthinkable happened. The client was performing an exercise with the cable machine when a screw holding the pulley inexplicably fell out, causing the client to fall backward and hit his head on the other side of the machine. Jimmy was not on hand to witness the incident.

Although embarrassed, the client claimed he felt fine and no other actions were taken by Jimmy's staff.

Consequences: A lawsuit was filed by the client claiming negligence on behalf of Jimmy Strawn and Westport Fitness Training. As Jimmy and his lawyer prepared their defense, a number of questions were posed.

Jimmy Strawn: Case Study 5 Questions

1. Which of the following types of insurance coverage would be the *most* relevant in this case?
   A) General liability
   B) Professional liability
   C) Worker's compensation
   D) Property

2. Which of the following documents would be the *most* relevant in Jimmy's defense?
   A) Preactivity health screening
   B) Waiver of liability
   C) Membership agreement
   D) Personal training agreement

3. Although Jimmy and his staff took no action, which of the following actions would have been appropriate immediately following the incident, given the information we have?
   A) Call 911
   B) Holding an all-staff meeting
   C) Contacting his lawyer immediately
   D) Initiating first aid protocol and complete incident report

4. Which of the following activities is *most* likely to have prevented the injury from occurring?
   A) Completing and documenting preventive maintenance procedures according to manufacturer's recommendations
   B) Training staff on proper spotting techniques
   C) Ensuring all participants sign a liability waiver
   D) Developing and using a comprehensive emergency protocol according to ACSM standards

5. Which of the following first aid procedures would have been appropriate in this situation?
   A) Check scene for safety, complete initial assessment, and provide appropriate care.
   B) Check scene for safety, call 911, and complete initial assessment.
   C) Call 911, check scene for safety, and provide appropriate care.
   D) Provide appropriate care and apply ice and direct pressure to injury.

6. Which of the following actions would *not* have been appropriate according to HIPAA guidelines?
   A) Completing incident report and sending to insurance carrier
   B) Obtaining video surveillance of incident and sending to insurance carrier
   C) Sending the injured party's membership agreement to insurance carrier
   D) Distributing injured party's medical information to all facility members

7. Which of the following ethical responsibilities (under ACSM's Code of Ethics) did Jimmy and his staff *fail* to uphold?
   A) Members should treat or train athletes with the objective of maintaining the integrity of competition and fair play.
   B) The College, and its members, should safeguard the public and itself against members who are deficient in ethical conduct.
   C) Members should not advise, aid, or abet any athlete to use prohibited substances or methods of doping.
   D) None of the above.

8. Which of the following knowledge areas did Jimmy *fail* to recognize prior to this incident?
   A) Knowledge of AED guidelines for implementation
   B) Knowledge of preventive maintenance schedules and audits
   C) Knowledge of preactivity screening, medical release, and waiver of liability for normal and at-risk participants

(Continued)

CASE STUDY 5: JIMMY STRAWN (Continued)

D) Knowledge of employment verification requirements mandated by state and federal laws

9. Jimmy's employees failed to implement any type of emergency protocol as part of this incident. How can Jimmy prevent this from occurring in the future?
   A) Develop and distribute a policy and procedures manual.
   B) Develop and distribute an emergency protocol.
   C) Hold regular emergency protocol training sessions with his staff.
   D) All of the above.

10. Which if the following would not be part of an appropriate emergency protocol for this incident?
   A) Assessing injury
   B) Checking scene

C) Activating EMS
D) Contacting friends and family of injured party

11. Given the legal and professional performance domains associated with the ACSM-EP, what areas should Jimmy have handled differently to better prepare himself and his business for this incident?

12. What are the requirements of an ACSM-EP in terms of incident reporting?

13. What responsibilities does an ACSM-EP have in terms of preventive maintenance, and how could those have reduced Jimmy's liability exposure in this incident?

14. What types of emergency procedures should have been implemented during this incident?

ACSM-EP

ANSWERS TO THE CASE STUDY CHALLENGES

MIKE CASE STUDY 1: ANSWERS

1. —B. No

   Explanation: Based on the ACSM algorithm, Mike does not need clearance to participate in moderate intensity exercise. He walks 3 times/wk for 30 min and has done so at a moderate intensity for the past 3 months, which satisfies the criteria for exercise participation. He has no known CV, renal, or metabolic disease and is not experiencing symptoms.

   Resource: Liguori G, senior editor. *ACSM'S Guidelines for Exercise Testing and Prescription*. 11th ed. Philadelphia (PA): Wolters Kluwer; 2021. Figure 2.2, Pg 35–36

2. —B. No

   Explanation: Based on the ACSM algorithm, Mike does not need clearance to participate in vigorous intensity exercise. He walks 3 times/wk for 30 min, which satisfies the criteria for exercise participation. He has no known CV, renal, or metabolic disease and is not experiencing symptoms.

   Resource: Liguori G, senior editor. *ACSM'S Guidelines for Exercise Testing and Prescription*. 11th ed. Philadelphia (PA): Wolters Kluwer; 2021. Figure 2.2, Pg 35–36

3. —Yes, he must be referred to a physician immediately due to the new recent symptoms of shortness of breath

   Explanation: Based on the ACSM algorithm, any symptom that might indicate a cardio-metabolic health issue (*e.g.*, breathlessness at rest) warrants a referral to a physician.

   Resource: Liguori G, senior editor. *ACSM'S Guidelines for Exercise Testing and Prescription*. 11th ed. Philadelphia (PA): Wolters Kluwer; 2021. Pg 33–36

4. —Ensure that the test area measures out to 1.5 mi. Inform Mike the purpose of the test and the need to pace himself properly over 1.5 mi. Start the test and give Mike feedback on time to help him pace. Once the test is complete, record the total time to the nearest hundredth of a minute. Finally, calculate estimated $\dot{V}O_{2max}$ using the following prediction equation for the 1.5-mi run test:

   $$\dot{V}O_{2max}(ml \cdot kg^{-1} \cdot min^{-1}) = 3.5 + 483/1.5\,mi\ time\,(min)$$

   Note: To calculate the time in hundredths of a minute, divide the results in seconds by 60 s. For example:

   If it takes Mike 11 min 15 s (11:15) to complete the 1.5-mi run, divide 15/60 = 0.25. Thus Mike's score = 11.25 min.

   Resource: Swain D, senior editor. *ACSM'S Resource Manual for Guidelines for Exercise Testing and Prescription*. 7th ed. Philadelphia (PA): Wolters Kluwer; 2014. 896 p.

(Continued)

MIKE CASE STUDY 1: ANSWERS (Continued)

5. —D. 38 mL · kg^{-1} · min^{-1}

$\dot{V}O_{2max}$(mL · kg^{-1} · min^{-1}) = 3.5 + 483/ 1.5 mi time (min)

= 3.5 + 483/14 min

= 38 mL · kg^{-1} · min^{-1}

Resource: Swain D, senior editor. *ACSM'S Resource Manual for Guidelines for Exercise Testing and Prescription*. 7th ed. Philadelphia (PA): Wolters Kluwer; 2014. 896 p.

6. —C. Fair

Explanation: Mike's $\dot{V}O_{2max}$ = 38 mL · kg^{-1} · min^{-1}. He is a 40-yr male. This places him in the Fair category.

Resource: Liguori G, senior editor. *ACSM'S Guidelines for Exercise Testing and Prescription*. 11th ed. Philadelphia (PA): Wolters Kluwer; 2021. Pg 89

7. —Testing should be completed only after Mike has participated in familiarization/ practice sessions. Mike should warm up by completing a number of submaximal repetitions of the bench press that will be used to determine the 1-RM. Determine the 1-RM (or any multiple of 1-RM) within four trials with rest periods of 3–5 min between trials. Select an initial weight that is within Mike's perceived capacity (~50%–70% of capacity). Resistance is progressively increased by 5%–10% for upper body exercise from previous successful attempts until Mike cannot complete the selected repetition(s); all repetitions should be performed at the same speed of movement and range of motion (ROM) to instill consistency between trials. The final weight lifted successfully is recorded as the absolute 1-RM or multiple-RM.

Resource: Liguori G, senior editor. *ACSM'S Guidelines for Exercise Testing and Prescription*. 11th ed. Philadelphia (PA): Wolters Kluwer; 2021.

8. —A. Excellent

Explanation: Mike performed 30 pushups and is a 40-yr male. This is considered Excellent.

Resource: Liguori G, senior editor. *ACSM'S Guidelines for Exercise Testing and Prescription*. 11th ed. Philadelphia (PA): Wolters Kluwer; 2021. Pg 100.

9. —B. Excellent

Explanation: To interpret Mike's 1-RM bench press result, we must calculate his relative bench press by dividing the weight he pressed by his body mass in pounds (lbs). Mike's body mass is 95.24 kg. You must convert kg to lbs (multiply by 2.2). 95.24 × 2.2 = 209 lbs.

Mike's 1-RM bench press was 225 lbs. 225 lbs/209 lbs = 1.07. Based on the normative data table (3.11) for upper body strength in the 11th ed *ACSM Guidelines for Exercise Testing and Prescription*, Mike's result would place him in the Excellent category.

Resource: Liguori G, senior editor. *ACSM'S Guidelines for Exercise Testing and Prescription*. 11th ed. Philadelphia (PA): Wolters Kluwer; 2021. Pg 96.

10. —A. Well above average

Explanation: Mike's 1RM leg press = 455 lbs. You will need to calculate Mike's relative leg strength to answer this question by dividing the weight he pressed by his body mass in pounds. Mike's leg press weight ratio = 455/209 lbs = 2.17. Based on the normative data table (3.12) in the 11th ed *ACSM Guidelines for Exercise Testing and Prescription*, Mike's result would place him in the well above average category.

Resource: Liguori G, senior editor. *ACSM'S Guidelines for Exercise Testing and Prescription*. 11th ed. Philadelphia (PA): Wolters Kluwer; 2021. Pg 98.

11. —C.

Explanation: The formula to calculate BMI = weight (kg)/height (m)^2.

Mike's weight = 95.24 kg. Height = 181 cm or 1.81 m

BMI = 95.24/(1.81)^2

BMI = 29.07 kg · m^{-2}

Resource: Liguori G, senior editor. *ACSM'S Guidelines for Exercise Testing* *and Prescription*. 11th ed. Philadelphia (PA): Wolters Kluwer; 2021. Pg 63.

12. —C. Overweight

Explanation: Mike's BMI = 29.07 kg · m^{-2} which falls in the overweight classification (25.0–29.9 kg · m^{-2}).

Resource: Liguori G, senior editor. *ACSM'S Guidelines for Exercise Testing and Prescription*. 11th ed. Philadelphia (PA): Wolters Kluwer; 2021. Pg 64.

13. —Cardiovascular exercise intensity can be monitored using HRR, $\dot{V}O_2R$, and RPE. ACSM uses the following parameters for moderate intensity exercise: 40%–59% HRR; 40%–59% $\dot{V}O_2R$, and RPE 12–13.

Resource: Liguori G, senior editor. *ACSM'S Guidelines for Exercise Testing and Prescription*. 11th ed. Philadelphia (PA): Wolters Kluwer; 2021. Pg 36

MR. MCCAIN CASE STUDY 2: ANSWERS

1. —B. No

Explanation: Mr. McCain is considered physically active as he has met the PA minimum requirements of 3 d/wk for 30 min for the past year. He does not have any symptoms/signs of CV, metabolic, or renal disease. He does not have known CV, metabolic or renal disease. Though he is hypertensive, this is considered a CVD risk factor and not CV disease. Based on the algorithm, he should begin a low-moderate intensity exercise and progress gradually following ACSM Guidelines.

Resource: Liguori G, senior editor. *ACSM'S Guidelines for Exercise Testing and Prescription*. 11th ed. Philadelphia (PA): Wolters Kluwer; 2021. Pg 35–36.

2. —Family History: Mr. McCain's father (first degree relative) died of a heart attack <50 yrs, Hypertension and LDL ≥130 mg dL^{-1}

Resource: Liguori, senior editor. *ACSM'S Guidelines for Exercise Testing and Prescription*. 11th ed. Philadelphia (PA): Wolters Kluwer; 2021. Pg 47.

3. —D. Stage 2 hypertension

Mr. McCain's resting BP was 140/84 mm Hg. Normal is <120 mm Hg (systolic) and <80 mm Hg (diastolic). Elevated is classified as 120–139 mm Hg (systolic) and <80 mm Hg (diastolic). Stage I hypertension is 130–139 mm Hg (systolic) or 80–89 mmHg (diastolic). Stage 2 hypertension is ≥140 mm Hg (systolic) or ≥90 mm Hg (diastolic). Thus, Mr. McCain's resting BP would place him in the category of stage 2 hypertension.

Resource: Whelton PK et al. 2017 ACC/AHA/AAPA/ABC/ACPM/AGS/APhA/ASH/ASPC/NMA/PCNA Guideline for the Prevention, Detection, Evaluation, and Management of High Blood Pressure in Adults. Hypertension.

4. —C. Good

Explanation: Mr. McCain's $\dot{V}O_{2max}$ is 45.5 mL kg^{-1} min^{-1} and age is 36 yr. Using Table 3.9 in the 11th ed of *ACSM's Guidelines for Exercise Testing and Prescription*, the fitness category is considered "Good."

Resource: Liguori G, senior editor. *ACSM'S Guidelines for Exercise Testing and Prescription*. 11th ed. Philadelphia (PA): Wolters Kluwer; 2021. Pg 91

5. —Mr. McCain should follow guidelines for hypertension, which include focusing weight reduction by increasing caloric expenditure coupled with reducing caloric intake

Frequency: Preferably aerobic or resistance exercise performed on most, preferably all, days of the week.

Intensity: Low, Moderate, or Vigorous with an emphasis on "Moderate." Moderate-intensity levels (40%–60% O_2R) is

(Continued)

ACSM-EP

MR. MCCAIN CASE STUDY 2: ANSWERS (Continued)

appropriate for aerobic activity; resistance training at 60%–80% of 1-RM

Time: 90–150 min per week or more

Type: Multi-modal exercise. Choose activities that are enjoyable and use large muscle groups (*e.g.*, walking, jogging, swimming) for aerobic; resistance training to include free weights or machine weights.

Resources: Pescatello L. et al. Physical activity to prevent and treat hypertension. On Behalf of the 2018 Physical Activity Guidelines Advisory Committee. *Med Sci Sports Exerc.* 2019;51(6):1314–23.

Liguori G, senior editor. *ACSM'S Guidelines for Exercise Testing and Prescription.* 11th ed. Philadelphia (PA): Wolters Kluwer; 2021. Pg 291.

6. —C. $28.7 \text{ mL} \cdot \text{kg}^{-1} \cdot \text{min}^{-1}$

To calculate % $\dot{V}O_2R$, use the formula $[(\dot{V}O_2max - 3.5) \times \text{desired intensity}]$

60% $\dot{V}O_2R = [(45.5 - 3.5) \times .60]$

60% $\dot{V}O_2R = 28.7 \text{ mL} \cdot \text{kg}^{-1} \cdot \text{min}^{-1}$

Resource: Liguori G, senior editor. *ACSM'S Guidelines for Exercise Testing and Prescription.* 11th ed. Philadelphia (PA): Wolters Kluwer; 2021. Pg 492

7. —C. 131–143 bpm

Mr. McCain's maximum HR during the GXT was 185 bpm. His resting HR = 65 bpm. Using the HRR formula = [Desired intensity ($HR_{max} - HR_{rest}$)] + HR_{rest}

Low end HR = $[.55(185 - 65)] + 65 = 131$ bpm

High end HR = $[.65(185 - 65)] + 65 = 143$ bpm

Resource: Liguori G, senior editor. *ACSM'S Guidelines for Exercise Testing and Prescription.* 11th ed. Philadelphia (PA): Wolters Kluwer; 2021. Pg 492.

8. —B. 396 kcal

Explanation: Mr. McCain weighs 202 lbs, which is 92 kg (202/2.2). His intensity is $28.7 \text{ mL} \cdot \text{kg}^{-1} \cdot \text{min}^{-1}$. Convert his relative $\dot{V}O_2$ to absolute $\dot{V}O_2$ to determine his caloric expenditure. (28.7 mL/kg/min × 92 kg)/1000 = 2.64 L/min. Assume, for every 1 LO_2 = 5 kcals expended.

2.64 L/min × 5 kcal/L = 13.2 kcal/min. He performed 30 min of exercise.

13.2 kcal/min × 30 min = 396 kcal

SARAH CASE STUDY 3: ANSWERS

1. —Sarah is physically active and has known metabolic disease (Type 1 DM). She is not experiencing any symptoms. Based on the algorithm, Sarah should seek medical clearance before continuing on with vigorous exercise

   Resource: Liguori G, senior editor. *ACSM'S Guidelines for Exercise Testing and Prescription.* 11th ed. Philadelphia (PA): Wolters Kluwer; 2021. Pg 35–36

2. —Sarah is physically active and has known metabolic disease (Type 1 DM). She is not experiencing any symptoms. Based on the algorithm, Sarah does not need medical clearance prior to participating in moderate intensity exercise

   Resource: Liguori G, senior editor. *ACSM'S Guidelines for Exercise Testing and Prescription.* 11th ed. Philadelphia (PA): Wolters Kluwer; 2021. Pg 35–36

3. —Sarah has no positive CVD risk factors. She has one negative risk factor; her HDL-C $\geq 60 \text{ mg} \cdot \text{dL}^{-1}$

   Resource: Liguori G, senior editor. *ACSM'S Guidelines for Exercise Testing and Prescription.* 11th ed. Philadelphia (PA): Wolters Kluwer; 2021. Pg 47

4. —To best answer this question, you must consider the client's goals, exercise experience, and the demands of their sport.

Sarah plays tennis, a sport involving quick changes of direction and speed. Some type of speed and agility test, such as the t-test, would be appropriate.

Though strength is relevant to tennis, Sarah has no experience in performing loaded squat and bench press patterns. After learning these movements and sufficient practice, inclusion of strength testing would be appropriate.

Tennis requires dynamic mobility and stability of multiple joint segments. A functional movement screen assessing shoulder, thoracic spine, hip, and ankle joint segments is warranted. In addition, an assessment of static glenohumeral ROM, including external (lateral), internal (medial), flexion, and extension would be prudent.

Tennis also requires anaerobic capacity, thus an anaerobic power and fatigue test, such as the Wingate, should be included in her testing line-up.

Vertical and horizontal power expression is relevant to the sport of tennis, thus a vertical jump test and a standing long jump would be reasonable.

Power of the upper body is also relevant to tennis. In which case, the seated medicine ball put, involving the participant propelling a medicine ball a maximal horizontal distance would be worthwhile.

Resource: Gordon B, senior editor. *ACSM's Resources for the Exercise Physiologist.* 3rd ed. Philadelphia (PA): Wolters Kluwer; 2021.

5. —Blood pressure and HR indications for ending a GXT include a drop in SBP ≥10 mm Hg with an increase in workload or if SBP decreases below the value obtained in the same position prior to testing. If SBP >250 mm Hg and/or DBP >115 mm Hg. If HR fails to increase, despite an increase in workload.

Resource: Liguori G, senior editor. *ACSM'S Guidelines for Exercise Testing and Prescription.* 11th ed. Philadelphia (PA): Wolters Kluwer; 2021. Pg 78

6. —Sarah should begin in the standard "down" position with hands pointing forward and under the shoulder, back straight. The push-up test for females uses the knee as the pivot point. Sarah must raise her body and return to the "down" position until the chin touches the mat or her chest is within one fist-width distance from the floor. Sarah should perform the maximal number of push-ups without rest. The test is terminated when she strains forcibly or is unable to maintain the proper technique within two repetitions.

Resource: Liguori G, senior editor. *ACSM'S Guidelines for Exercise Testing and Prescription.* 11th ed. Philadelphia (PA): Wolters Kluwer; 2021. Pg 99

7. —"Normal" glenohumeral IR ROM is 70°–90°. Sarah's right glenohumeral IR is considered limited. Her left IR is normal.

Resource: Liguori G, senior editor. *ACSM'S Guidelines for Exercise Testing and Prescription.* 11th ed. Philadelphia (PA): Wolters Kluwer; 2021. Pg 103

8. —The three skinfold sites used on Sarah include the following:
   i) Triceps: on the posterior midline of the upper arm, hallway between the acromion and olecranon processes.
   ii) Suprailiac: in line with the natural angle of the iliac rest taken in the anterior axillary line immediately superior to the iliac crest.
   iii) Thigh: on the anterior midline of the thigh, midway between the proximal border of the patella and the inguinal crease.

Resource: Gordon, B, senior editor. *ACSM's Resources for the Exercise Physiologist.* 3rd ed. Philadelphia (PA): Wolters Kluwer; 2021. Chapter 7

9. —Skinfold testing relies on the assumption that 1/3 of an individual's fat is located subcutaneously, which is not always the case. Additionally, measurement error, whether related to the lack of experience by the evaluator or an improperly calibrated caliper can occur.

(Continued)

ACSM-EP

SARAH CASE STUDY 3: ANSWERS (Continued)

In severely obese individuals, the skin-fold thickness may exceed the maximum opening of the calipers.

Resource: Gordon B, senior editor. *ACSM's Resources for the Exercise Physiologist.* 3rd ed. Philadelphia (PA): Wolters Kluwer; 2021. Chapter 7

MRS. KELLY CASE STUDY 4: ANSWERS

1. —C. 34 kg · m^{-2}

   Explanation: Her BMI is 34 kg · m^{-2} placing her in the class I obesity category.

   Converting her body mass of 210 lbs to kg = 210/2.2 = 95 kg

   Convert her height of 5'6" to m = 66" × .0254 = 1.67 m

   BMI = 95/(1.67)^2 = 34 kg · m^{-2}

2. —B. Increase total volume of cardiovascular exercise as tolerated until she meets the ACSM recommended amount of a minimum of 150 min of moderate-to-vigorous intensity activity each week.

   Explanation: She is currently walking, and increasing the time she is active in small increments will provide mastery experiences to increase her self-efficacy. Burning more calories will help her lose weight, and doing so slowly will aid in prevention of further injury to her knee. Small changes may also be more realistic and safe for her to achieve (small changes model).

   Resource: Hargens T, senior editor. *ACSM's Resources for the Personal Trainer.* 6th ed. Philadelphia (PA): Wolters Kluwer; 2021. Chapter 7.

3. —D. Preparation

   Explanation: Preparation, because she is currently trying to be active by walking her dog but is not meeting the guidelines. She is coming to you for help with a plan.

4. —B. Health belief model

   Explanation: The health belief model states that people are likely to change a behavior if that current behavior poses a perceived serious potential health problem, the threat is severe, and the person perceives themselves to be susceptible to the threat.

   Resource: Hargens T, senior editor. *ACSM's Resources for the Personal Trainer.* 6th ed. Philadelphia (PA): Wolters Kluwer; 2021. Chapter 7.

5. —B. Client-centered approach

   Explanation: The client-centered approach is a counseling style that "takes the client's perspective into account, features collaboration between the client and the practitioner, and includes genuine respect for the client's opinions."

   Resource: Hargens T, senior editor. *ACSM's Resources for the Personal Trainer.* 6th ed. Philadelphia (PA): Wolters Kluwer; 2021. Chapter 7.

6. —A. Include Mrs. Kelly in a small group resistance training session with women of similar age and interests

   Explanation: According to Bandura, providing vicarious experiences—watching others who are similar to you change their behavior—will increase a client's self-efficacy.

   Resource: Liguori G, senior editor. *ACSM'S Guidelines for Exercise Testing and Prescription.* 11th ed. Philadelphia (PA): Wolters Kluwer; 2021. Pg 445.

7. —A. Enlist social support (*e.g.*, working out with a friend)

   Explanation: "Enlisting social support, *i.e.*, walking with a neighbor" can help maintainers avoid boredom.

   Resource: Liguori G, senior editor. *ACSM'S Guidelines for Exercise Testing and Prescription.* 11th ed. Philadelphia (PA): Wolters Kluwer; 2021. Pg 454.

8. —A. Relapse prevention strategies

    Explanation: The relapse prevention strategies are a combination of behavioral skill training, cognitive intervention, and lifestyle change

    Resource: Nigg C. *ACSM's Behavioral Aspects of Physical Activity and Exercise.* Philadelphia (PA): Lippincott Williams & Wilkins; 2014:107

9. —Provide guidance to Mrs. Kelly on overcoming specific barriers to physical activity. For example, provide her with workouts she can perform during travel, and encouraging her to fit in her activity when and where she can while taking care of her nephew will help keep her active until she can return to her normal life routine. Using a planning worksheet can help her think through (coping planning) and plan around her various barriers.

    Reducing her level of anxiety regarding committing to a regular exercise program is asking her to pay attention to her feelings about finally becoming more active (dramatic relief). It also addresses the cognitive portion of the RPM. To help her with the behavioral aspect of the RPM, you can develop activities she can participate in when traveling. To help her with her overall lifestyle change, she needs to see herself as an active person (social liberation).

    Resource: Nigg C. *ACSM's Behavioral Aspects of Physical Activity and Exercise.* Philadelphia (PA): Lippincott Williams & Wilkins; 2014:107.

10. —Mrs. Kelly has elevated total cholesterol, borderline elevated LDL-C, decreased HDL-C, and elevated triglyceride and blood glucose levels. Although controlled by her medication, she also has high BP. Her BMI is 33.9 kg m^{-2} placing her in the class I obesity category. By using motivational interviewing skills, she will understand the importance to lower her disease risk and BMI. Implementing goal setting principles that are specific, measurable, achievable, realistic, and time-oriented will help her achieve her initial goal.

    Resources: Nigg C. *ACSM's Behavioral Aspects of Physical Activity and Exercise.* Philadelphia (PA): Lippincott Williams & Wilkins; 2014:76–77,137.

    Liguori G, senior editor. *ACSM's Guidelines for Exercise Testing and Prescription.* 11th ed. Philadelphia (PA): Wolters Kluwer; 2021. Pg 453, 457–458.

JIMMY STRAWN CASE STUDY 5: ANSWERS

1. —A. General liability

    Resource: Gordon B, senior editor. *ACSM's Resources for the Exercise Physiologist.* 3rd ed. Philadelphia (PA): Wolters Kluwer; 2021. Chapter 14.

2. —B. Waiver of liability

    Resource: Gordon, B, senior editor. *ACSM's Resources for the Exercise Physiologist.* 3rd ed. Philadelphia (PA): Wolters Kluwer; 2021.

3. —D. Initiating first aid protocol and complete incident report

    Resource: Gordon B, senior editor. *ACSM's Resources for the Exercise Physiologist.* 3rd ed. Philadelphia (PA): Wolters Kluwer; 2021. Chapter 14.

4. —A. Completing and documenting preventive maintenance procedures according to manufacturer's recommendations

    Sanders, ME. *ACSM's Health/Fitness Facilities Standards and Guidelines.* 5th ed. Champaign (IL): Human Kinetics, 2018.

ACSM-EP

(Continued)

5. —A. Check scene for safety, complete initial assessment, and provide appropriate care

   Resource: Gordon B, senior editor. *ACSM's Resources for the Exercise Physiologist.* 3rd ed. Philadelphia (PA): Wolters Kluwer; 2021. Chapter 14

6. —D. Distributing injured party's medical information to all facility members

   Resource: Health Insurance Portability and Accountability Act of 1996 (HIPAA)

7. —D. None of the above

   Resource: Liguori G, senior editor. *ACSM'S Guidelines for Exercise Testing and Prescription.* 11th ed. Philadelphia (PA): Wolters Kluwer; 2021.

8. —B. Knowledge of preventive maintenance schedules and audits

   Resource: Sanders ME. *ACSM's Health/ Fitness Facilities Standards and Guidelines.* 5th ed. Champaign (IL): Human Kinetics; 2018.

9. —D. All of the above

   Resource: Gordon B, senior editor. *ACSM's Resources for the Exercise Physiologist.* 3rd ed. Philadelphia (PA): Wolters Kluwer; 2021. Chapter 16

10. —D. Contacting friends and family of injured party

    Resource: Gordon B, senior editor. *ACSM's Resources for the Exercise Physiologist.* 3rd ed. Philadelphia (PA): Wolters Kluwer; 2021. Chapter 16

11. —The areas include policies and procedures manual, emergency procedure training, complete preventive maintenance as manufacturer's required, incident report training, safety procedures and supplies, understanding of insurance coverage differences for contractors versus employees, and installation of proper signage for equipment use.

    Resource: Sanders, ME. *ACSM's Health/ Fitness Facilities Standards and Guidelines.* 5th ed. Champaign (IL): Human Kinetics, 2018.

12. —Develop a written incident report that includes name and contact information for injured party and witnesses, description of event and injuries, time and day of incident, and any actions taken by the staff. Complete this report for any injury, regardless of severity and keep on file. To train all qualified subordinate staff on proper incident report completion

    Resource: Sanders, ME. *ACSM's Health/ Fitness Facilities Standards and Guidelines.* 5th ed. Champaign (IL): Human Kinetics, 2018.

13. —An ACSM-EP needs to be familiar with all preventive maintenance schedules as recommended by the manufacturer(s), to complete the preventive maintenance, and to document preventive maintenance procedures when completed.

    Resource: Sanders, ME. *ACSM's Health/ Fitness Facilities Standards and Guidelines.* 5th ed. Champaign (IL): Human Kinetics, 2018.

14. —Emergency procedures include incident report completion, first aid assessment by staff, first aid provided (if needed) by staff, and evaluation of emergency medical services personnel involvement. Interview injured party and document all relevant information on the scene conditions, individuals present, extent of injury, and the incident itself.

    Resource: Sanders, ME. *ACSM's Health/ Fitness Facilities Standards and Guidelines.* 5th ed. Champaign (IL): Human Kinetics, 2018.

PART 3

ACSM Certified Clinical Exercise Physiologist® (ACSM-CEP®) Certification

Samuel A. Headley, PhD, FACSM, ACSM-CEP, EIM3
Associate Editor

DOMAIN NUMBER	I	II	III	IV	V	VI
DOMAIN NAME	PATIENT ASSESSMENT	EXERCISE TESTING	EXERCISE PRESCRIPTION	EXERCISE TRAINING AND LEADERSHIP	EDUCATION AND BEHAVIOR CHANGE	LEGAL AND PROFESSIONAL RESPONSIBILITIES

OUTLINE OF THIS PART:

DOMAIN I: PATIENT ASSESSMENT

A. Assess a patient's medical record for information related to their visit.

Domain I Subdomain A: What you need to know

Knowledge of:

A) the procedure to obtain patient's medical history through available documentation.

B) the necessary medical records needed to properly assess a patient, given their diagnosis and/or reason for referral.

C) the procedure to obtain physician referral and medical records required for program participation.

D) information and documentation required for program participation.

E) the epidemiology, pathophysiology, progression, risk factors, key clinical findings, and treatments of chronic diseases.

F) the techniques (*e.g.*, lab results, diagnostic tests) used to diagnose chronic diseases, their indications, limitations, risks, normal and abnormal results.

G) medical charting, terminology, and common acronyms.

Skill in:

A) interpreting information from medical records in patient care and/or exercise prescription.

B) assessing various vital signs.

C) assessing participant physician referral and/or medical records to determine program participation status.

Domain I Subdomain A: Multiple Choice Questions

1. Which of the following procedures provides the *least* sensitivity and specificity in the diagnosis of coronary artery disease?
   A) Coronary angiography
   B) Echocardiography
   C) Electrocardiography
   D) Radionuclide imaging

2. Which of the following is the thickest, middle layer of the artery wall that is composed predominantly of smooth muscle cells and is responsible for vasoconstriction and vasodilation?
   A) Endothelium
   B) Intima
   C) Media
   D) Adventitia

3. Orthopnea is _____.
   A) Dyspnea caused by physical exertion
   B) Dyspnea at rest in a recumbent position that is relieved by sitting upright or standing
   C) The same as orthostatic hypotension
   D) Dyspnea that occurs going from a recumbent position to a standing position

4. Which of the following is characterized by an inflammation and edema of the trachea and bronchial tubes, hypertrophy of the mucous glands that narrows the airway, arterial hypoxemia that leads to vasoconstriction of smooth muscle in the pulmonary arterioles and venules, and in the presence of continued vasoconstriction results in pulmonary hypertension?
   A) Emphysema
   B) Bronchitis
   C) Pulmonary hypertension
   D) Asthma

5. Which of the following statements concerning the surgical treatment of coronary artery disease is *true*?
   A) A coronary artery stent carries a lower rate of revascularization than does PTCA.

B) Atherectomy is a prerequisite requirement for PTCA.
   C) Venous grafts are significantly superior to arterial grafts in terms of patency.
   D) Long-term outcome of laser angioplasty is unknown and thus rarely used.

6. Which of the following is not true for an individual who suffered a cerebral vascular accident and wishes to return to work?
   A) Patients should be educated on avoidance and precautions.
   B) Assessment of muscular strength and endurance are needed.
   C) They should not be encouraged to return to work.
   D) Exercise programs should be specific to occupational requirements.

7. Which of the following is a reversible pulmonary condition caused by some type of irritant (*e.g.*, dust, pollen) and characterized by bronchial airway narrowing, dyspnea, coughing, and, possibly, hypoxia and hypercapnia?
   A) Emphysema
   B) Bronchitis
   C) Asthma
   D) Pulmonary vascular disease

B. Interview patient regarding medical history for their visit and reconcile medications.

Domain I Subdomain B: What you need to know

Knowledge of:

A) establishment of rapport through health counseling techniques (*e.g.*, the patient-centered approach), and nonjudgmental positive regard in creation of collaborative partnership.
B) use of open-ended inquiry, active listening and attention to nonverbal behavior, interest and empathy.
C) information and documentation required for program participation.
D) the procedure to obtain informed consent from patient to meet legal requirements.
E) commonly used medications in patients with chronic diseases, their mechanisms of action, and side effects.

F) medical charting, terminology and common acronyms.

Skill in:

A) administering informed consent.
B) interviewing patient for medical history pertinent to the reason for their visit and reconciling medications.
C) active listening and usage of health counseling techniques.
D) data collection during baseline intake assessment.
E) proficiency in medical charting.

Domain I Subdomain B: Multiple Choice Questions

1. During a medical emergency, which of the following medications is an endogenous catecholamine that can be used to increase blood flow to the heart and brain?

   A) Lidocaine
   B) Oxygen
   C) Atropine
   D) Epinephrine

2. Which of the following medications reduces myocardial ischemia by lowering myocardial oxygen demand, is used to treat typical and variant angina, but has *not* been shown to reduce post-myocardial infarction (MI) mortality?
   A) β-adrenergic blockers
   B) Niacin
   C) Aspirin
   D) Nitrates

3. Which of the following medications does *not* affect exercise HR response?
   A) Angiotensin-converting enzyme (ACE) inhibitors and angiotensin II blockers
   B) Calcium channel blockers
   C) Thyroid medications
   D) β-blockers

4. Medications may directly alter the ECG response during exercise and result in false-positive tests. Assuming no change in underlying disease status, the drug *most* likely to have this effect is _____.
   A) Lidocaine (Xylocaine)
   B) Propranolol (Inderal)
   C) Digitalis (Lanoxin)
   D) Reserpine (Serpasil)

5. Compared with data obtained during a previous graded exercise test when no medications were taken, a patient now taking propranolol (Inderal) would have which of the following response to the same submaximal exercise intensity during a second test?
   A) A higher RPP
   B) A larger QRS duration
   C) A lower HR
   D) Greater ST-segment depression

6. A cardiac patient is taking a β-blocker medication. During an exercise test, you would expect _____.
   A) An ST-segment depression because β-blockers depress the ST segment on the resting ECG
   B) An increase in the anginal threshold compared with a test without the medication
   C) No change in HR or BP compared with a test without the medication
   D) A slight decrease or no effect on BP compared with a test without the medication

C. Obtain and assess resting biometric data (e.g., height, weight, ECG, arterial oxygen saturation, blood glucose, body composition, spirometry).

Domain I Subdomain C: What you need to know

Knowledge of:

A) best practice-based intake assessment tools and techniques to assess and interpret clinical and health measures (*e.g.*, height, weight, anthropometrics, body mass index, resting energy expenditure).

B) medical therapies for chronic diseases and their effect on resting vital signs and symptoms.

C) normal cardiovascular, pulmonary and metabolic anatomy and physiology.

D) techniques for assessing signs and symptoms (*e.g.*, peripheral pulses, blood pressure, edema, pain).

E) 12-lead and telemetry ECG interpretation for normal sinus rate and rhythm or abnormalities (*e.g.*, arrhythmias, blocks, ischemia, infarction).

F) ECG changes associated with, but not limited to, drug therapy, electrolyte abnormalities, myocardial injury and infarction, congenital defects, pericarditis, pulmonary embolus, and the clinical significance of each.

Skill in:

A) administering and interpreting resting biometric data to determine baseline health status.

B) preparing a patient and ECG electrode application for resting ECGs.

C) assessing vital signs and symptoms at rest.

D) assessing ankle brachial index using a hand-held Doppler

Domain I Subdomain C: Multiple Choice Questions

1. Which of the following medications works by opposing the action of the catecholamines.
   A) β-adrenergic blockers
   B) Niacin
   C) Aspirin
   D) Nitrates

2. The cardiac rehabilitation's medical director orders a pre-rehabilitation ECG on a 50-year-old man. The exercise physiologist performing the ECG notes the machine error message reads artifact in the precordial lead V_4. To correct the artifact, an exercise physiologist would check which of the following lead positions for adhesive contact?
   A) Fourth intercostal space, left sternal border
   B) Fourth intercostal space, right sternal border
   C) Midaxillary line, fifth intercostal space
   D) Midclavicular line, fifth intercostal space

3. A 55-year-old cardiac rehabilitation patient returned from vacation with the following complaints: elevation in BP, slight chest pain, shortness of breath with chest wheezing, and dryness and burning of the mouth and throat. Based on this information, the exercise physiologist would suspect that the patient was exposed to which of the following environments?
   A) Extreme cold
   B) Extreme heat
   C) High altitude
   D) High humidity

4. Which of the following tests would give the best confirmation of diabetes?
   A) Fasting blood glucose test
   B) Oral glucose tolerance test
   C) Glycolated hemoglobin (HbA1C)
   D) Total blood count

5. While monitoring the ECG of a cardiac rehabilitation patient, a progressive lengthening of the PR interval until a dropped QRS complex is observed. Based on this observation, what kind of AV block are you observing?
   A) First degree
   B) Mobitz type I
   C) Mobitz type II
   D) Third degree

6. You are asked to review an ECG strip for evidence of myocardial ischemia and/or injury. On what areas of the ECG should you focus?
   A) Q wave
   B) PR interval
   C) ST segment
   D) P wave

7. In an ECG recording, the presence of certain combinations of ST-segment abnormalities (*i.e.*, elevation and/or depression) and significant Q waves may be suggestive of what condition?
   A) Acute MI
   B) Left ventricular hypertrophy
   C) Right bundle-branch block
   D) Ventricular aneurysm

8. Why is it important to choose the appropriate BP cuff size?
   A) A cuff too small will give a lower reading for both the systolic and diastolic pressures.
   B) If cuff size encircles <80% of the upper arm, measurement will be inaccurate.
   C) When deflating the cuff, you will not be able to maintain a deflation rate of 2–3 mm Hg $\cdot$ s^{-1}.
   D) Both B and C

9. Which of the following is not a characteristic of ventricular tachycardia?
   A) Wide QRS complex (≥120 ms)
   B) AV dissociation (P waves and QRS complexes have no relationship)
   C) Flutter waves at a rate of 250–350 atrial depolarizations per minute
   D) Three or more consecutive ventricular beats at 100 bpm

10. Which type of AV block occurs with a fixed PR interval that is associated with a non-conduced P waves?
    A) First degree
    B) Second degree, Mobitz type I
    C) Second degree, Mobitz type II
    D) Third degree

11. Which of the following ECG interpretations involves a QRS complex duration that exceeds 0.11 s and a P wave precedes the QRS complex if it is present?
    A) AV conduction delay
    B) Normal cardiac function
    C) Supraventricular aberrant conduction
    D) Acute MI

12. ST-segment elevation may occur in all of the following except _____.
    A) Coronary artery spasm
    B) A ventricular aneurysm
    C) An acute MI
    D) Subendocardial ischemia

D. Determine a sufficient level of monitoring/supervision based on a preparticipation health screening.

Domain I Subdomain D: What you need to know

Knowledge of:

A) normal physiologic responses to exercise.

B) abnormal responses/signs/symptoms to exercise associated with different pathologies (*e.g.*, cardiovascular, pulmonary, metabolic).

C) pertinent areas of a patient's medical history (*e.g.*, any symptoms since their procedure, description of discomfort/pain, orthopedic issues).

D) indications and contraindications to exercise testing and training.

E) current published guidelines for treatment of cardiovascular, pulmonary and metabolic pathologies (*e.g.*, American College of Cardiology/American Heart Association [ACC/AHA] Joint Guidelines, Global Initiative for Chronic Obstructive Lung Disease [GOLD], American Diabetes Association [ADA]).

F) industry recognized preparticipation health screening practices (*e.g.*, the Physical Activity Readiness Questionnaire for Everyone [PAR-Q+], ACSM's preparticipation screening algorithm).

G) medical therapies for chronic diseases and their effect on the physiologic response to exercise.

H) the timing of daily activities (*e.g.*, medications, dialysis, meals, glucose monitoring) and their effect on exercise in patients with chronic diseases.

I) abnormal signs and symptoms in apparently healthy individuals and those with chronic disease.

J) methods used to obtain a referral for clinical exercise physiology services.

Skill in:

A) implementing industry-recognized preparticipation health screening practices.

B) administering informed consent.

C) selecting an exercise test based on a patient's disease, condition and ability.

D) determining risk and level of monitoring of patient using health history, medical history, medical records, and additional diagnostic assessments.

E) modifying exercise/physical activity program in response to medication use, timing, and side effects.

Domain I Subdomain D: Multiple Choice Questions

1. Which of the following statements regarding contraindications to graded exercise testing is accurate?
   A) Some individuals have risk factors that outweigh the potential benefits from exercise testing and the information that may be obtained.
   B) Absolute contraindications refer to conditions under which exercise testing should not be performed until the condition has stabilized.
   C) Relative contraindications refer to unfavorable conditions under which exercise testing might be tested if the potential benefit from exercise testing outweighs the relative risk.
   D) All of the above statements are true.

2. Which of the following cardiac indices increases curvilinearly with the work rate until it reaches near maximum at a level equivalent to approximately 50% of aerobic capacity, increasing only slightly thereafter?
   A) Stroke volume
   B) HR
   C) Cardiac output
   D) Systolic blood pressure (BP)

3. Which of the following statements are false concerning stroke volume in healthy adults?
   A) A greater preload will increase stroke volume.
   B) Increased arterial BP and greater ventricular outflow resistance will reduce stroke volume.
   C) During exercise, stroke volume increases to 50% to 60% of maximal capacity, after which increases in cardiac output are largely caused by further increases in HR.
   D) Stroke volume is equal to the ratio of end-diastolic volume to end-systolic volume.

E. Assess patient goals, needs and objectives based on health and exercise history, motivation level, and physical activity readiness.

Domain I Subdomain E: What you need to know

Knowledge of:

A) patient-centered health counseling techniques with nonjudgmental positive regard.

B) assessment of patient goals and exercise history through use of open-ended inquiry, active listening and attention to nonverbal behavior, and reflective listening.

C) the effects of a sedentary lifestyle, including extended periods of physical inactivity and approaches to counteract these changes.

D) behavior modification tools and techniques to assess patient's expectations, goals, and motivation level (*e.g.*, health literacy, identification of real and perceived barriers, decisional balance).

E) common barriers to exercise compliance and adherence (*e.g.*, physical/disease state, environmental, demographic, vocation).

F) known demographic factors related to likelihood of adherence and maintenance of exercise (*e.g.*, age, gender, socioeconomic status, education, ethnicity).

G) characteristics associated with poor adherence to healthy behaviors (*e.g.*, low self-efficacy, poor social support).

H) psychological issues associated with acute and chronic illness (*e.g.*, anxiety, depression, social isolation, suicidal ideation).

I) validated tools for measurement of psychosocial health status.

J) a variety of behavioral assessment tools (*e.g.*, SF-36, health-related quality of life, Chronic Respiratory Disease Questionnaire) and strategies for their use.

K) recognizing adverse effects of exercise in apparently healthy persons or those with chronic disease.

Skill in:

A) active listening and behavior modification techniques.

B) counseling techniques and strategies to overcome real and perceived barriers.

C) applying health behavior theories and strategies to strengthen patient barriers self-efficacy and optimize compliance and adherence in support of achievement of goals.

D) adapting/modifying an exercise program based on unique needs of a patient.

E) administering commonly used screening tools to evaluate mental health status.

Domain I Subdomain E: Multiple Choice Questions

1. Which of the following is classified as a characteristic of sedentary behavior?
   A) Individuals adopt a lying or sitting posture
   B) Individuals have an energy expenditure less than 3 METS
   C) Individuals have an energy expenditure less than 1.5 METS
   D) A and C
   E) A and B

DOMAIN II: EXERCISE TESTING

A. Select, administer, and interpret submaximal aerobic exercise tests (e.g., treadmill, step test, 6-minute walk).

Domain II Subdomain A: What you need to know

Knowledge of:

A) tests to assess submaximal aerobic endurance.

B) the acute and chronic responses to aerobic exercise on the function of the cardiovascular, respiratory, musculoskeletal, neuromuscular, metabolic, endocrine, and immune systems in trained and untrained individuals.

C) the mechanisms underlying the acute and chronic responses to aerobic exercise on the function of the cardiovascular, respiratory, musculoskeletal, neuromuscular, metabolic, endocrine, and immune systems in trained and untrained individuals.

D) the effect of chronic diseases on acute and chronic responses to aerobic exercise.

E) standard and/or disease-specific endpoints for submaximal aerobic exercise tests in apparently healthy individuals and those with chronic disease.

F) typical submaximal aerobic test results and physiological values in trained and untrained individuals and those with and without chronic diseases.

G) abnormal signs and symptoms in apparently healthy individuals and those with chronic disease.

H) abnormal readings and results from exercise testing equipment (*e.g.*, treadmill, ergometers, electrocardiograph, spirometer, metabolic cart, sphygmomanometer) that may indicate equipment malfunction.

I) commonly used medications in patients with chronic diseases, their mechanisms of action and side effects.

Skill in:

A) selecting the appropriate exercise test based on a patient's disease, condition and ability.

B) administering and interpreting of submaximal aerobic exercise tests.

C) modifying submaximal aerobic test and/or interpretation of results in response to medication use, timing, and side effects.

Domain II Subdomain A: Multiple Choice Questions

1. What percentage of the peak work rate from the incremental exercise test should be used to evaluate the intensities an individual with chronic obstructive pulmonary disease (COPD) is likely to experience during everyday life?
   A) 75%–90%
   B) 80%–90%
   C) 75%–85%
   D) 70%–90%

2. From the options given which of the following tests can evaluate the endurance of the upper body muscles
   A) Curl-up test
   B) 1-RM bench press test
   C) 1-RM leg press test
   D) Push-up test

B. Select, administer and interpret tests to assess musculoskeletal fitness, mobility, and balance.

Domain II Subdomain B: What you need to know

Knowledge of:

A) tests to assess muscular strength, muscular endurance, flexibility, and mobility.

B) the acute and chronic responses to resistance exercise on the function of the cardiovascular, respiratory, musculoskeletal, neuromuscular, metabolic, endocrine, and immune systems in trained and untrained individuals.

C) tests to assess function and balance.

D) the acute and chronic responses to flexibility and mobility exercise on the function of the cardiovascular, respiratory, musculoskeletal, neuromuscular, metabolic, endocrine, and immune systems.

E) the mechanisms underlying the acute and chronic responses to resistance exercise on the function of the cardiovascular, respiratory, musculoskeletal, neuromuscular, metabolic, endocrine, and immune systems in trained and untrained individuals.

F) the effects of chronic diseases and their treatments on acute and chronic responses to resistance exercise, and an individual's flexibility and mobility.

G) standard and/or disease-specific endpoints for muscular strength, endurance, functional, and balance testing in apparently healthy individuals and those with chronic disease.

H) typical muscular strength, muscular endurance, functional. and balance test results and physiological values in trained and untrained individuals and those with and without chronic diseases.

I) commonly used medications in patients with chronic diseases, their mechanisms of action and side effects.

Skill in:

A) selecting an exercise test based on a patient's disease, condition, and ability.

B) administering and interpreting tests to assess muscular strength and endurance.

C) administrating and interpreting functional and balance tests.

D) modifying musculoskeletal fitness, mobility, and balance tests and/or interpretation of results in response to medication use, timing, and side effects.

Domain II Subdomain B: Multiple Choice Questions

1. Which of the following populations would benefit *most* (from a bone health perspective)from regular muscular strength and endurance training?
   A) Postmenopausal women
   B) Athletes <14 year of age
   C) Stroke survivors
   D) Hypertensive adults

2. Which of the following statements regarding BP and resistance exercise (weightlifting) is correct?

   A) People with even mild CVD should never perform resistance exercise.
   B) BP elevations are highest during isometric muscular actions.
   C) BP elevations during resistance exercise are independent of the muscle mass involved.
   D) Typically, BP elevations seen during maximal resistance exercise are less than those observed during maximal aerobic exercise.

C. Select, prepare, and administer maximal, symptom-limited exercise tests.

Domain II Subdomain C: What you need to know

Knowledge of:

A) contraindications to symptom-limited, maximal exercise testing, and factors associated with complications (*e.g.*, probability of coronary heart disease, abnormal blood pressure).
B) medical therapies for chronic diseases and their effect on the physiologic response to exercise.
C) current practice guidelines/recommendations (*e.g.*, AHA, Arthritis Foundation, National Multiple Sclerosis Society) for the prevention, evaluation, treatment, and management of chronic diseases.
D) the timing of daily activities (*e.g.*, medications, dialysis, meals, glucose monitoring) and their effect on exercise in patients with chronic diseases.
E) cardiovascular, pulmonary and metabolic pathologies, their clinical progression, diagnostic testing, and medical regimens/procedures to treat.
F) normal and abnormal endpoints (*i.e.*, signs/symptoms) for termination of exercise testing.
G) abnormal signs and symptoms in apparently healthy individuals and those with chronic disease.
H) medical therapies for chronic diseases and their effect on resting vital signs and symptoms.
I) commonly used medications in patients with chronic diseases, their mechanisms of action, and side effects.

J) procedures to prepare a patient for ECG monitoring, including standard and modified lead placement.
K) tools to guide exercise intensity (*e.g.*, heart rate, perceived exertion, dyspnea scale, pain scale).
L) the use of effective communication techniques (*e.g.*, active listening and attention to nonverbal behavior, open-ended questioning, reflective listening skills) to address any concerns with the exam procedures.
M) tests to assess maximal exercise tolerance.
N) the physiologic responses during incremental exercise to maximal exertion in trained and untrained individuals and those with and without chronic diseases.
O) standard and/or disease-specific endpoints for maximal exercise testing in apparently healthy individuals and those with chronic disease.
P) typical maximal exercise test results and physiological values in trained and untrained individuals and those with and without chronic diseases.
Q) medical therapies for chronic diseases and their effect on clinical measurements and the physiologic response to maximal exercise.

Skill in:

A) administering a symptom-limited, maximal exercise test.
B) preparing a patient for ECG monitoring during exercise.
C) assessing vital signs and symptoms at rest and during exercise.
D) interpreting ECG rhythms and 12-lead ECGs.

Domain II Subdomain C: Multiple Choice Questions

1. Which of the following techniques can be used to diagnose coronary artery disease and assess heart wall motion abnormalities, ejection fraction, and cardiac output?
   A) Electrocardiography
   B) Radionuclide imaging
   C) Echocardiography
   D) Cardiac spirometry

2. Healthy, untrained individuals have an anaerobic threshold at approximately what percentage of their maximal volume of oxygen consumed per unit of time ($\dot{V}O_{2max}$)?
   A) 25%
   B) 55%
   C) 75%
   D) 95%

3. Which of the following is an absolute indication to terminate a symptom-limited maximal exercise test?
   A) Achievement of ≥85% of the age-predicted maximal heart rate (HR_{max})
   B) Signs of poor perfusion (cyanosis or pallor)
   C) Systolic BP ≥250 mm Hg
   D) Development of bundle-branch block

4. All of the following statements regarding the clinical exercise physiologist administering clinical exercise tests are true except _____.
   A) The clinical exercise physiologist will review and interpret the results of the test and report them to the supervising physician.
   B) The clinical exercise physiologist must have the knowledge to recognize and treat complications of exercise testing.
   C) The clinical exercise physiologist must have knowledge of cardiac arrhythmias and the ability to recognize and treat serious arrhythmias.
   D) The clinical exercise physiologist may administer clinical exercise tests without the personal supervision of a physician, but a qualified physician must be in the immediate vicinity and available for all emergencies.

5. Data obtained from a clinical exercise test can be useful for all of the following *except* _____.

   A) Determining a return to work date prior to a patient undergoing CABG surgery
   B) Predicting prognosis in patients with known heart disease
   C) Developing an exercise prescription for a patient in cardiac rehabilitation
   D) Evaluating preoperative risk

6. Which of the following gives information about the degree of stenosis that could be present in the arteries
   A) Coronary angiography
   B) Echocardiography
   C) Electrocardiography
   D) Radionuclide imaging

7. Which of the following treadmill protocols would be appropriate for an individual with intermittent claudication?
   A) Bruce
   B) Modified Åstrand
   C) Naughton
   D) Balke and Ware

8. False-negative test results limit the diagnostic value of an exercise test. The incidence of false negatives is related to all but one of the following. Which is *not* related to false-negative results?
   A) Insufficient level of stress
   B) Single vessel coronary artery disease
   C) Monitoring an insufficient number of ECG leads
   D) Lack of metabolic determination (*i.e.*, $\dot{V}O_{2max}$)

9. Which of the following would you not expect to occur with increased workload?
   A) Increased $\dot{V}O_2$
   B) Increased total peripheral resistance
   C) Increased cardiac output
   D) Increased mean arterial pressure

10. Which of the following is generally true of the hemodynamic exercise response in a patient who has received a cardiac transplant when compared to age-matched healthy individuals?
    A) Exercising HR is usually elevated.
    B) BP is attenuated at rest and during exercise.
    C) HR returns to rest faster.
    D) HR returns to rest slower.

ACSM-CEP

D. Evaluate and report results from a symptom-limited maximal exercise test to medical providers and in the medical record as required.

Domain II Subdomain D: What you need to know

Knowledge of:

A) the effects of chronic diseases on acute responses to maximal exercise.

B) standard and/or disease-specific endpoints for maximal exercise testing in apparently healthy individuals and those with chronic disease.

C) abnormal signs and symptoms in apparently healthy individuals and those with chronic disease during maximal exercise testing.

D) typical maximal exercise test results and physiological values in trained and untrained individuals and those with and without chronic diseases.

E) medical therapies for chronic diseases and their effect on clinical measurements and the physiologic response to maximal exercise.

F) the interpretation of maximal exercise test measures (*e.g.*, ECG response, oxygen saturation, rate-pressure product, claudication) and prognostic tools (*e.g.*, Duke Treadmill Score) in context with the indication for the test, termination reason, and the patient's medical history.

Skill in:

A) interpreting and reporting results from a symptom-limited, maximal exercise test.

Domain II Subdomain D: Multiple Choice Questions

1. The best measurement of exercise capacity (METs) is obtained by which of the following?
   A) Using exercise time on a standard protocol to estimate peak METs
   B) Using standard ACSM equations to calculate METs from peak workload
   C) Using the Borg RPE scale
   D) Using open-circuit indirect spirometry to determine maximal oxygen uptake ($\dot{V}O_{2max}$)

2. Following termination of a graded exercise (stress) test, a 12-lead ECG is _____.
   A) Monitored immediately and then every 1–2 min for 5 min of recovery or until exercise-induced changes are at baseline
   B) Monitored immediately and then at 2 and 5 min after the test
   C) Monitored immediately only
   D) Monitored and recorded only if any signs or symptoms arise during recovery

3. An individual's maximal exercise test is terminated secondary to symptoms of myocardial ischemia. Which of the following variables monitored during the test would be the most reliable estimate of ischemic threshold when prescribing exercise for this individual?
   A) Rating of perceived exertion (RPE)
   B) HR_{max}
   C) Rate-pressure product (RPP)
   D) Maximal metabolic equivalent (MET) level achieved

4. What is the best test to help determine ejection fraction at rest and during exercise?
   A) Angiogram
   B) Thallium stress test
   C) Single-photon emission computed tomography test
   D) Multiple-gated acquisition (MUGA) (blood pool imagery) study

E. Identify relative and absolute contraindications for test termination and report to medical personnel as needed.

Domain II Subdomain E: What you need to know

Knowledge of:

A) absolute contraindications and endpoints for terminating exercise testing.

Skill in:

A) interpreting and reporting results from a symptom-limited, maximal exercise test.

B) assessing vital signs and symptoms at rest and during exercise.

C) interpreting ECG rhythms and 12-lead ECGs.

Domain II Subdomain E: Multiple Choice Questions

1. When conducting a symptom-limited maximal exercise test, relative indications for terminating the test include _____.
   A) Moderate to severe angina
   B) Subject's request to stop
   C) Drop in systolic BP >10 mm Hg (persistently below baseline) despite an increase in workload, in the absence of other evidence of ischemia
   D) Signs of poor perfusion (*i.e.*, cyanosis or pallor)

DOMAIN III: EXERCISE PRESCRIPTION

A. Develop individualized exercise prescription to support patient needs and goals for various exercise environments (e.g., home/community based, facility based, virtual).

Domain III Subdomain A: What you need to know

Knowledge of:

A) appropriate mode, volume, and intensity of exercise to produce favorable outcomes in apparently healthy individuals and those with chronic disease.
B) the FITT-VP (frequency, intensity, time, type, volume, progression) principle for aerobic, muscular fitness/resistance training and flexibility exercise prescription.
C) the benefits and risks of aerobic, resistance, and flexibility exercise training in apparently healthy individuals and those with chronic disease.
D) the effects of physical inactivity and methods to counteract these changes.
E) normal and abnormal physiologic responses to exercise in healthy individuals and those with chronic diseases.
F) the timing of daily activities (*e.g.*, medications, dialysis, meals, glucose monitoring) and their effect on exercise training in patients with chronic diseases.
G) disease-specific strategies or tools (*e.g.*, breathing techniques, assistive devices, prophylactic nitroglycerin) to improve exercise tolerance in patients with chronic disease.
H) appropriate modifications to the exercise prescription in response to environmental conditions in apparently healthy individuals and those with chronic disease.
I) current practice guidelines/recommendations (*e.g.*, U.S. Department of Health and Human Services, American College of Sports Medicine, Arthritis Foundation) for exercise prescription in apparently healthy individuals and those with chronic disease.
J) applying metabolic calculations.

K) proper biomechanical technique for exercise (*e.g.*, gait assessment, proper weight lifting form).
L) muscle strength/endurance and flexibility modalities and their safe application and instruction.
M) principals and application of exercise session organization.
N) known demographic factors related to likelihood of adherence and maintenance of exercise (*e.g.*, age, gender, socioeconomic status, education, ethnicity, vocation).
O) psychological issues associated with acute and chronic illness (*e.g.*, anxiety, depression, social isolation, suicidal ideation).
P) goal setting (*e.g.*, SMART goals), reviewing, and constructive feedback in identifying barriers and reinforcing positive changes.
Q) risk factor reduction programs and alternative community resources (*e.g.*, dietary counseling, weight management, smoking cessation, stress management, physical therapy/back care).
R) incorporating health behavior theories into clinical practice.

Skill in:

A) interpreting functional and diagnostic exercise testing with applications to exercise prescription.
B) interpreting muscular strength/endurance testing with applications to exercise prescription.
C) developing an exercise prescription based on a participant's clinical status and goals.
D) applying metabolic calculations.

E) applying strategies to reduce risk of adverse events during exercise (*e.g.*, gait belt, blood glucose monitoring).

F) individualizing home exercise programs.
G) optimizing patient compliance and adherence of exercise prescription.

Domain III Subdomain A: Multiple Choice Questions

1. If a healthy young man who weighs 80 kg exercises at an intensity of 45 mL · kg^{-1} · min^{-1} for 30 min, five times per week, how long (assuming an isocaloric diet) would it take him to lose 10 lb?
   A) 9 wk
   B) 11 wk
   C) 13 wk
   D) 15 wk

2. Which of the following would be an adequate initial exercise prescription for a patient who has had a heart transplant?
   A) High intensity, short duration, small muscle groups, and high frequency
   B) High intensity, long duration, small muscle groups, and high frequency
   C) Moderate intensity, 6 d · wk^{-1}, large muscle groups, and moderate duration
   D) Low intensity, 3 d · wk^{-1}, large muscle groups, and moderate duration

3. Which behavioral change model is often used in cardiac rehabilitation and diabetes management programs because it suggests that individuals who perceive they are susceptible to serious disease are more likely to engage in behaviors to prevent the health problem from occurring?
   A) Motivational interviewing
   B) Social cognitive theory
   C) Disease observation model
   D) Health Belief Model

4. Which of the following statements *best* describes the exercise precautions for patients with an automatic implantable cardioverter defibrillator (AICD)?
   A) Persons with AICD must be monitored closely during exercise, keeping the heart rate (HR) 10 beats or more below the activation rate for a shock.
   B) Persons with AICD are not at risk for an inappropriate shock because most AICDs are set to an HR of 300 bpm.
   C) Persons with AICD can inactivate the AICD before high-intensity exercise to avoid the risk of shock.

   D) Persons with AICD can exercise at or above the cutoff HR but only if monitored by instantaneous ECG telemetry.

5. Moderate aerobic exercise is recommended for most adults when prescribing exercise. What is considered to be moderate intensity in regard to aerobic training?
   A) 40%–59% heart rate reserve (HRR)/ $\dot{V}O_{2max}$
   B) 39%–60% HRR/$\dot{V}O_{2max}$
   C) 45%–75% HRR/$\dot{V}O_{2max}$
   D) 55%–80% HRR/$\dot{V}O_{2max}$

6. During which times should the most caution be taken when beginning an exercise program with an individual with diabetes?
   A) Early morning and late evening
   B) Late morning
   C) Afternoon
   D) Evening

7. Which of the following cold-weather activities has been shown to increase HR up to 97% HR$_{max}$ and systolic BP up to 200 mm Hg, resulting in a potentially dangerous increase in risk of morbidity and mortality for individuals with cardiovascular disease (CVD)?
   A) Ice skating
   B) Shoveling snow
   C) Building snowman
   D) Walking on ice

8. What is the relative oxygen consumption rate for walking on a treadmill at 3.5 mph with a 10% grade?
   A) 18.17 mL · kg^{-1} · min^{-1}
   B) 27.96 mL · kg^{-1} · min^{-1}
   C) 29.76 mL · kg^{-1} · min^{-1}
   D) 31.28 mL · kg^{-1} · min^{-1}

9. A patient weighing 200 lb sets the treadmill at 4.0 mph with a 5% grade. At peak exercise, his BP is 150/90 mm Hg, HR is 150 bpm, and respiratory quotient is 1.0. What is his estimated absolute energy expenditure?
   A) 1.07 L · min^{-1}
   B) 2.17 L · min^{-1}
   C) 4.28 L · min^{-1}
   D) 8.56 L · min^{-1}

10. Patients enrolled in an outpatient cardiac rehabilitation program can begin upper body resistance training at ≥5–10 lb (or <50% of maximal voluntary contraction [MVC]) approximately how soon after their coronary artery bypass surgery?
    A) 4–6 wk
    B) 6–8 wk
    C) 10–12 wk
    D) Only after they have been cleared by their surgeon

11. In patients with a new implantable cardioverter defibrillator (ICD), mild upper body extremity range of motion (ROM) activities can be initiated how soon after device implantation?
    A) After the first 72 h
    B) After the first 24 h
    C) Within the first 24 h
    D) As soon as the patent's pain tolerance permits

12. What is the total energy expenditure for a 70-kg man doing an exercise session composed of 5 min of warm-up at 2.0 METs, 20 min of treadmill running at 9 METs, 20 min of leg cycling at 8 METs, and 5 min of cool-down at 2.5 METs?
    A) 162 kcal
    B) 868 kcal
    C) 444 kcal
    D) 1,256 kcal

13. Both the American College of Sports Medicine (ACSM)/American Heart Association (AHA) Primary Physical Activity Recommendation and the Primary Physical Activity Recommendations from the *2018 Physical Activity Guidelines Committee Report* suggest that healthy adults should participate in which of the following exercise prescriptions for aerobic activity?
    A) 20 min · d^{-1}, five times a week (*i.e.*, 100 min) of moderate intensity exercise or 75 min · wk^{-1} of low intensity exercise
    B) 30 min · d^{-1}, five times a week or 150 min · wk^{-1} of moderate intensity exercise
    C) 20 min · d^{-1}, three times a week (*i.e.*, 60 min) of moderate intensity exercise
    D) 30 min · d^{-1}, five times a week or 150 min · wk^{-1} of vigorous intensity exercise

14. The progressive overload principle is defined as _____.
    A) Employing controlled movements during a specific ROM

B) Performing less sets per muscle group and increasing the number of days per week muscle groups are trained
    C) Performing more sets per muscle group and increasing the number of days per week muscle groups are trained
    D) Performing a one repetition maximum (1-RM) test every 6 wk

15. Which of the following is the minimum that will improve muscular strength, particularly among novice participants?
    A) One set 8–12 repetitions of a resistance training exercise
    B) Two sets 8–12 repetitions of a resistance training exercise
    C) Three sets of 8–12 repetitions a resistance training exercise
    D) Four sets of 8–12 repetitions a resistance training exercise

16. At a set workload (*e.g.*, 4 METs), myocardial oxygen consumption of a patient with coronary artery disease is reduced following endurance training as evidenced by a decrease in _____.
    A) Systolic ejection period
    B) RPE
    C) HR
    D) Whole-body oxygen consumption

17. When prescribing exercise for patients with atherosclerosis, which of the following is *true*?
    A) Training HR among patients who are status post-MI are altered by α-blocking agents.
    B) Patients with peripheral arterial disease should exercise to leg pain level 3 (on 4-point scale), with intermittent rest periods.
    C) Most patients with stable angina who are cleared to participate in outpatient exercise programs (*i.e.*, YMCA) can exercise safely with moderate angina levels (2+).
    D) During the initial phase (1–3 d after the event) of inpatient programs, activities should be restricted to moderate intensity (3–5 METs).

18. Long-term conditioning results in adaptations of the cardiovascular system. When measured at the same submaximal exercise intensity, these adaptations result in a decrease in _____.
    A) Stroke volume
    B) HR

C) Cardiac output

D) Arteriovenous oxygen difference

19. Myocardial oxygen consumption is highly correlated with RPP. Which variables are used to determine RPP?

A) Systolic BP and stroke volume

B) Mean arterial pressure and HR

C) Systolic pressure and HR

D) Pulse pressure and HR

20. Which of the following would be the *best* marker of ischemic threshold?

A) HR

B) BP

C) Oxygen uptake

D) RPP

21. Long-term participation by healthy persons in activities such as running, cycling, and swimming results in the following adaptations during maximum exercise *except* _____.

A) Increased oxidative capacity of a given mass of muscle

B) Increased venous return

C) Increased HR

D) Increased blood flow through active muscles

22. Which method of determining exercise intensity is mostly recommended for individuals with autonomic neuropathy?

A) HRR

B) BP

C) $\dot{V}O_2R$

D) RPE

B. Communicate the exercise prescription, including the use of exercise equipment, and the importance of promptly reporting any adverse reactions or symptoms.

Domain III Subdomain B: What you need to know

Knowledge of:

A) normal and abnormal physiologic responses to exercise in healthy individuals and those with chronic diseases.

B) the timing of daily activities (*e.g.*, medications, dialysis, meals, glucose monitoring) and their effect on exercise training in patients with chronic diseases and how to communicate this information with patient.

C) lay terminology for explanation of exercise prescription.

D) the operation of various exercise equipment/ modalities.

E) proper biomechanical technique for exercise (*e.g.*, gait assessment, proper weight lifting form).

F) muscle strength/endurance and flexibility modalities and their safe application and instruction.

G) principals and application of exercise session organization.

H) proper protocol to report adverse symptoms per facility policy.

Skill in:

A) communicating exercise prescription, exercise techniques, and organization of exercises.

Domain III Subdomain B: Multiple Choice Questions

1. What does flow-resistive training (a type of breathing retraining) teach patients with pulmonary disease?

A) To effectively breathe through a progressively smaller airway

B) Coordinate breathing with activities of daily living

C) Increase respiratory muscle endurance and strength

D) Increase ventilatory threshold

2. An increase in maximal attainable RPP following successful CABG surgery for severe angina suggests _____.

A) Decreased myocardial oxygen demand

B) Increased cardiac output during submaximal exercise

C) Increased maximum coronary blood flow

D) Increased extraction of oxygen by the myocardium

C. Explain and confirm patient understanding of exercise intensity and measures to assess exercise intensity (e.g., target heart rate, RPE, signs/symptoms, talk test).

Domain III Subdomain C: What you need to know

Knowledge of:

A) tools to guide exercise intensity (*e.g.*, heart rate, RPE, dyspnea scale, pain scale, talk test).

B) abnormal signs and symptoms during exercise training in apparently healthy individuals and those with chronic disease.

C) clear communication using patient learning style and/or health literacy to explain exercise intensity assessment.

D) clear communication through effective communication techniques (*e.g.*, active listening and attention to nonverbal behavior, open-ended questioning, reflective listening skills).

Skill in:

A) teaching methods used to guide exercise intensity.

Domain III Subdomain C Multiple Choice Questions

1. According to *ACSM's Guidelines for Exercise Testing and Prescription*, 11th ed., moderate intensity exercise is defined as _____.
   A) 30%–<40% HRR or oxygen consumption reserve ($\dot{V}O_2R$), 2–<3 METs, RPE 9–11, an intensity that causes slight increases in HR and breathing
   B) ≥60% HRR or $\dot{V}O_2R$, ≥6 METs, RPE ≥14, an intensity that causes substantial increases in HR and breathing
   C) 40%–59% HRR or $\dot{V}O_2R$, 3–<6 METs, RPE 12–13, an intensity that causes noticeable increases in HR and breathing
   D) 35%–<50% HRR or $\dot{V}O_2R$, 2–<4 METs, RPE 10–12, an intensity that causes moderate increases in HR and breathing

D. Evaluate and modify the exercise prescription based on the patient's compliance, signs/symptoms, and physiologic response to the exercise program, as needed.

Domain III Subdomain D: What you need to know

Knowledge of:

A) physiologic effects due to changes in medical therapies for chronic diseases and their impact on exercise training.

B) typical responses to aerobic, resistance and flexibility training in apparently healthy individuals and those with chronic disease.

C) the timing of daily activities (*e.g.*, medications, dialysis, meals, glucose monitoring) and their effect on exercise in patients with chronic diseases.

D) disease-specific strategies or tools (*e.g.*, breathing techniques, assistive devices, prophylactic nitroglycerin) to improve exercise tolerance in patients with chronic disease.

E) abnormal signs and symptoms during exercise training in apparently healthy individuals and those with chronic disease.

F) mode, volume, and intensity of exercise to produce favorable outcomes in apparently healthy individuals and those with chronic disease.

G) commonly used medications in patients with chronic diseases, their mechanisms of action and side effects.

H) modifications to the exercise prescription in response to environmental conditions in apparently healthy individuals and those with chronic disease.

I) systems for tracking participant progress in both preventive and rehabilitative exercise programs.

J) participant progress in a preventive and rehabilitative exercise program given gender, age, clinical status, pre-program fitness level, specifics of the exercise program (*e.g.*, walking only vs. comprehensive monitored program) and rate of program participation.

Skill in:

A) helping patients identify barriers and providing strategies to overcome them.

B) assessing adequacy of patient's progress in a preventive or rehabilitative exercise program given age, sex, gender, clinical status, specifics of the exercise program and rate of program participation.

C) developing an individualized exercise prescription.

D) using patient feedback and developing individualized exercise prescription and/or care plan.

E) active listening.

F) modifying an exercise prescription specifically to meet a patient's individual needs and goals.

Domain III Subdomain D: Multiple Choice Questions

1. Individuals with diabetes should follow exercise guidelines to avoid unnecessary risks. The following list of recommendations should include all of the following *except*_____.
   A) Avoiding injection of insulin into an exercising muscle
   B) Exercising with a partner
   C) Exercising only when temperature and humidity are moderate
   D) Avoiding exercise during peak insulin activity

2. An exercise physiologist monitoring the ECG of a cardiac rehabilitation patient observes QT-interval shortening and ST-segment scooping during exercise. Based on this observation, the physiologist can suspect that the patient is treated with which of the following medications?
   A) β-blockers
   B) Calcium channel blockers
   C) Potassium
   D) Digitalis

3. Jane, a 47-year-old female with no prior history of regular exercise recently completed a 12-wk exercise training program. Her routine consisted of walking and/or bike riding three times per week at approximately 6–7 METS for 30 min. Originally, Jane found that going up the stairs was rather difficult, often leaving her short of breath. Jane is now able to walk up multiple flights of stairs with ease. Her increase in exercise volume (went from being inactive to performing 540–630 MET · min^{-1} · wk^{-1}) and aerobic capacity (increased peak oxyten uptake by 15%) over 12 weeks is an example of what type of relationship?
   A) Linear relationship
   B) Dose–response relationship
   C) Principle of adaptation relationship
   D) Inverse–linear relationship

4. For individuals with heart failure, what intensity and duration should be used for their exercise program?
   A) RPE 9–13; 30–60 min · d^{-1}
   B) RPE 11–14; 15–30 min · d^{-1}
   C) RPE 9–13; 15–30 min · d^{-1}
   D) RPE 11–14; 30–60 min · d^{-1}

DOMAIN IV: EXERCISE TRAINING AND LEADERSHIP

A. Discuss and explain exercise training plan, patient and clinician expectations and goals.

Domain IV Subdomain A: What you need to know

Knowledge of:

A) health counseling techniques (*e.g.*, the patient-centered approach) and nonjudgmental positive regard in creation of collaborative partnership.

B) effective communication techniques, while using clear, patient-friendly terms (*e.g.*, active listening, body language, motivational interviewing).

C) factors related to health literacy skills and capacity.

D) cardiovascular, pulmonary and metabolic pathologies, their clinical progression.

E) diagnostic testing and medical regimens/procedures to treat.

F) the FITT-VP principle (frequency, intensity, time, type, volume, progression) for aerobic, muscular fitness/resistance training, and flexibility exercise prescription.

G) the timing of daily activities (*e.g.*, medications, dialysis, meals, glucose monitoring) and their effect on exercise training in patients with chronic diseases.

H) disease-specific strategies or tools (*e.g.,* breathing techniques, assistive devices, prophylactic nitroglycerin) to improve exercise tolerance in patients with chronic disease.

I) exercise training concepts specific to industrial or occupational rehabilitation, such as work hardening, work conditioning, work fitness, and job coaching.

J) commonly used medication for cardiovascular, pulmonary, and metabolic diseases.

Skill in:

A) identifying unique needs of those with chronic diseases in exercise prescription.

B) communicating the exercise prescription and related exercise programming techniques.

C) educating patients following the observation of problems with comprehension and performance of their exercise program.

D) applying techniques to reduce risks of adverse events during exercise (*e.g.,* gait belt, blood glucose monitoring).

E) educating participants on the use and effects of medications.

F) communicating with participants from a wide variety of educational backgrounds.

G) using patient feedback to develop individualized exercise prescription and/or care plan.

H) active listening.

Domain IV Subdomain A: Multiple Choice Questions

1. For previously sedentary individuals, a 20%–30% reduction in all-cause mortality can be obtained from physical activity (PA) with a daily energy expenditure of _____.
   A) 50–80 kcal $\cdot$ d^{-1}
   B) 80–100 kcal $\cdot$ d^{-1}
   C) 150–200 kcal $\cdot$ d^{-1}
   D) >400 kcal $\cdot$ d^{-1}

2. The exercise physiologist is orienting a 60-year-old patient entering cardiac rehabilitation after having CABG 3 wk ago. All of the following statements are correct *except* _____.
   A) The patient should avoid upper body resistance training because of sternal and leg wounds for 4–6 months.
   B) The clinician should observe for infection or discomfort along the incision.
   C) The patient should be monitored for chest pain, dizziness, and dysrhythmias.
   D) The patient should avoid high-intensity exercise early in the rehabilitation period.

3. For patients with congestive heart failure, which of the following statements is *true*?
   A) Patients may not exceed a workload of 5 METs.
   B) Warm-up and cool-down periods should be limited to 5 min.

C) Patients should expect no significant improvement in exercise capacity.
   D) Peripheral adaptations are largely responsible for an increase in exercise tolerance.

4. Studies show the least physically active populations to include all of the following *except* _____.
   A) Obese
   B) Elderly
   C) Less educated
   D) Upper middle class

5. The primary effects of chronic exercise training on blood lipids include _____.
   A) Decreased TG and increased HDL
   B) Decreased total cholesterol and LDL
   C) Decreased HDL and increased LDL
   D) Decreased total cholesterol and increased HDL

6. When working with an individual with a cerebrovascular accident (stroke), which of the following should be avoided
   A) Addressing the comorbidities that are likely to be present
   B) Assessment of muscular strength and endurance prior to program initiation
   C) The Valsalva maneuver when performing resistance exercise.
   D) Using the treadmill at a slow speed including the use of a harness

B. Identify, adapt, and instruct in cardiorespiratory fitness, muscular strength and endurance, flexibility, coordination and agility exercise modes.

Domain IV Subdomain B: What you need to know

Knowledge of:

A) the selection, operation, and modification of exercise equipment/modalities based on the disease, condition and ability of the individual.

B) proper biomechanical technique for exercise (*e.g.*, gait, weight lifting form).

C) exercise techniques to reduce risk and maximize the development of cardiorespiratory fitness, muscular strength, and flexibility.

D) mode, volume and intensity of exercise to produce favorable outcomes in apparently healthy individuals and those with chronic disease.

E) disease-specific strategies or tools (*e.g.*, breathing techniques, assistive devices, prophylactic nitroglycerin) to improve exercise tolerance in patients with chronic disease.

F) counseling techniques to optimize participant's disease management, risk reduction, and goal attainment.

G) modifications to the exercise prescription in response to environmental conditions in apparently healthy individuals and those with chronic disease.

H) the benefits and risks of aerobic, resistance, and flexibility training in apparently healthy individuals and those with chronic disease.

Skill in:

A) identifying unique needs and goals of a patient and adapting/modifying an exercise program.

B) supervising and leading patients during exercise training.

C) communicating the exercise prescription and related exercise programming techniques.

D) educating patients following the observation of problems with comprehension and performance of their exercise program.

Domain IV Subdomain B: Multiple Choice Questions

1. The progressive ascent to higher altitudes will result in which two acute physiological responses?
   A) Increased arterial oxygen levels and increased cardiac output
   B) Increased arterial oxygen levels and decreased cardiac output
   C) Decreased arterial oxygen levels and decreased cardiac output
   D) Decreased arterial oxygen levels and increased cardiac output

2. Which exertional heat illness occurs when the body cannot sustain the level of needed to support skin blood flow for thermoregulation and blood flow for metabolic requirements of exercise?
   A) Heat cramps
   B) Syncope
   C) Heat exhaustion
   D) Heat stroke

C. As indicated, provide patient monitoring (e.g., pulse oximetry, biometric data) and supervision during exercise.

Domain IV Subdomain C: What you need to know

Knowledge of:

A) normal and abnormal exercise responses, signs and symptoms associated with different pathologies (*i.e.*, cardiovascular, pulmonary, metabolic, orthopedic/musculoskeletal, neuromuscular, neoplastic, immunologic, and hematologic disorders).

B) normal and abnormal 12-lead and telemetry ECG interpretation.

C) exercise program monitoring (*e.g.*, telemetry, oximetry, glucometry).

D) disease-specific strategies or tools (*e.g.*, breathing techniques, assistive devices, prophylactic nitroglycerin) to improve exercise tolerance in patients with chronic disease.

E) the benefits and risks of aerobic, resistance and flexibility training in apparently healthy individuals and those with chronic disease.

F) the components of a patient's medical history necessary to screen during program participation.

G) commonly used medications in patients with chronic diseases, their mechanisms of action and side effects.

H) the timing of daily activities with exercise (*e.g.*, medications, meals, insulin/glucose monitoring).

I) how medications or missed dose(s) of medications impact exercise and its progression.

J) psychological issues associated with acute and chronic illness (*e.g.*, depression, social isolation, suicidal ideation).

K) health counseling techniques and nonjudgmental positive regard.

Skill in:

A) monitoring and supervising patients during exercise training.

B) interpreting ECG rhythms and 12-lead ECGs.

C) recognizing adverse effects of exercise in apparently healthy persons or those with pathologies of acute and/or chronic disease.

D) applying and interpreting tools for clinical assessment (*e.g.*, telemetry, oximetry and glucometry, perceived rating scales).

E) modifying exercise/physical activity programming in response to medication use, timing, and side effects.

Domain IV Subdomain C: Multiple Choice Questions

1. A supraventricular ectopic rhythm that results from a focus of automaticity located in the bundle of His is an example of _____.
   A) Ventricular arrhythmia
   B) Junctional arrhythmia
   C) Atrioventricular (AV) block
   D) Premature ventricular contraction

2. Cardiac impulses originating in the sinoatrial node and then spreading to both atria, causing atrial depolarization, are represented on the electrocardiogram (ECG) as a _____.
   A) P wave
   B) QRS complex
   C) ST segment
   D) T wave

3. As a CEP you are called upon to work with an individual with chronic kidney disease not on dialysis. Which of the following are things you must consider?

   A) The major cause of death in this population is cardiovascular disease and therefore care must be taken to focus on cardiovascular risk factor modification
   B) Since these patients are high risk, medical clearance should be sought prior to initiating an exercise program
   C) When performing an exercise test on individuals with predialysis CKD, standard procedures can be followed.
   D) B and C only
   E) A, B, and C

4. Sounds heard during measurement of BP are produced by _____.
   A) The closing of the mitral valve
   B) The closing of the aortic valve and pulmonary valves
   C) The contraction of the ventricle
   D) Turbulent blood flow

D. Evaluate the patient's contraindications to exercise training and associated risk/benefit and modify the exercise/activity program accordingly.

Domain IV Subdomain D: What you need to know

Knowledge of:

A) the contraindications to exercise training and factors associated with complications in apparently healthy individuals and those with chronic disease.

B) the benefits and risks of aerobic, resistance, and flexibility training in apparently healthy individuals and those with chronic disease.

C) abnormal signs and symptoms in apparently healthy individuals and those with chronic disease.

D) the acute and chronic responses to exercise training on the function of the cardiovascular, respiratory, musculoskeletal, neuromuscular, metabolic, endocrine and immune systems in trained and untrained individuals.

E) cardiovascular, pulmonary and metabolic pathologies, diagnostic testing and medical management regimens and procedures.

ACSM-CEP

Skill in:

A) identifying contraindications to exercise training.

B) modifying the exercise program based on participant's signs and symptoms, feedback and exercise responses.

Domain IV Subdomain D: Multiple Choice Questions

1. Which of the following is a pulmonary condition caused by destruction of the lung parenchyma and can be trigged by smoking?
   A) Emphysema
   B) Bronchitis
   C) Asthma
   D) Pulmonary vascular disease

2. Exercise has been shown to reduce mortality in people with coronary artery disease. Which of the following mechanisms is *not* responsible?
   A) The effect of exercise on CVD risk factors
   B) Reduced myocardial oxygen demand at rest and at submaximal workloads
   C) Reduced platelet aggregation
   D) Decreased endothelial-mediated vasomotor tone

3. Which of the following treatment strategies is most commonly used in patients with multiple vessel disease that is not responding to other treatments?
   A) Percutaneous transluminal coronary angioplasty (PTCA)
   B) Coronary artery stent
   C) Coronary artery bypass graft (CABG) surgery
   D) Pharmacologic therapy

4. Which of the following is most likely to represent nonischemic or atypical chest pain?
   A) Pain in one or both arms or shoulders
   B) Pain provoked by cold weather or excitement
   C) Pain that is substernal across the mid thorax area
   D) Pain in the left submammary or hemithorax area

5. Bilateral ankle edema that is most evident at night is a characteristic sign of _____.
   A) Congestive heart failure
   B) Pulmonary hypertension
   C) Metabolic syndrome
   D) Coronary artery disease

6. Which should be lowered as an effective strategy in limiting the progression and promoting regression of atherosclerosis?
   A) Low-density lipoprotein (LDL) cholesterol
   B) High-density lipoprotein (HDL) cholesterol
   C) Triglycerides (TGs)
   D) Blood platelets

7. Which of the following is *not* associated with exercise-induced myocardial ischemia?
   A) Angina pectoris
   B) ST-segment depression
   C) Impaired left ventricular function
   D) Decreased RPP

E. Evaluate, document and report patient's clinical status and response to exercise training in the medical records.

Domain IV Subdomain E: What you need to know

Knowledge of:

A) the techniques (*e.g.*, lab results, diagnostic tests) used to diagnose different pathologies, their indications, limitations, risks, normal and abnormal results.

B) the acute and chronic responses to exercise training on the function of the cardiovascular, respiratory, musculoskeletal, neuromuscular, metabolic, endocrine, and immune systems in trained and untrained individuals.

C) normal and abnormal exercise responses, signs, and symptoms associated with different pathologies (*i.e.*, cardiovascular, pulmonary, metabolic, orthopedic/musculoskeletal, neuromuscular, neoplastic, immunologic, and hematologic disorders).

D) how chronic diseases may affect the acute and chronic responses exercise training.

E) abnormal signs or symptoms which may be associated with worsening of a chronic disease.

F) proper medical documentation according to generally accepted principles and individual facility standards.

G) regulations relative to documentation and protecting patient privacy (*e.g.*, written and electronic medical records, Health Insurance Portability and Accountability Act [HIPAA]).

Skill in:

A) summarizing patient's exercise sessions, outcomes and clinical status into patient's medical record.
B) proficiency in medical charting.

Domain IV Subdomain E: Multiple Choice Questions

1. A 35-year-old female client asks the exercise physiologist to estimate her energy expenditure. She weighs 110 lb and pedals the cycle ergometer at 50 rpm with a resistance of 2.5 kp for 60 min. The physiologist should report which of the following caloric values?
   A) 250 cal
   B) 510 cal
   C) 770 cal
   D) 1,700 cal

2. Greater oxygen delivery is provided to the myocardium in all of the following situations *except* _____.
   A) Severe coronary artery disease
   B) Increase HR
   C) Increase coronary blood flow
   D) Increase cardiac output

3. While at rest, physically inactive men compared to physically active men of the same weight and age typically have a _____.
   A) Higher BP
   B) Higher metabolic rate
   C) Higher cardiac output
   D) Lower stroke volume

4. A reversible or transient perfusion defect on a myocardial perfusion imaging test is diagnostic for which of the following?
   A) MI
   B) Transient ischemic attack (TIA), or "mini-stroke"
   C) Exertional myocardial ischemia
   D) Angina pectoris

F. Discuss clinical status and response to exercise training with patients and adapt and/or modify the exercise program, as indicated.

Knowledge of:

A) common barriers to exercise compliance and adherence (*e.g.*, physical, environmental, demographic).
B) effective communication techniques (*e.g.*, active listening, body language).
C) techniques to adapt/modify exercise program based on a patient's needs.
D) assess patient's individual progress based on known cardiorespiratory fitness, muscular strength, and flexibility improvements expected within a given population.

E) assess patient's tolerance to exercise modality and suggest comparable alternative modalities.

Skill in:

A) communicating health information based on a patient's learning style and health literacy.
B) modifying the exercise program based on participant's signs and symptoms, feedback and exercise responses.
C) summarizing patient's exercise sessions, outcomes and clinical status into patient's medical record.

Domain IV Subdomain F: Multiple Choice Questions

1. You have noted that a dialysis patient complains of dizziness when performing exercise immediately after a hemodialysis session. Which of the following would be viable solutions to this problem to enhance physical activity in this patient?
   A) Encourage the patient to exercise during the first half of the dialysis session
   B) Encourage the patient to exercise during the last phase of the dialysis session
   C) Encourage the patient to exercise on the non-dialysis days
   D) A and C
   E) B and C

ACSM-CEP

G. Promptly report new or worsening symptoms and adverse events in the patient's medical record and consult with the responsible health care provider.

Domain IV Subdomain G: What you need to know

Knowledge of:

A) proper medical documentation according to generally accepted principles and individual facility standards.

B) the scope of practice of health care professionals (*e.g.*, physical therapist, nurse, dietician, psychologist).

C) abnormal signs and symptoms during exercise training in apparently healthy individuals and those with chronic disease.

D) the effects of chronic diseases on the acute and chronic responses to exercise training.

Skill in:

A) assessing normal and abnormal response to exercise.

B) educating patients following the observation of problems with comprehension and performance of their exercise program.

C) evaluating and prompt reporting of a patient's adverse response to an exercise program in accordance with a facility policy and procedures.

Domain IV Subdomain G: Multiple Choice Questions

1. During a training session with an apparently healthy individual, the CEP noticed that the individual's heart rate began to fluctuate dramatically. Which of the following would be an appropriate response
   A) Ignore this observation and carry on the training session normally
   B) Stop the training session immediately and get medical clearance before continuing
   C) Check to make sure that the device is working properly and if so then advise the individual to get medical clearance before continuing any more exercise sessions
   D) Stop the individual, check their blood pressure, and resume exercise

2. Assume that in another situation as described above the individual begins to complain of dizziness and shortness of breath. What should the CEP do under those circumstances?
   A) Ignore this observation and carry on the training session normally
   B) Stop the training session immediately and get the individual evaluated by a healthcare professional as soon as possible.
   C) Check to make sure that the device is working properly and if so then advise the individual to get medical clearance before continuing any more exercise sessions
   D) Stop the individual, check their blood pressure, and resume exercise

DOMAIN V: EDUCATION AND BEHAVIOR CHANGE

A. Continually evaluate patients using observation, interaction, and industry-accepted tools, to identify those who may benefit from counseling or other mental health services using industry-accepted screening tools.

Domain V Subdomain A: What you need to know

Knowledge of:

A) establishment of rapport through use of open-ended questions, active listening and attention to nonverbal behavior, interest and empathy.

B) the psychological issues associated with acute and chronic illness (*e.g.*, anxiety, depression, social isolation, hostility, aggression, suicidal ideation).

C) theories of health behavior change (*e.g.*, Social Cognitive Theory [SCT], Health Belief Model [HBM], Transtheoretical Model [TTM]).

D) industry accepted screening tools to evaluate mental health status (*e.g.*, SF-36, Beck Depression Index).

E) signs and symptoms of failure to cope during personal crises (*e.g.*, job loss, bereavement, illness).

F) accepted methods of referral to behavioral health or other specialist as needed.

Skill in:

A) administering commonly used screening tools to evaluate mental health status.

B) applying and interpreting psychosocial assessment tools.

C) identifying patients who may benefit from behavioral health services.

Domain V Subdomain A: Multiple Choice Questions

1. In the "readiness to change model," which stage is it recommended to use multiple resources to stress the importance of a desired change?

   A) Precontemplation
   B) Contemplation
   C) Preparation
   D) Instruction

B. Assess patient's understanding of their disease and/or disability and conduct education to teach the role of lifestyle in the prevention, management, and treatment of the disease.

Domain V Subdomain B: What you need to know

Knowledge of:

A) active listening, open-ended questioning, reflective listening skills.

B) patient-centered health counseling techniques (*e.g.*, Five-A's Model, Motivational Interviewing).

C) factors related to health literacy skills and capacity.

D) barriers to exercise compliance (*e.g.*, physical/disease state, psychological environmental, demographic).

E) social ecological model.

F) psychological issues associated with acute and chronic illness (*e.g.*, anxiety, depression, suicidal ideation).

G) theories of health behavior change (*e.g.*, Social Cognitive Theory, Health Belief Model, Transtheoretical Model).

H) tools to determine a patient's knowledge and their readiness to change (*e.g.*, scoring rulers, decisional balance).

I) the benefits and risks of aerobic, resistance, flexibility, and balance training in apparently healthy individuals and those with chronic disease.

J) the health benefits of a physically active lifestyle, the hazards of sedentary behavior, and current recommendations from U.S. national reports on physical activity (*e.g.*, U.S. Surgeon General, National Academy of Medicine).

K) abnormal signs and symptoms during rest and exercise in apparently healthy individuals and those with chronic disease.

L) the epidemiology, pathophysiology, progression, risk factors, key clinical findings, and treatments of chronic disease.

M) education content and program development based on participant's medical history, needs, and goals.

N) medical therapies and commonly used medications for chronic diseases and their effect on resting vital signs, clinical measurements, and the response to exercise.

O) disease-specific strategies and tools to improve exercise tolerance (*e.g.*, breathing techniques, insulin pump use, prophylactic nitroglycerin).

P) risk factor reduction strategies (*e.g.*, healthy nutrition, weight management/BMI, body composition, smoking cessation, stress management, back care, substance abuse).

Skill in:

A) assessing a patient's educational needs.

B) communicating health information based on a patient's learning style and health literacy.

C) developing educational materials and programs on disease and the role of lifestyle intervention.

D) teaching health information to patient's in individual and group settings.

E) communicating exercise techniques, prescription and progression.

ACSM-CEP

Domain V Subdomain B: Multiple Choice Questions

1. If an individual is in the action stage of the "stages of motivational readiness," he or she _____.
   A) Has been physically active on a regular basis for <6 month
   B) Participates in some exercise but does so irregularly
   C) Intends to start exercising in the next 6 month
   D) Has been physically active on a regular basis for >6 month

2. In the stages of change model, the _____ stage includes individuals who are inactive but are thinking about becoming active.
   A) Precontemplation
   B) Contemplation
   C) Action
   D) Maintenance

3. Which of the following factors is believed to have the strongest influence on feelings of self-efficacy?
   A) Encouragement from others
   B) SMART goals
   C) The environment
   D) Personal (mastery) experience

C. Apply health behavior change techniques (e.g., Motivational Interviewing, Cognitive Behavioral Therapy [CBT], Health Coaching) based upon assessment of readiness to change according to Transtheoretical Model (TTM).

Domain V Subdomain B: What you need to know

Knowledge of:

A) active listening, open-ended questioning, reflective listening skills.
B) barriers to exercise compliance and adherence (*e.g.*, physical/disease state, psychological environmental, demographic, vocational).
C) known demographic factors related to likelihood of adherence and maintenance of exercise (*e.g.*, age, gender, socioeconomic status, education, ethnicity).
D) characteristics associated with poor adherence to healthy behaviors.
E) health counseling techniques (*e.g.*, the patient-centered approach).
F) goal setting (*e.g.*, SMART goals), reviewing, and constructive feedback in support of patient for best likelihood of achievement of goals.

G) theories of health behavior change (*e.g.*, Social Cognitive Theory [SCT], Health Belief Model [HBM], Transtheoretical Model ([TTM]).)
H) application of behavior-change techniques (*e.g.*, motivational interviewing, cognitive-behavioral therapy, health coaching).
I) eliciting change talk by patient through motivational interviewing technique.
J) development of self-efficacy (task and barriers) in exercise behaviors.

Skill in:

A) effective use of behavior-change techniques.
B) active listening of patient feedback and consideration with decision making of exercise prescription and/or care plan.
C) promoting patient engagement in process of fitness and health improvement.
D) creating clear communication using medical terminology suitable for patient's health literacy and/or learning style.

Domain V Subdomain C: Multiple Choice Questions

1. The process by which one maintains long-term behavior change by anticipating potentially high-risk situations and devising strategies to cope with these situations is called
   A) Decisional balance
   B) Self-efficacy
   C) Relapse prevention
   D) Processes of change

2. Social Ecology Theory (sometimes known as the ecological perspective) emphasizes multiple influences on behavior. These include:
   A) Intrapersonal factors
   B) Interpersonal factors
   C) Environmental factors
   D) A, B, and C
   E) A and B only

ACSM-CEP

D. Promote adherence to healthy behaviors through a patient centered approach (e.g., addressing barriers, engaging in active listening, expressing interest and empathy, increasing self-efficacy, teaching relapse prevention techniques and identifying support).

Domain V Subdomain D: What you need to know

Knowledge of:

A) establishment of rapport through use of open-ended questions, active listening and attention to nonverbal behavior, interest, and empathy.

B) health counseling techniques (*e.g.*, the patient-centered approach) and nonjudgmental positive regard in creation of collaborative partnership.

C) theories of health behavior change (*e.g.*, Social Cognitive Theory [SCT], Health Belief Model [HBM], Transtheoretical Model [TTM]].

D) barriers to exercise compliance and adherence (*e.g.*, physical/disease state, psychological environmental, demographic, vocational).

E) known demographic factors related to likelihood of adherence and maintenance of exercise (*e.g.*, age, sex, gender, socioeconomic status, education, ethnicity).

F) tools for measuring clinical exercise tolerance (*e.g.*, heart rate, glucometry, subjective rating scales), and consideration of affect regulation in determining exercise prescription.

G) risk factor reduction programs and alternative community resources (*e.g.*, wellness coaching, smoking cessation, physical therapy/back care, dietary counseling).

H) goal setting (*i.e.*, SMART goals), reviewing, and constructive feedback in support of pa-

tient for best likelihood of achievement of goals.

I) eliciting change talk by patient through motivational interviewing technique.

J) development of self-efficacy (task and barriers) in exercise behaviors.

K) promotion of patient intrinsic motivation (*e.g.*, supporting feelings of autonomy and competence, positive feedback, enjoyment) in facilitating long-term adherence to exercise.

L) community resources (exercise and/or health support) available for participant use following program conclusion and/or discharge.

M) relapse prevention techniques (*e.g.*, proactive problem solving, managing lapses, maintaining high self-efficacy in health behaviors, identifying social support).

N) guidance of social support (*e.g.*, reassurance, nurturance, supportive exercise groups).

Skill in:

A) effective use of behavior-change techniques.

B) active listening and receptiveness to patient feedback in decision making of exercise prescription and/or care plan.

C) effective communication with participants from a wide variety of backgrounds.

D) promoting patient engagement in process of fitness and health improvement.

Domain V Subdomain D: Multiple Choice Questions

1. Self-efficacy can be improved by observing others perform the activity. This is known as:
   A) Vicarious experience or modeling
   B) Imitation
   C) Mastery experiences
   D) Self-regulation

2. When implementing a physical activity program, it is important to focus on individuals' initial feelings of self-efficacy and to help to increase their outcome expectations through shaping early successes. Which of the following will not help with this?
   A) Providing regular feedback and support
   B) Teaching clients how to monitor their own physical activity levels
   C) Helping participants set realistic goals
   D) Having physical activity goals be the same for each participant

3. Which of the following are not included in relapse preparation plans:
   A) Exercise by yourself so you can set the time and location
   B) Plan to exercise as soon as possible after a break in routine
   C) Identify alternate activities that can be performed in the place of a usual activity
   D) Modifying goals to avoid discouragement

ACSM-CEP

4. Select the option that is not included in the Health Belief Model:
   A) Perceived barriers
   B) Perceived benefits
   C) Perceived severity
   D) Perceived loss

5. When setting goals, it is recommended that the goal should be specific. Which of the following is an example of a specific goal?
   A) I will stop smoking soon
   B) I will try to increase my fruit and vegetable intake
   C) I must do more exercise
   D) None of the above

6. Which of the following is an example of an INTRINSIC reward?
   A) Accumulating participation points
   B) Winning a prize for perfect attendance
   C) Enjoyment
   D) Buying new exercise clothes

7. According to the Theory of Reasoned Action, _____ to perform a behavior is the central determinant of whether or not an individual engages in that behavior.
   A) Attitude
   B) Intention
   C) Subjective norms
   D) Perceived behavioral control

8. Jane is thinking about joining a local running group. The group meets twice per week and one of the times conflicts with another leisure-time activity she enjoys. To figure out whether she will join the running group, Jane writes down all of the positive and negative factors associated with making this new change in her life. In doing so, Jane is engaging in:
   A) Decisional balance
   B) Outcome expectation
   C) Relapse prevention
   D) None of the above

9. Rapport refers to the positive relationship that counselors establish with their clients or patients. Which of the following are recommended way to build rapport?
   A) Ask open-ended questions
   B) Convey interest and empathy
   C) Remember that the counselor is the expert in this situation
   D) A and B are both correct.

10. Which of the following is not included in motivational interviewing which is a patient-centered counseling technique:
    A) Helping individuals explore and resolve any ambivalence to change
    B) active listening
    C) reflective statements
    D) confronting resistance to change

11. Which of the following would not be considered a symptom of an anxiety disorder?
    A) Intense worry, fear, or dread
    B) Difficulty sleeping
    C) Loss of interest in previously enjoyed activities
    D) Sympathetic nervous system activation

DOMAIN VI: LEGAL AND PROFESSIONAL RESPONSIBILITIES

A. Evaluate the exercise environment and perform regular inspections of any emergency equipment and practice emergency procedures (e.g., crash cart, activation of emergency procedures) per industry and regulatory standards and facility guidelines.

Domain VI Subdomain A: What you need to know

Knowledge of:

A) government and industry standards and guidelines (*e.g.,* American Association of Cardiovascular and Pulmonary Rehabilitation [AACVPR], American College of Sports Medicine [ACSM], Academy of Nutrition and Dietetics, Health Insurance Portability and Accountability Act [HIPAA], Joint Commission: Accreditation, Health Care, Certification [JCAHO], Occupational Health and Safety Act [OHSA], Americans with Disabilities Act, American Diabetes Association [ADA]).

B) the operation and routine maintenance of exercise equipment.

C) current practice guidelines/recommendations for facility layout and design.

D) standards of practice during emergency situations (*e.g.,* American Heart Association, American Red Cross).

E) local and institutional procedures for activation of the emergency medical system.

F) standards for inspection of emergency medical equipment.

G) risk-reduction strategies, universal precautions, basic life support, emergency equipment, and standard emergency procedures.

Skill in:

A) adhering to legal guidelines and documents.

B) implementing facility safety policies and procedures.

C) applying basic life support procedures (*e.g.*, Cardiopulmonary resuscitation [CPR], automated external defibrillator [AED]).

D) the use of medical terminology

Domain VI Subdomain A: Multiple Choice Questions

1. Which of the following is correct related to emergency preparedness in facilities performing exercise testing.
   A) All personnel involved with exercise testing and supervision in a clinical exercise setting should be certified in basic CPR
   B) A skills and practice session with the AED is recommended every 3–6 months
   C) There should be a physician immediately available at all times when maximal sign or symptom-limited exercise testing is performed on high-risk individuals.
   D) A and B only
   E) A, B, and C

2. Which of the following is the proper emergency response for a patient who has experienced a cardiac arrest but now is breathing and has a palpable pulse?
   A) Continue the exercise test to determine why the patient had this response.
   B) Place the patient in the recovery position with the head to the side to prevent airway obstruction.
   C) Place the patient in a comfortable seated position.
   D) Start phase I cardiac rehabilitation.

3. Which of the following statements regarding an emergency plan is *true*?
   A) The emergency plan does not need to be written down as long as everyone understands it.

   B) As long as everyone knows his or her individual responsibilities during an emergency, a list of each staff member's responsibilities is not needed.
   C) All emergency situations must be documented with dates, times, actions, people involved, and outcomes.
   D) There is no need to practice emergencies as long as the staff members fully understand their responsibilities.

4. Which of the following statements is (are) true in relation to emergency risk management
   A) Facilities offering exercise services must have written emergency response system policies and procedures that are reviewed and rehearsed regularly and include documentation of these activities
   B) Exercise facilities in the health/fitness or community setting must have as part of their written emergency response system a public access defibrillation program
   C) Exercise facilities must have in place a written system for sharing information with users and employees or independent contractors regarding the handling of potentially hazardous materials including the handling of bodily fluids by the facility's staff in accordance with the standards of OSHA.
   D) A, B, and C
   E) A and B only

B. Follow industry-accepted scopes of practice, ethical, legal (e.g., data privacy, informed consent), and business standards.

Domain VI Subdomain B: What you need to know

Knowledge of:

A) professional liability and common types of negligence seen in exercise rehabilitation and exercise testing environments.

B) the legal implications of documented safety procedures, the use of incident documents, and ongoing safety training.

C) the scope of practice of healthcare professionals (*e.g.*, physical therapist, nurse, dietician, psychologist).

D) current practice guidelines/recommendations (*e.g.*, National Heart, Lung, and Blood Institute, Arthritis Foundation, National Multiple Sclerosis Society) for the prevention, evaluation, treatment, and management of chronic diseases.

E) regulations relative to documentation and protecting patient privacy (*e.g.*, written and electronic medical records, Health Insurance Portability and Accountability Act [HIPAA]).

Skill in:

A) proficiency in medical charting.
B) applying industry and regulatory standards.
C) adhering to legal guidelines and documents.
D) the use of medical terminology.

Domain VI Subdomain B: Multiple Choice Questions

1. Which of the following statements about confidentiality is *not* correct?
   A) All records must be kept by the program director/manager under lock and key.
   B) Data must be available to all individuals who need to see it.
   C) Data should be kept on file for at least 1 year before being discarded.
   D) Sensitive information (*e.g.*, participant's name) needs to be protected.

DOMAIN I

Domain I Subdomain A: Multiple Choice Answers

1. —C. Electrocardiography

   Electrocardiography is the least sensitive and specific of all these tests. Directly visualizing the coronary arteries using coronary angiography provides the highest sensitivity and specificity. Radionuclide imaging and echocardiography have about the same sensitivity and specificity.

2. —C. Media

   The media contains most of the smooth muscle cells, which maintain arterial tone. The endothelium comprises a single layer of cells that forms a tight barrier between blood and the arterial wall to resist thrombosis, promote vasodilation, and inhibit smooth muscle cells from migration and proliferation into the intima. The intima is the very thin, innermost layer of the artery wall and is composed mainly of connective tissue with some smooth muscle cells. The adventitia is the outermost layer of the arterial wall and consists of connective tissue, fibroblasts, and a few smooth muscle cells. Adventitia is highly vascularized and provides the media and intima with oxygen and other nutrients.

3. —B. Dyspnea at rest in a recumbent position that is relieved by sitting upright or standing.

   Orthopnea refers to dyspnea occurring at rest in the recumbent position that is relieved promptly by sitting upright or standing. Paroxysmal nocturnal dyspnea refers to dyspnea that begins usually 2–5 h after the onset of sleep, which may be relieved by sitting on the side of the bed or standing to get out of bed. Both conditions are symptoms of left ventricular dysfunction.

4. —B. Bronchitis

   Signs and symptoms of bronchitis include chronic cough, mucus production, and mucous gland enlargement that involves the large airways. The body attempts to heal by depositing collagen in the airway walls. The effects include further airway narrowing, an increase in airway resistance decreasing ventilation to the lung, increased perfusion resulting in ventilation–perfusion mismatch, arterial hypoxemia, and pulmonary arterial hypertension. Common clinical symptoms of emphysema are shortness of breath or coughing, sputum production notable in the morning, hypoxemia, and eventual cor pulmonale. Emphysema primarily involves abnormalities of the lung parenchyma and smaller airways. Asthma is an episodic reversible condition that is characterized by increased airway reactivity to various stimuli resulting in widespread reversible narrowing of the airways. Pulmonary hypertension is a mean pulmonary artery pressure at rest >25 mm Hg or >30 mm Hg with exercise.

5. —A. A coronary artery stent carries a lower rate of revascularization than does PTCA.

   Restenosis occurs within 6 months in approximately 30%–50% of patients who have had a PTCA, whereas a stent has about a 25% failure rate and the drug-eluting stent having a restenosis rate in the low single digits. Atherectomy can be used along with

PTCA and is useful when the PTCA catheter cannot pass through the artery, but atherectomy is not a prerequisite for PTCA. Internal mammary artery grafts are preferred over saphenous venous grafts because of superior patency (90% vs. <50% at 10 year). About 25%–50% of patients will experience a restenosis within 6 months of laser angioplasty.

6. —C. They should not be encouraged to return to work

Exercise programs consisting of aerobic and resistance training specific to provide muscular strength and endurance appropriate for their previous occupation and improve their ability to work, self-efficacy, and comfort with working after their illness, as long as adjustments are appropriately made.

7. —C. Asthma

Bronchitis is inflammation of the main air passages to the lungs. Bronchitis can be acute or chronic. Acute bronchitis is characterized by a cough, with or without the production of sputum, and can last several days or weeks. Chronic bronchitis, a type of chronic obstructive pulmonary disease, is characterized by the presence of a productive cough that lasts for 3 months or more per year for at least 2 year. Emphysema usually refers to a long-term, progressive disease of the lungs that causes shortness of breath. Emphysema is called an obstructive lung disease because the destruction of lung tissue around the alveoli makes these air sacs unable to hold their functional shape upon exhalation. Pulmonary vascular disease is a category of disorders that affect the blood circulation in the lungs. Examples include pulmonary arterial hypertension and pulmonary edema.

Domain I Subdomain B: Multiple Choice Answers

1. —D. Epinephrine

Epinephrine is an endogenous catecholamine that optimizes blood flow to the heart and brain by increasing aortic diastolic pressure and preferentially shunting blood to the internal carotid artery. Lidocaine is an antiarrhythmic agent that can decrease automaticity in the ventricular myocardium as well as raise the fibrillation threshold. Supplemental oxygen ensures adequate arterial oxygen content and greatly enhances tissue oxygenation. Atropine is a parasympathetic blocking agent used to treat bradyarrhythmias.

2. —D. Nitrates

Nitrates relax peripheral venous vessels, which decrease preload, attenuate myocardial oxygen demand, and alleviate ischemia. Nitrates do not reduce the risk of post-MI mortality. β-adrenergic blockers reduce myocardial ischemia by lowering myocardial oxygen demand. These agents lower BP, control ventricular arrhythmias, and significantly reduce first-year mortality rates in patients after MI by 20%–35%. Niacin lowers low-density lipids by inhibiting secretion of lipoproteins from the liver. Aspirin is a platelet inhibitor.

3. —A. Angiotensin-converting enzyme (ACE) inhibitors and angiotensin II blockers.

ACE inhibitor and angiotensin II receptor blockers: ↔ HR (R and E) Calcium channel blockers: ↑ or ↑ or ↔ HR (R and E) β-blockers: ↓ HR (R and E) thyroid medications: ↑ HR (R and E).

4. —C. Digitalis (Lanoxin)

Digitalis can modify the ST–T contour and slow AV conduction. Digitalis may produce characteristic scooping of the ST–T complex. The ST segment and T wave are fused together, and it can be impossible to tell where one ends and the other begins. This may occur when digitalis is in the therapeutic range. With digitalis toxicity, digitalis can cause virtually any arrhythmia and all degrees of AV.

5. —C. A lower HR

Inderal is a β-blocker that diminishes the effect of norepinephrine and epinephrine and lowers HR.

6. —B. An increase in the anginal threshold compared with a test without the medication

β-blockers increase the anginal threshold by reducing myocardial oxygen demand at rest and during exercise. This occurs through a reduction in chronotropic (HR) and inotropic (strength of contraction) responses. BP is also reduced at rest and during exercise by a reduction in cardiac output (reduced chronotropic and inotropic response) and a reduction in total peripheral resistance. β-blockers do not produce ST-segment changes on the resting ECG.

Domain I Subdomain C: Multiple Choice Answers

1. — A. β-adrenergic blockers

   These medications reduce heart rate and therefore myocardial oxygen demand. The work by blocking the action of the catecholamines on the β-adrenergic receptors.

2. —D. Midclavicular line, fifth intercostal space

   The proper anatomic location of V4 is the midclavicular line, fifth intercostal space. Precordial leads V1 and V2 are located at the fourth intercostal space, right and left sternal borders. There is no precordial lead site at the midaxillary line, fifth intercostal space.

3. —A. Extreme cold

   Exposure to cold causes vasoconstriction (higher BP response); lowers the anginal threshold in patients with angina; can provoke angina at rest (variant or Prinzmetal angina); and can induce asthma, general dehydration, and dryness or burning of the mouth and throat.

4. —C. Glycolated hemoglobin (HbA1C)

   HbA1C is a blood chemistry test that reflects glucose levels in the blood over a 2–3 month period. Levels ≥6.5% are diagnostic for diabetes.

5. —B. Mobitz type I

   Second-degree AV block is subdivided into two types: Mobitz type I and Mobitz type II. Mobitz type I also is known as the Wenckebach phenomenon. In this condition, the conduction of the impulse through the AV junction becomes increasingly more difficult, resulting in a progressively longer PR interval, until a QRS complex is dropped following a P wave. This indicates that the AV junction failed to conduct the impulse from the atria to the ventricles. This pause allows the AV node to recover, and the following P wave is conducted with a normal or slightly shorter PR interval.

6. —C. ST segment

   ST segments are considered to be sensitive indicators of myocardial ischemia or injury. A Q wave is a negative deflection of a QRS complex preceding an R wave. A "pathologic" Q wave is an indication of an old transmural MI. The PR interval is the time that it takes from the initiation of an electrical impulse in the sinoatrial node to the initiation of electrical activity in the ventricles. The T wave indicates ventricular repolarization.

7. —A. Acute MI

   An ECG is an excellent tool for detecting cardiac rhythm and conduction abnormalities, chamber enlargements, ischemia, and infarction. In an ECG recording, ST-segment elevation with an absence of R waves that are replaced by Q waves is a sign of acute MI.

8. —B. If cuff size encircles < 80% of the upper arm, measurement will be inaccurate.

   While choosing too small of a cuff will lead to an inaccurate reading, it will tend to overestimate systolic and diastolic pressures. The deflation rate is not dependent on cuff size but technique by technician.

9. —C. Flutter waves at a rate of 250–350 atrial depolarizations per minute

   Ventricular tachycardia is characterized by three or more consecutive ventricular beats per minute or faster, a wide QRS complex (≥120 ms), AV dissociation (the P waves and QRS complexes have no relationship), and a QRS complex that does not have the morphology of bundle-branch block. Atrial flutter is characterized by flutter waves at a rate of 250–350 atrial depolarizations per minute.

10. —C. Second degree: Mobitz type II

    PR interval remains fixed until a P wave fails to conduct.

11. —C. Supraventricular aberrant conduction

    QRS complex is ≥0.11 s; widened QRS usually with unchanged initial vector; P present or absent but with relationship to QRS.

12. —D. Subendocardial ischemia

    The most common ECG change with subendocardial ischemia is ST-segment depression, not ST-segment elevation. ST-segment depression indicates insufficient blood flow (*i.e.*, ischemia) to the heart muscle.

Domain I Subdomain D: Multiple Choice Answers

1. —D. All of the previously mentioned statements are true

   All of these statements are true regarding contraindications to exercise testing.

2. —A. Stroke volume

   During exercise, stroke volume increases curvilinearly with work rate until it reaches near maximum at a level equivalent to approximately 50% of aerobic capacity, increasing only slightly thereafter. The left ventricle is able to contract with greater force during exercise because of a greater end-diastolic volume and enhanced mechanical ability of muscle fibers to produce force.

3. —D. Stroke volume is equal to the ratio of end-diastolic volume to end-systolic volume

Domain I Subdomain E: Multiple Choice Answers

1. —D. Both A&C

   Sedentary behavior is defined by both a posture (lying or sitting) and energy expenditure (<1.5 METS).

DOMAIN II

Domain II Subdomain A: Multiple Choice Answers

1. —B. 80%–90%

   To evaluate the work-related activity levels that are likely to be incorporated into everyday life, a constant work rate test using 80%–90% of the peak work achieved during the incremental exercise test is ideal, especially when the test is performed on a treadmill.

2. —D. Push-up test

   This is a simple field test involving the maximum number of continuous repetitions. It gives an indication of upper body endurance.

Domain II Subdomain B: Multiple Choice Answers

1. —A. Postmenopausal women

   A reduction in the risk of osteoporosis, low back pain, hypertension, and diabetes are associated with resistance training. In addition, the benefits of increased muscular strength, bone density, enhanced strength of connective tissue, and the increase or maintenance of lean body mass may also occur. These adaptations are beneficial for all ages, including middle-aged and older adults, and, in particular, postmenopausal women who may experience a more rapid loss of bone mineral density.

2. —B. BP elevations are highest during isometric muscular actions

   During isometric contractions, constant-rather than rhythmic-force is generated by the skeletal muscle fibers. This constant force exerts pressure on the blood vessels, which results in occlusion (or blocking) of blood flow through the vessels. Because of this vascular resistance and the heart's efforts to overcome it, BP is highest during isometric contractions. Because of the associated cardiovascular challenges, isometric contractions should be avoided, particularly among those with known CVD.

Domain II Subdomain C: Multiple Choice Answers

1. —C. Echocardiography

   In the diagnosis of coronary artery disease, electrocardiography, radionuclide imaging, and echocardiography are commonly used by themselves or with other tests. However, echocardiography uses sound waves to assess heart wall motion, abnormalities, ejection fraction, systolic and diastolic function, and cardiac output. Other important diagnostic studies for coronary artery disease include coronary angiography.

2. —B. 55%

   The anaerobic threshold is normally expressed as a percentage of an individual's $\dot{V}O_{2max}$. For example, if $\dot{V}O_{2max}$ occurs at 6 mph on a treadmill test and a sharp rise in blood lactate concentration above resting levels is seen at

3 mph, then the anaerobic threshold is said to be 50% $\dot{V}O_{2max}$. In well-trained athletes, anaerobic threshold typically occurs at 70%–80% $\dot{V}O_{2max}$. In untrained individuals, it occurs much sooner at 50%–60% $\dot{V}O_{2max}$. This is because the adaptations from regular aerobic exercise have not occurred (*e.g.*, increased mitochondria and capillary density).

3. —B. Signs of poor perfusion (cyanosis or pallor)

The development of a bundle-branch block and a systolic BP of ≥250 mm Hg are relative indications to terminate a symptom-limited maximal exercise test. The achievement of ≥85% age-predicted HR_{max} would indicate the termination of an exercise test with a predetermined intensity goal, which diminishes the sensitivity of the test. Signs of poor perfusion are an absolute indication to terminate the test.

4. —A. The clinical exercise physiologist will review and interpret the results of the test and report them to the supervising physician

The clinical exercise physiologist will not review and interpret the results of the test; this is done by the physician. The physician does not have to be directly present in the exercise testing room but must be available for emergencies. The clinical exercise physiologist must possess the cognitive skills to recognize and treat exercise testing complications and/or serious arrhythmias.

5. —A. Determining a return to work date prior to a patient undergoing CABG surgery.

Data from a clinical exercise test performed after a cardiac event or procedure is useful in developing return to work guidelines for patients. Due to the somewhat unpredictable nature of post-CABG recovery (*i.e.*, possible postoperative complications, individual variability in recovery, etc.), it is not appropriate to use data from a clinical exercise test

performed prior to surgery to predict a return to work date.

6. —A. Coronary angiography

This enables an assessment of the degree of coronary blockage that exists. It is an invasive procedure that has been used successfully for some time.

7. —C. Naughton

The Naughton protocol is appropriate for diseased populations. It is more gradual with increases in intensity and it uses a lower speed than other common protocols (*e.g.*, Bruce protocol). The speed remains constant (2 mph) throughout the test. The grade starts at 0% and increases every 2 min. Small increments in grade allow claudication times to be stratified according to peripheral arterial disease severity.

8. —D. Lack of metabolic determination (*i.e.*, $\dot{V}O_{2max}$)

Sufficient physiological stress is needed to reach an ischemic threshold. There can be compensation by collateral circulation with single vessel disease. Sufficient ECG leads (*e.g.*, 12-lead) are required to monitor a complete view of the heart. However, not determining $\dot{V}O_{2max}$ is not a cause for a false negative.

9. —B. Increased peripheral resistance

During increasing aerobic activity, there is a volume load on the heart and cardiovascular system, which causes a *decrease* in peripheral vascular resistance. This volume load results in a rise in systolic BP and no change or a slight decrease in diastolic BP. An increase in O_2, cardiac output, and mean arterial pressure is typically seen with an increased workload.

10. —D. HR returns to rest slower

Because a transplanted heart is denervated, it lacks direct autonomic control of HR. Without parasympathetic innervation, HR is slower to return to preexercise levels.

Domain II Subdomain D: Multiple Choice Answers

1. —D. Using open-circuit indirect spirometry to determine maximal oxygen uptake ($\dot{V}O_{2max}$)

Exercise time on a standard protocol and the ACSM equations are both useful for estimating the attained MET level during clinical exercise testing. However, the analysis of expired gases obtained during indirect spirometry is the best method for accurately measuring exercise capacity.

2. —A. Monitored immediately and then every 1–2 min for 5 min of recovery or until exercise-induced changes are at baseline

The 12-lead ECG should be recorded immediately after exercise and then every 1–2 min for 5 min or until exercise-induced ECG changes are at baseline.

ACSM-CEP

3. —C. Rate-pressure product (RPP)

The RPP should be used to prescribe exercise for this individual because it is a repeatable estimate of the ischemic threshold. RPP is also a more reliable estimate of ischemic threshold than external workload, which is why it is the best choice.

4. —D. Multiple-gated acquisition (MUGA) (blood pool imagery) study

MUGA study may be performed to assess resting and exercise cardiac function related to cardiac output, ejection fraction, and wall motion. In this test, technetium-99 m is injected into the bloodstream, where it attaches to red blood cells. Areas where the blood pools, such as the ventricles, are visualized by the technetium emissions.

Domain II Subdomain E: Multiple Choice Answers

1. —C. Drop in systolic blood pressure >10 mm Hg (persistently below baseline) despite an increase in workload, in the absence of other evidence of ischemia.

Although all of the options are absolute indicators to terminate a symptom limited test. If benefits of exercise testing outweigh the risks, this contraindication may be superseded.

DOMAIN III

Domain III Subdomain A: Multiple Choice Answers

1. —C. 13 wk

The steps are as follows:

a. Convert relative O_2 to absolute O_2 by multiplying relative O_2 ($mL \cdot kg^{-1} \cdot min^{-1}$) by his body weight.

b. The young man weights 80 kg. Therefore,

$$\begin{aligned} \text{Absolute } \dot{V}O_2 &= \text{relative } \dot{V}O_2 \times \\ &\quad \text{body weight} \\ &= 45 \text{ mL} \cdot kg^{-1} \cdot min^{-1} \times \\ &\quad 80 \text{ kg} \\ &= 3{,}600 \text{ mL} \cdot min^{-1} \end{aligned}$$

c. To get $L \cdot min^{-1}$, divide $mL \cdot min^{-1}$ by 1,000.

$$3{,}600 \text{ mL} \cdot min^{-1}/1{,}000 = 3{,}60 \text{ L} \cdot min^{-1}$$

d. Multiply $3.60 \text{ L} \cdot min^{-1}$ by the constant 5.0 to get $kcal \cdot min^{-1}$.

$$3.60 \text{ L} \cdot min^{-1} \times 5.0 = 18.0 \text{ kcal} \cdot min^{-1}$$

e. Multiply $18.0 \text{ kcal} \cdot min^{-1}$ by the total number of minutes that he exercises (~30 min five times wk^{-1} = 150 total min) to get the total caloric expenditure.

$$18.0 \text{ kcal} \cdot min^{-1} \times 150 \text{ min} = 2{,}700 \text{ kcal} \cdot wk^{-1}$$

f. Divide by 3,500 to get pounds of fat.

$$2{,}700 \text{ kcal} \cdot wk^{-1}/3{,}500 \text{ kcal} \cdot 1b^{-1} \text{ of fat} = 0.7714 \text{ 1b of fat} \cdot wk^{-1}$$

g. Divide 10 lb by 0.7714 to get how many weeks it will take him to lose 10 lb of fat.

$$10 \text{ 1b of fat}/0.7714 = 12.96 \text{ wk or approximately } 13.0 \text{ wk}$$

2. —C. Moderate intensity, 6 d $\cdot$ wk^{-1}, large muscle groups, and moderate duration

Patients who have had heart transplant should exercise at an RPE of between 11 and 16 (moderate) and not use a target HR prescription. Duration should include a prolonged warm-up and cooldown. In addition, resistance training can be used in moderation after 8–12 wk (follow sternotomy special considerations).

3. —D. Health Belief Model

The Health Belief Model (HBM) is centered on the idea that an individual will be more likely to engage in corrective behaviors if they meet the following criteria: (a) Believe they are susceptible to disease, (b) believe the disease has serious consequences, (c) believe taking action reduces their susceptibility to the condition or its severity, (d) believe benefits of taking action outweigh the costs, (e) believe they can successfully perform actions, and (f) believe they are exposed to factors that prompt action.

4. —A. Persons with AICD must be monitored closely during exercise, keeping the heart rate (HR) 10 beats or more below the activation rate for a shock.

There are many benefits of chronic exercise for a patient with an AICD. Several precautions need to be taken, however, including monitoring the HR and knowing the rate at which the AICD is set to shock the patient. The rate for activation is preset and varies for each patient.

5. —A. 40%–59% heart rate reserve (HRR)/$\dot{V}O_{2max}$

   Moderate intensity for aerobic training would be 40%–59% of a person's HRR and/or $\dot{V}O_{2max}$. Vigorous intensities would be 60%–89% HRR/$\dot{V}O_{2max}$, and light/low intensities would range from 30% to 39% HRR/$\dot{V}O_{2max}$.

6. —A. Early morning and late evening

   Exercising early in the morning may result in elevated blood glucose levels after exercise. Avoid exercise prior to bed to avoid hypoglycemia when sleeping. This is due to the release of the counter regulatory hormones epinephrine and glucagon.

7. —B. Shoveling snow

   Shoveling snow can quickly create a potential crisis for an individual with CVD due to a triad of common physiological responses. Snow shoveling raises the HR up to 97% HR_{max} and systolic BP up to 200 mm Hg. Also, cold outdoor temperatures cause whole body and facial cooling, which can lower the threshold for the onset of angina during exercise. Additionally, activities in cold temperatures that involve the upper body and increase metabolism further increase the risk for individuals with CVD.

8. —C. 29.76 mL $\cdot$ kg^{-1} $\cdot$ min^{-1}

   The steps are as follows:
   a. Choose the ACSM's walking formula.
   b. Write down your knowns and convert the values to the appropriate units.

   $$3.5 \text{ mph} \times 26.8 = 93.8 \cdot \text{min}^{-1}$$
   $$10\% \text{ grade} = 0.10$$

   c. Write down the ACSM's walking formula.

   $$\text{walking (kg}^{-1} \cdot \text{min}^{-1}) = (0.1 \times \text{speed}) + (1.8 \times \text{speed} \times \text{fractional grade}) + 3.5 \text{ (mL} \cdot \text{kg}^{-1} \cdot \text{min}^{-1})$$

   d. Substitute the known values for the variable name.

   $$\text{mL} \cdot \text{kg}^{-1} \cdot \text{min}^{-1} = (0.1 \times 93.8) + (1.8 \times 93.8 \times 0.1) + 3.5 \text{ mL} \cdot \text{kg}^{-1} \cdot \text{min}^{-1} = 9.8 + 16.884 + 3.5$$

   e. Solve for the unknown.

   $$\text{mL} \cdot \text{kg}^{-1} \cdot \text{min}^{-1} = 9.38 + 16.884 + 3.5 \text{ gross walking } \dot{V}O = 29.76 \text{ mL} \cdot \text{kg}^{-1} \cdot \text{min}^{-1}$$

9. —B. 2.17 L $\cdot$ min^{-1}

   The steps are as follows:
   a. Choose the ACSM's walking formula.
   b. Write down your knowns and convert the values to the appropriate units.

   $$5\% \text{ grade} = 0.05$$
   $$4.0 \text{ mph} = 107.2 \text{ m} \cdot \text{min}^{-1}$$
   $$200 \text{ 1b} = 90.91 \text{ kg}$$

   c. Write down the ACSM's walking formula.

   $$\text{walking (kg}^{-1} \cdot \text{min}^{-1}) = (0.1 \times \text{speed}) + (1.8 \times \text{speed} \times \text{fractional grade}) + 3.5 \text{ (mL} \cdot \text{kg}^{-1} \cdot \text{min}^{-1})$$

   d. Substitute knowns.

   $$\dot{V}O_2 = (0.1 \times 107.2) + (1.8 \times 107.2 \times 0.05) + 3.5$$

   e. Solve.

   $$\dot{V}O_2 = 23.87 \text{ mL} \cdot \text{kg}^{-1} \cdot \text{min}^{-1}$$
   $$\dot{V}O_2 = 23.83 \times 90.01 \text{ kg}/1{,}000$$
   $$\dot{V}O_2 = 2.17 \text{ L} \cdot \text{min}^{-1}$$

10. —C. 10–12 wk

    Because of the median sternotomy used to provide access for cardiovascular surgery, it is common to provide ROM and weight load restrictions for upper limb movement. These instructions are conveyed at discharge and may vary somewhat. However, they are usually set at 5–10 lb or <50% MVC for 10–12 wk postoperatively.

11. —B. After the first 24 h

    Mobilization of the upper extremities may be useful in preventing joint complications after ICD implantation. Guidelines suggest that gentle ROM activities begin after the first 24 h to reduce the risk of lead displacement.

12. —C. 444 kcal

    First, determine the MET level for each activity.

    Warm-up is 2.0 METs × 5 min = 10 METs

    Treadmill is 9.0 METs × 20 min = 180 METs

    Cycle is 8.0 METs × 20 min = 160 METs

    Cool-down is 2.50 METs × 5 min = 12.5 METs

    Then, determine the total number of MET for all activities. 10 + 180 + 160 + 12.5 = 362.5. Multiply 362.5 METs by 3.5 (because 1 MET = 3.5 mL $\cdot$ kg^{-1} $\cdot$ min^{-1}), which is equal to 1,268.75 mL $\cdot$ kg^{-1}.

Multiply 1,268.75 mL · kg^{-1} by body weight (70 kg), which is equal to 88,812.5 mL. Divide that number by 1,000 (because 1,000 mL = 1 L), which is equal to 88.81 L. Multiply 88.81 L by 5 (because 5 kcal = 1 L of oxygen consumed), which is equal to 444 kcal.

13. —B. 30 min · d^{-1}, five times a week or 150 min · wk^{-1} of moderate-intensity exercise

The ACSM/AHA Primary Physical Activity Recommendations suggest that all healthy individuals aged 18–65 year should participate in moderate-intensity, aerobic PA for a minimum of 30 min on 5 d of the week or vigorous intensity, aerobic activity for a minimum of 20 min on 3 d of the week. The Primary Physical Activity Recommendations from the *2018 Physical Activity Guidelines Committee Report* suggest that all Americans should participate in an amount of energy expenditure equivalent to 150 min · wk^{-1} of moderate-intensity aerobic activity or 75 min · wk^{-1} of vigorous-intensity aerobic activity.

14. —C. Performing more sets per muscle group and increasing the number of days per week muscle groups are trained.

The progressive overload principle incorporates more repetitions per muscle group while increasing the number of days per week muscle groups are trained.

15. —A. One set 8–12 repetitions of a resistance training exercise.

Novices will improve with even one set. If they are gradually exposed to multiple sets, they will show even greater improvement.

16. —C. HR

Myocardial oxygen consumption is increased by a number of variables, including increased HR. A decreased HR at a given intensity

(4 METs) would reduce myocardial oxygen consumption. The other three choices do not directly affect myocardial oxygen demand.

17. —B. Patients with peripheral arterial disease should exercise to leg pain level 3 (on 4-point scale), with intermittent rest periods. Weight-bearing endurance exercise has been shown to increase the time for the onset of pain in patients with PAD. The effect intensity is described as to the point of moderate pain (3) on a 4-point scale.

18. —B. HR

Adaptations to long-term aerobic activity include an increased oxidative capacity of the exercised muscles, increased blood flow through active muscles, and increased venous blood flow return to the heart. These adaptations (*i.e.*, increased aerobic fitness) result in a decreased HR at the same level of submaximal exercise intensity.

19. —C. Systolic pressure and HR

For example, HR is 80 bpm, systolic pressure is 140.

20. —D. RPP

RPP (HR × systolic BP) is a measure or indicator of the stress put on the cardiac muscle (myocardial oxygen demand), making it a better indicator of the ischemic threshold compared to HR or BP alone. Oxygen uptake is not a direct measure of ischemia.

21. —C. Increased HR

HR during maximal exercise will not increase with adaptations from long-term PA. HR during maximal exercise is related to age.

22. —D. RPE

RPE, because individuals with autonomic neuropathy may show blunted HR and BP responses to exercise.

Domain III Subdomain B: Multiple Choice Answers

1. —A. To effectively breathe through a progressively smaller airway

Flow-resistive training involves breathing through a progressively smaller airway or opening. Paced breathing helps to coordinate breathing with activities of daily living. Respiratory muscle training increases respiratory muscle endurance and strength. Ventilatory threshold is the breakpoint in

ventilation during exercise and likely reflects a balance between lactate production and removal.

2. —C. Increased maximum coronary blood flow

RPP is an indicator of myocardial oxygen demand. An increase in maximal RPP indicates that there is improved/increased blood flow to the coronary arteries.

Domain III Subdomain C: Multiple Choice Answers

1. —C. 40%–<59% HRR or $\dot{V}O_2R$, 3–<6 METs, RPE 12–13, an intensity that causes noticeable increases in HR and breathing

   ACSM defines moderate-intensity exercise as an exercise workload of 40%–<60% HRR or $\dot{V}O_2R$, 3–<6 METs, RPE 12–13, at an intensity that causes noticeable increases in HR and breathing. This level of exercise may be suitable for a cardiac rehabilitation patient who has completed many of the prescribed exercise sessions with an estimated or actual peak oxygen consumption ($\dot{V}O_{2peak}$) of ≥8 METs.

Domain III Subdomain D: Multiple Choice Answers

1. —C. Exercising only when temperature and humidity are moderate

   Recommended precautions for the exercising patient with diabetes include wearing proper footwear, maintaining adequate hydration, monitoring blood glucose level regularly, always wearing a medical identification bracelet or other form of identification, avoiding injecting insulin into exercising muscles, always exercising with a partner, and avoiding exercise during peak insulin activity. There is no reason why a patient with diabetes cannot exercise at any time if proper precautions are followed.

2. —D. Digitalis

   Digitalis is used to treat heart failure and certain arrhythmias. Shortening of the QT interval and a "scooping" of the ST–T complex characterize the effects of digitalis on the ECG.

3. —B. Dose–response relationship

   The dose–response relationship shows that an increase in the volume of exercise results in an increase in health and fitness benefits.

4. —D. RPE 11–14; 30–60 min $\cdot$ d^{-1}

   Individuals with heart failure should exercise 3–5 d $\cdot$ wk^{-1} at an intensity of 11–14 on a 6–20 RPE scale. They should increase up to 30 min $\cdot$ d^{-1} and then to 60 min $\cdot$ d^{-1} by free or treadmill walking or the use of a cycle ergometer.

DOMAIN IV

Domain IV Subdomain A: Multiple Choice Answers

1. —C. 150–200 kcal $\cdot$ d^{-1}

   A minimal caloric threshold of 150–200 kcal of PA per day is associated with a significant 20%–30% reduction in risk of all-cause mortality, and this should be the initial goal for previously sedentary individuals.

2. —A. The patient should avoid upper body resistance training because of sternal and leg wounds for 4–6 months

   Avoiding tension on the upper body typically is recommended for 8–12 wk, not for 2–4 months. All of the other precautions are appropriate.

3. —D. Peripheral adaptations are largely responsible for an increase in exercise tolerance

   Physical conditioning in patients with heart failure and moderate-to-severe left ventricular dysfunction results in improved functional capacity and quality of life and reduced symptoms. Peripheral adaptation (increased skeletal muscle oxidative enzymes and improved mitochondrial size and density) is responsible for the increase in exercise tolerance.

4. —D. Upper middle class

   Obese and older adult persons are often less physically active because of various physical or medical limitations (*e.g.*, osteoarthritis, frailty). The less educated are often not aware of the important health and fitness benefits of being physically active on a regular basis. For healthy adults, stroke volume is calculated by subtracting end-systolic volume from end-diastolic volume.

5. —A. Decreased TG and increased HDL

   Chronic exercise training has its greatest benefit on lowering TG and increasing HDL. Changes in total cholesterol or LDL cholesterol are influenced more by dietary habits and body weight than by exercise training.

6. —C. They should avoid the Valsalva maneuver to avoid excessive elevation in BP.

Domain IV Subdomain B: Multiple Choice Answers

1. —D. Decreased arterial oxygen levels and increased cardiac output

   Higher altitudes (2,400–4,000 m or 7,874–13,123 ft) have a decreased atmospheric pressure, which reduces the partial pressure of oxygen in the inspired air. This change will result in a physiological decrease in arterial oxygen levels and the immediate compensatory response includes increased ventilation and cardiac output.

2. —C. Heat exhaustion

   Heat exhaustion is often associated with fatigue and peripheral vascular dilation resulting in hypotension, blood pooling, and cardiovascular insufficiency. This blood pooling reduces intravascular heat transport from the core to the skin and diminishes thermoregulation. Heat cramps are muscle spasms that may occur in association with strenuous activity, syncope is a temporary loss of consciousness, and heat stroke is caused by hyperthermia of >40°C or 104°F.

Domain IV Subdomain C: Multiple Choice Answers

1. —B. Junctional arrhythmia

   A junctional arrhythmia is a supraventricular ectopic rhythm that results from a focus of automaticity located in the bundle of His. A ventricular arrhythmia could be a premature ventricular complex (PVC) in which one of the ventricles depolarizes first and then spreads to the other ventricle or ventricular fibrillation, which is often triggered by the simultaneous conduction of ischemic ventricular cells within multiple locations of the ventricles. An AV block results when supraventricular impulses are delayed in the AV node. A premature ventricular contraction occurs when the ventricles are prematurely depolarized.

2. —A. P wave

   The cardiac impulse originating in the sinoatrial node that spreads to both atria causing atrial depolarization is indicated on the ECG as a P wave. Atrial repolarization usually is not seen on the ECG because it is obscured by the ventricular electrical potentials. Ventricular depolarization is represented on the ECG by the QRS complex. Ventricular repolarization is represented on the ECG by the ST segment, the T wave, and, at times, the U wave.

3. —E. CKD patients are at high risk of dying from premature cardiovascular disease. When tested, standard procedures can be followed but these patients should receive medical clearance prior to initiating an exercise program.

4. —D. Turbulent blood flow

   When measuring BP, blood flows in spurts as the pressure in the artery rises above the pressure in the cuff and then drops back down beyond the cuffed region of the arm. This results in turbulence that produces the audible sounds (Korotkoff sounds).

Domain IV Subdomain D: Multiple Choice Answers

1. —A. Emphysema

   Emphysema is a pulmonary condition that is caused by destruction of the lung parenchyma. Smoking is implicated in the development of this condition.

2. —D. Decreased endothelial-mediated vasomotor tone

   The mechanisms responsible for a reduction in deaths from coronary artery disease include its effect on other risk factors, reduced myocardial oxygen demand both at rest and at submaximal workloads (resulting in an increased ischemic and anginal threshold), reduced platelet aggregation, and improved endothelial-mediated vasomotor tone.

3. —C. Coronary artery bypass graft (CABG) surgery

   CABG surgery usually is reserved for patients who have a poor prognosis for survival or are unresponsive to pharmacologic treatment, stents, or PTCA. Such patients include those with angina, left main coronary artery stenosis, multiple vessel disease, and left ventricular dysfunction.

4. —D. Pain in the left submammary or hemithorax area

   Chest pain in the left submammary or hemithorax area is generally not ischemic in origin. Atypical or nonischemic chest pain may be caused by many conditions other than angina pectoris including musculoskeletal conditions, costochondritis, abdominal gas, or infection.

5. —A. Congestive heart failure

   Bilateral ankle edema that is most evident at night is a characteristic sign of congestive heart failure (or bilateral chronic venous insufficiency). Unilateral edema of a limb often results from venous thrombosis or lymphatic blockage in the limb. Generalized edema (known as anasarca) occurs in those with the nephrotic syndrome, severe heart failure, or hepatic cirrhosis.

6. —A. Low-density lipoprotein (LDL) cholesterol

   Lowering total cholesterol and LDL cholesterol has proved to be effective in reducing and even reversing atherosclerosis. The goal is to reduce the availability of lipids to the injured endothelium. In primary prevention trials, lowering total cholesterol and LDL cholesterol has been shown to reduce the incidence and mortality of coronary artery disease.

7. —D. Decreased RPP

   RPP is a measure of the stress put on the cardiac muscle (myocardial oxygen demand) based on the number of times it needs to beat per minute and the arterial BP that it is pumping against (HR × systolic BP). A decreased RPP indicates less myocardial oxygen demand. An *increased* RPP can be associated with exercise-induced myocardial ischemia.

Domain IV Subdomain E: Multiple Choice Answers

1. —B. 510 cal

   The steps are as follows:
   a. Choose the ACSM's leg cycling formula.
   b. Write down your knowns and convert the values to the appropriate units.

   $$110 \text{ lb}/2.2 = 50 \text{ kg}$$
   $$50 \text{ rpm} \times 6 \text{ m} = 300 \text{ m} \cdot \text{min}^{-1}$$
   $$2.5 \text{ kp} = 2.5 \text{ kg}$$
   $$60 \text{ min of cycling}$$

   c. Write down the ACSM leg cycling formula.

   $$\text{Leg cycling (mL} \cdot \text{kg}^{-1} \cdot \text{min}^{-1}) = (1.8 \times \text{work rate/body weight}) + 3.5 + 3.5 \text{ (mL} \cdot \text{kg}^{-1} \cdot \text{min}^{-1})$$

   d. Calculate the work rate.

   $$\text{Work rate} = \text{kg} \cdot \text{m} \cdot \text{min}^{-1}$$
   $$= 2.5 \text{ kg} \cdot 300 \text{ m} \cdot \text{min}^{-1}$$
   $$= 750 \text{ kg} \cdot \text{m} \cdot \text{min}^{-1}$$

   e. Substitute the known values for the variable name.

   $$\text{mL} \cdot \text{kg}^{-1} \cdot \text{min}^{-1} = (1.8 \times 750/50) + 3.5 + 3.5$$

   f. Solve for the unknown.

   $$\text{mL} \cdot \text{kg}^{-1} \cdot \text{min}^{-1} = 27 + 3.5 + 3.5$$
   $$\text{Gross leg cycling } \dot{V}O_2 = 34 \text{ mL} \cdot \text{kg}^{-1} \cdot \text{min}^{-1}$$

   g. To find out how many calories she expends, we must first convert her oxygen consumption to absolute terms.

   $$\text{Absolute } \dot{V}O_2 = \text{relative } \dot{V}O_2 \times \text{body weight}$$
   $$= 34 \text{ mL} \cdot \text{kg}^{-1} \cdot \text{min}^{-1}$$
   $$= 1{,}700 \text{ mL} \cdot \text{min}^{-1}$$

   h. Convert $\text{mL} \cdot \text{min}^{-1}$ to $\text{L} \cdot \text{min}^{-1}$ by dividing by 1,000.

   $$1{,}700 \text{ mL} \cdot \text{min}^{-1}/1{,}000 = 1.7 \text{ L} \cdot \text{min}^{-1}$$

   i. Next, we must see how many calories she expends in 1 min by multiplying her absolute O_2 (in $\text{L} \cdot \text{min}^{-1}$) by the constant 5.0.

   $$1.7 \text{ L} \cdot \text{min}^{-1} \times 5.0 = 8.5 \text{ kcal} \cdot \text{min}^{-1}$$

   j. Finally, multiply the number of calories she expends in 1 min by the number of minutes that she cycles.

   $$8.5 \text{ kcal} \cdot \text{min}^{-1} \times 60 \text{ min} = 510 \text{ total calories}$$

2. —A. Severe coronary artery disease

   Severe coronary artery disease will result in less oxygen delivery to the myocardium because of blockage(s), which will reduce or limit oxygenated blood flow to the myocardium.

ACSM-CEP

3. —D. Lower stroke volume

Regular aerobic activity typically increases stroke volume at rest. Increased aerobic fitness usually results in a lower resting HR (HR_{rest}). The lower HR prolongs diastole (ventricular filling), increasing end-diastolic volume, and enables more blood to be ejected with each beat. So, physically inactive men will typically have a lower stroke volume compared to physically active men of the same age and weight.

4. —C. Exertional myocardial ischemia

A reversible perfusion defect is caused by decreased uptake of the radionuclide isotope by the myocardium due to the relative reduction of blood flow to the ischemic tissue during exercise. This may or may not be accompanied by symptoms of angina pectoris. This abnormality is not seen when myocardial perfusion is evaluated at rest.

Domain IV Subdomain F: Multiple Choice Answers

1. —D. Dialysis patients should be encouraged to exercise on non-dialysis days

However, another time efficient alternative is to have them exercise during dialysis. This is called intradialytic exercise. Patients do better when the exercise is performed during the first half of the treatment. If exercise is performed late in the dialysis session, some individuals complain of dizziness because of the fluid shifts that occur during dialysis.

Domain IV Subdomain G: Multiple Choice Answers

1. —C. Check to make sure that the device is working properly and if so then advise the individual to get medical clearance before continuing any more exercise sessions.

2. —B. Stop the training session immediately and get the individual evaluated by a healthcare professional as soon as possible.

DOMAIN V

Domain V Subdomain A: Multiple Choice Answers

1. —A. Precontemplation

Patients express lack of interest in making change. Moving patients through this stage involves the use of multiple resources to stress the importance of the desired change. This can be achieved through written materials, educational classes, physician and family persuasion, and other means.

Domain V Subdomain B: Multiple Choice Answers

1. —A. Has been physically active on a regular basis for <6 months

Stages of motivational readiness describe five categories of readiness to change or maintain behavior. As applied to PA or exercise, they are precontemplation (stage 1), contemplation (stage 2), preparation (stage 3), action (stage 4), and maintenance (stage 5). The action stage is when the person is engaged in PA or exercise that meets the current ACSM's recommendations for PA but has not maintained this program for 6 month or more.

2. —B. Contemplation

In the contemplation stage, individuals are thinking about becoming active but they have not yet begun to change their behavior (this happens in the preparation stage).

3. —D. Personal experience

Personal experience is the strongest influence on feelings of self-efficacy. Specifically, past success performing a behavior (known as personal mastery experience) leads to increased self-efficacy for that behavior.

Domain V Subdomain C: Multiple Choice Answers

1. —C. Relapse prevention

The relapse prevention model aims to assist individuals in long-term maintenance of behavior change by anticipating potentially high-risk situations (*e.g.*, travel, bad weather, illness) and devising strategies to cope with these high-risk situations. This model distinguishes between a lapse (temporary slip, *e.g.*, missing one exercise session) and relapse (return to former behavior patterns).

2. —D. A, B, and C

The social ecological model addresses multiple factors that influence a person's physical activity levels. This includes intrapersonal factors (*e.g.*, age, sex, motivational level, self-efficacy); interpersonal factors (*e.g.*, social networks, cultural influences, work-place policies), and environmental factors (*e.g.*, presence of sidewalks, interesting scenery). This approach recognizes that no single factor alone accounts for how much physical activity we do, they all interrelate to determine how much physical activity a person achieves.

Domain V Subdomain D: Multiple Choice Answers

1. —A. Vicarious experience or modeling

Individuals increase their self-efficacy by watching others successfully accomplish the behavior. This is especially important in group settings (*e.g.*, cardiac rehab) and when the person feels that they can relate to the individual they are observing.

2. —D. Having physical activity goals be the same for each participant

It is important that goals are individualized to each participant, relative to their exercise history and current level of fitness. There is no "one size fits all" approach to physical activity goals.

3. —A. Exercise by yourself so you can set the time and location

Making plans or exercising with others leverages social support and creates a sense of accountability that can be helpful in avoiding relapse.

4. —D. Perceived loss

According to the Health Belief model, a person will engage in preventative health practices, such as exercise, based upon their beliefs about health problems (perceived severity and perceived susceptibility), and the relative balance between perceived benefits of action and barriers to action. Other components of the model include self-efficacy and cues to action.

5. —D. None of the above

None of these are specific goals. An example of a specific goal is "I would like to lose 15 lb," or "I will take a 20 min walk after dinner 3 days a week."

6. —C. Enjoyment

Extrinsic rewards are tangible and are usually given to the person doing the activity; as such, they are typically not from within the person. In contrast, an intrinsic reward is intangible and comes from within (*e.g.*, enjoyment, satisfaction).

7. —B. Intention

Intention is the sole and immediate predictor of behavior. Behavioral intention mediates the effect of attitude, subjective normative beliefs, and perceived behavioral control toward the behavior.

8. —A. Decisional balance

Decisional balance involves the comparison of the benefits of making a behavior change versus the costs (*i.e.*, pros and cons). Individuals are more likely to be active when they perceive that the benefits (*e.g.*, better sleep) will outweigh the perceived costs (*e.g.*, time taken away from other activities).

9. —D. A and B are both correct

Asking open-ended questions encourages clients/patients to share their thoughts and feelings. Demonstrating empathy and interest helps the client/patient feel like they are being understood, which is important for trust building and rapport. In a counseling relationship, the client/patient and counselor should work together.

10. —D. Confronting resistance to change

With motivational interviewing, the counselor should demonstrate active, reflective listening and help the client explore their own motivation for change and ambivalence to change in a nonconfrontational manner.

11. —C. Loss of interest in previously enjoyed activities

Loss of interest in previously enjoyed activities is a symptom of depression, not anxiety. However, these two disorders can often coexist. Anxiety disorders are characterized by persistent, excessive fear or worry in situations that are not threatening. Anxiety disorders can manifest emotionally (*e.g.*, fear, worry, panic) and physically (*e.g.*, racing heart rate, sweating, insomnia).

ACSM-CEP

DOMAIN VI

Domain VI Subdomain A: Multiple Choice Answers

1. —E. All listed items are recommended.

2. —B. Place the patient in the recovery position with the head to the side to prevent airway obstruction

   The proper response to a patient who has experienced a cardiac arrest yet is breathing and has a pulse is to call to the emergency medical system immediately; place the patient in the recovery position, with the head to the side to avoid an airway obstruction; and then stay with the patient and continue to monitor their vital signs.

3. —C. All emergency situations must be documented with dates, times, actions, people involved, and outcomes.

The emergency plan must be written down and available in all testing and exercise areas. The plan should list the specific responsibilities of each staff member, required equipment, and predetermined contacts for an emergency response. All emergencies must be documented with dates, times, actions, people involved, and results. The plan should be practiced with both announced and unannounced drills periodically. All staff members, including nonclinical staff members, should be trained in the emergency plan.

4. —D. A, B, and C are correct

   All of the statements are correct based upon standard guidelines.

Domain VI Subdomain B: Multiple Choice Answers

1. —C. Data should be kept on file for at least 1 year before being discarded

   There is no accepted minimal or maximal amount of time that data should be stored.

Clearly, however, data must be stored in a confidential (lock-and-key) manner, and discretion must be used when sharing data.

There are a total of 10 individual case studies in this section: Grant, Seamus, Keith, Steve, Nancy, Joe, Mr. Kyle, Sheryl, Jim, and Kimberly, as well as two case studies that cover brief scenarios on patient privacy and emergency preparedness. Additionally, this section includes 13 ECG case studies.

CASE STUDY 1: GRANT
Author: Trent A. Hargens, PhD, FACSM
Author's Certifications: ACSM-CEP, EIM3

You are a certified clinical exercise physiologist (CEP) at a wellness center with a physician-referred exercise program. Grant is a 42-year-old male who works as a computer information technology specialist. His physician has referred Grant to the facility and has already cleared him for all exercise activity. He currently weighs 250 lb and is 6 ft 1 in. tall, and his waist circumference (WC) is 40.5 in. Bioelectrical impedance estimated a body fat percentage of 35.5%. His resting heart rate (HR_{rest}) was 72 bpm, and his average resting blood pressure (BP) was 128/86 mm Hg. Results from his most recent (within 1 month) blood measures were the following: Total cholesterol = 209 mg $\cdot$ dL^{-1}, high-density lipoprotein cholesterol (HDL-C) = 36 mg $\cdot$ dL^{-1}, low-density lipoprotein cholesterol (LDL-C) = 115 mg $\cdot$ dL^{-1}, triglycerides = 292 mg $\cdot$ dL^{-1}, and glucose = 112 mg $\cdot$ dL^{-1}. Grant reports on his health history questionnaire that he is not on any medications and no symptoms suggestive of cardiovascular, metabolic, or pulmonary disease. His 67-year-old father has been on BP medication for the previous 20 years and was recently diagnosed with Type 2 diabetes mellitus (DM).

During your initial consultation with Grant, he reports that he spends most of his workdays sitting behind the computer and that he walks his dog around the neighborhood two to three times per week for approximately 10 min. He has been doing this since his dog was a puppy several years ago. He also reports that it was not his idea to join your wellness center. His doctor, who told him that he needs to improve his lifestyle, referred him to the program. He expresses to you that he is not very motivated about the program, but pressure from his doctor and his family are why he is here. He feels that his current health status is just "part of getting old."

Grant: Case Study 1 Questions

1. Grant's body mass index (BMI) is
   A) 27.6 kg $\cdot$ m^{-2}
   B) 33.1 kg $\cdot$ m^{-2}
   C) 40.1 kg $\cdot$ m^{-2}
   D) 61.4 kg $\cdot$ m^{-2}

2. According to the most recent edition of the *American College of Sports Medicine's* (ACSM) *Guidelines For Exercise Testing and Prescription* (GETP), which of the following would not be part of the decision-making

(Continued)

CASE STUDY 1: GRANT (Continued)

process for referral to a health care provider prior to initiating a moderate-to-vigorous intensity exercise program for Grant?

A) Current lipid values
B) Dog walking
C) Report of signs and symptoms
D) Health history concerning diagnosed cardiovascular, metabolic, or renal disease

3. According to the most recent edition of the *ACSM's GETP*, what is recommended prior to his beginning exercise at a light-to-moderate intensity in your facility?

A) Signed informed consent form only
B) Signed informed consent form and additional medical clearance from physician
C) Signed informed consent form and graded exercise test (GXT)
D) Signed informed consent form, additional medical clearance from physician, and GXT with physician supervision

4. Based on what Grant has expressed during his initial consultation, he is in which stage of change?

A) Precontemplation
B) Contemplation
C) Preparation
D) Action

5. According to the most recent edition of *ACSM's GETP*, which of the following would classify Grant as having fasting blood glucose level?

A) Grant would be classified as having normal fasting blood glucose.
B) Grant would be classified as having impaired fasting glucose (IFG).
C) Grant would be classified as having insulin-dependent DM.
D) Grant would be classified as having noninsulin-dependent DM.

6. What do you believe should be the primary goal for Grant as he begins his exercise program?

7. As exercise capacity increases, Grant will need an adjustment in his exercise prescription. What would be an appropriate progression in his frequency, intensity, time, and type (FITT) of activity?

CASE STUDY 2: SEAMUS
Author: Emily M. Miele, PhD
Author's Certifications: ACSM-EP, EIM3

You are a CEP in an outpatient hospital setting. Seamus is a 48-year-old male who gets referred to you by his endocrinologist. Upon reviewing his intake information, you find that he has Type 2 DM with an HbA1C of 6.8 and is currently taking insulin glargine 18 units in the morning and 18 units in the evening. He currently weighs 325 lb at a height of 5'10". Seamus is a supervisor for a utility company and spends the majority of his workday in the car driving to various job sites and dispatching calls over the phone. He has not regularly exercised since playing football in college. He tells you that he knows he should be exercising regularly and is ready to start a program with you, despite having many failed attempts over the past few years. He quit smoking 4 years ago. Seamus also takes a β-blocker for hypertension and his resting blood pressure during your initial intake is 134/82 mm Hg.

Seamus: Case Study 2 Questions

1. What does his HbA1C reflect?
A) Fasting plasma glucose
B) Glucose tolerance
C) Blood glucose control over the last 2–3 months
D) Waist to hip ratio

2. Which of the following is/are component(s) of the medical history that should be obtained during the initial interview?
   A) Cardiovascular disease risk factors and the presence of any other complications associated with diabetes
   B) Exercise history and habitual level of activity
   C) History of symptoms such as chest discomfort, palpitations, shortness of breath, dizziness
   D) All of the above

3. According to the most recent edition of the *ACSM's GETP* and based on Seamus' current medications, when should his blood sugar be tested and reported to you?
   A) He does not need to test his blood sugar
   B) Before exercise only
   C) Before and after exercise only
   D) Before, occasionally during, and after exercise

4. According to the Transtheoretical Model (TTM), what stage of behavior change is Seamus currently in?
   A) Preparation
   B) Maintenance
   C) Precontemplation
   D) Contemplation
   E) Action

5. What is an appropriate target goal for reduction of body weight in the first 3–6 months of the exercise program for Seamus?
   A) Weight loss should not be a goal for Seamus.
   B) 2.5–5.75 lb
   C) 9.75–32.5 lb
   D) 50–75.25 lb

6. When performing an exercise test for the purpose of designing an exercise Rx for Seamus, should he take his regularly scheduled β-blocker dose?
   A) Yes
   B) No

7. Based on Seamus' medical history and according to recommendations in the most recent edition of the *ACSM's GETP*, what values of SBP and DBP, respectively, are appropriate during exercise?
   A) SBP ≤200 mm · Hg and/or DBP ≤ 120 mm · Hg
   B) SBP ≤220 mm · Hg and/or DBP ≤ 105 mm · Hg
   C) SBP ≤180 mm · Hg and/or DBP ≤ 110 mm · Hg
   D) SBP ≤230 mm · Hg and/or DBP ≤ 90 mm · Hg

8. Which of the following is/are signs or symptoms of <u>hypoglycemia</u> that you would instruct Seamus to report to you during exercise?
   A) Shakiness
   B) Visual disturbances
   C) Abnormal Sweating
   D) All of the above
   E) A and C only

9. Due to better blood glucose control since starting his exercise program with you, Seamus' physician takes him off of insulin and prescribes metformin and glipizide (a sulfonylurea) to control his blood sugar. Should his blood glucose still be monitored around exercise due to increased risk of hypoglycemia?
   A) Only if he reports symptoms
   B) Only for afternoon exercise
   C) Yes
   D) No

10. A few weeks into the exercise program, Seamus informs you that he noticed his blood sugar has been low when he checks it upon waking up in the morning. What should you advise in this scenario?
    A) Advise Seamus to skip his nighttime diabetes medication doses and monitor his blood glucose more closely.
    B) Advise Seamus to reduce his morning diabetes medication doses and monitor his blood glucose more closely.
    C) Advise Seamus not to do anything as this is not a concern.
    D) Advise Seamus to report these changes this to his physician and inform his physician of his current exercise routine.

11. Before beginning exercise, Seamus tests his blood glucose and gets a reading of 85 mg/dL. What recommendations would you make, in regards to his exercise session for that day?

12. How should you initiate and progress a resistance training program for Seamus, in terms of frequency, intensity, sets, and repetitions?

CASE STUDY 3: KEITH
DOMAIN II: EXERCISE PRESCRIPTION
Author: David E. Verrill, MS
Author's Certifications: ACSM-CEP, EIM3

You are a CEP employed in the medical fitness program at a local health/fitness facility. You have a new client, Keith, joining your program. He is a 57-year-old male who currently weighs 193 lb and is 66 in. tall (BMI = 31.2 $kg \cdot m^{-2}$). His body composition by skinfolds was estimated at 32% body fat, and his waist (abdominal) circumference was 42 in. He is a current smoker (smokes one pack a day). His HR_{rest} was 72 bpm, and his resting BP was 142/88 mm Hg. Fasting blood values were measured 2 weeks ago as the following: Total cholesterol = 227 $mg \cdot dL^{-1}$; HDL-C = 33 $mg \cdot dL^{-1}$; triglycerides = 156 $mg \cdot dL^{-1}$; glucose = 132 $mg \cdot dL^{-1}$; and HbA1C = 7.2%. He has been walking his "older" dog daily for the last 4 weeks but reports no other physical activity. He reports no symptoms of exercise intolerance except SOB when walking up hills. His brother died of a fatal heart attack at age 60 years. Currently, he is only taking a diuretic (hydrochlorothiazide [HCTZ], 25 mg once daily) to control his BP. He also takes rosuvastatin (Crestor) 10 mg once daily and metformin (Glucophage XR) 1,500 mg once daily. He has recently joined your medical fitness program to increase his fitness level and manage his body weight, dyslipidemia, diabetes, and hypertension safely.

Your client recently had a modified Bruce (5% grade) maximal exercise test ordered by his physician due to his SOB concerns. The physician interpreted the test as equivocal, as he did not reach 85% of predicted maximal heart rate (HR_{max}). The test interpretation also indicated ~0.5–1 mm of ST depression in the lateral leads at peak exercise only, but no symptoms of ischemia. His HR_{max} and peak BP were 132 bpm and 224/94 mm Hg, respectively. His maximal oxygen consumption was estimated to be 23.1 $mL \cdot kg^{-1} \cdot min^{-1}$ (6.6 METs). His physician ordered a pulmonary function test with the following results: Forced expiratory volume in one second ($FEV_{1.0}$) = 2.1 L (54% predicted) and his forced vital capacity (FVC) = 3.2 L (64% predicted) immediately following bronchodilator administration. His $FEV_{1.0}$/FVC ratio = 0.66.

Based on these clinical findings, his physician has cleared him to exercise in a medically supervised health and fitness program.

Keith: Case Study 3 Questions

1. According to the most recent edition of the *ACSM's GETP*, when prescribing exercise, the optimal intensity of exercise for aerobic fitness benefits for this client would be set at
   A) Light; 30%–<40% of heart rate reserve (HRR)
   B) Light to moderate; 30%–<60% of HRR
   C) Moderate to vigorous; 40%–≥60% of HRR
   D) Vigorous; ≥60% of HRR

2. According to the most recent edition of the *ACSM's GETP*, the recommended frequency of exercise to achieve health benefits would optimally be
   A) 1–2 $d \cdot wk^{-1}$
   B) 2–3 $d \cdot wk^{-1}$
   C) 3–4 $d \cdot wk^{-1}$
   D) ≥5 $d \cdot wk^{-1}$

3. Metformin (Glucophage) is a
   A) Sulfonylureas drug for Type 1 DM
   B) Meglitinide drug for Type 2 DM
   C) Biguanide drug for Type 2 DM
   D) Glucagon-like peptide 1 receptor agonist drug for Type 2 DM

4. Based on your client's fasting blood levels,
   A) He currently has his medical conditions under adequate control.
   B) He may need to see his physician for follow-up of his current medication dosages.
   C) He may be noncompliant with taking his medications.
   D) Both B and C

5. Given the health information provided, your client very likely has
   A) Metabolic syndrome
   B) Pulmonary disease

C) Peripheral vascular disease
D) All of the above
E) Only A and B of the above

6. An appropriate target heart rate (THR) for your client on his *first* day of exercise would be
A) 96–102 bpm
B) 99–115 bpm
C) 115–124 bpm
D) 124–130 bpm

7. The use of ACSM's metabolic calculations for the treadmill would suggest which of the following workloads as appropriate for an initial workload for exercise training?
A) 5.0 mph and 4% grade
B) 1.5 mph and 2% grade
C) 3.0 mph and 2% grade
D) 3.3 mph and 7% grade

8. Muscle strengthening and flexibility exercises for this client should include _____ d · wk^{-1} at a _____ intensity.
A) 4–5; moderate
B) 6–7; light

C) 2–3; moderate
D) 1–2; vigorous

9. Resistance exercise training has been shown to
A) Enhance insulin sensitivity.
B) Diminish glucose tolerance.
C) Decrease total fat-free mass (FFM).
D) Increase insulin resistance.

10. According to the most recent edition of the *ACSM's GETP*, what would your recommended weekly MET-minute exercise prescription be for your client?
A) ≥100–500 MET-min · wk^{-1}
B) ≥2,000–4,000 MET-min · wk^{-1}
C) ≥500–1,000 MET-min · wk^{-1}
D) ≤200–400 MET-min · wk^{-1}

11. What questions or recommendations will you have for your client prior to developing his exercise prescription?

12. What would you tell your client about the exercise benefits for those with his medical conditions?

CASE STUDY 4: STEVE
Author: Joselyn M. Rodriguez, MSH

You are a CEP in an outpatient cardiopulmonary rehabilitation department at a hospital. Steve is a 66-year-old male patient who currently weighs 145 lb and is 70 in. in height. He was referred by his physician to participate in your monitored phase II cardiac rehabilitation program. Steve is a current smoker. He has smoked two packs a day for the past 50 years. He stated that his father was a smoker and suffered a stroke at the age of 54 years. During his initial evaluation, several measurements were attained and a recent report of fasting blood levels was discussed.

WC: 38 in.

Resting vitals: HR$_{rest}$ = 78 bpm, resting BP = 150/82 mm Hg (left arm) and 144/76 mm Hg (right arm)

Peripheral capillary oxygen saturation (SpO$_2$): 93% (on room air)

Fasting blood levels:

Glucose (mg · dL^{-1})	89
Total cholesterol (mg · dL^{-1})	195
LDL (mg · dL^{-1})	129
HDL-C (mg · dL^{-1})	43
Triglycerides (mg · dL^{-1})	147

He is currently taking an angiotensin-converting enzyme (ACE) inhibitor (ramipril), a platelet inhibitor (clopidogrel), and a statin (pravastatin) to treat his hypertension, prevent formation of clots, and treat his dyslipidemia, respectively. He states that he has not been exercising for several years due to cramping and burning sensation in his calf muscles with exertion. He was recently hospitalized for an inferior wall myocardial infarction (MI), for which he was submitted

(Continued)

CASE STUDY 4: STEVE (Continued)

to a cardiac catheterization and had his RCA stented. Steve was administered a physician-supervised modified treadmill GXT 1 week after his event. The GXT consisted of walking at a constant speed of 2.0 mph, increasing the grade 2.0% every 2 min. Steve's test was terminated due to sharp bilateral burning pain in his calf muscles (4 on the intermittent claudication [IC] scale at the sixth minute). Note: IC scale is a 1–4 scale. His maximum HR and BP were measured at 110 bpm and 182/78 mm Hg, respectively. His ankle/brachial systolic pressure index (ABI) at the completion of the test was 0.66 versus his ABI of 0.76 at rest (pretest). Steve had no silent or clinical signs of myocardial ischemia during the duration of the GXT. His estimated maximal oxygen consumption was 3.6 METs using ACSM's walking treadmill metabolic calculations (having stopped the test at 2.0 mph and 4.0% after completing this stage).

Steve: Case Study 4 Questions

1. Steve was administered a 12-lead ECG during his recent hospitalization. Which leads would display ST elevation for an inferior wall MI?
   A) I, aVL, V_5, V_6
   B) V_1–V_4
   C) II, III, aVF
   D) None of the above

2. Steve's medical history, fasting blood levels, and GXT results indicate that he most likely has
   A) Congestive heart failure.
   B) Chronic obstructive pulmonary disease (COPD).
   C) Peripheral arterial disease (PAD).
   D) Aortic stenosis.

3. Prior to ending Steve's GXT as a result of a rating of 4 on the IC scale, he experienced bilateral calf pain/burning that he rated as a 3 on the IC scale at minute 4. As a CEP, how would you go about determining exercise intensity for Steve?
   A) <10 beats below is maximum HR
   B) 40%–59% HRR or $\dot{V}O_2R$, allowing him to walk until he reaches an IC pain rating of 3
   C) RPE of 16
   D) Cannot be determined from the data given

4. What type of modality would be most appropriate for this patient?
   A) Water aerobics
   B) Interval training exercise bike protocol
   C) Rowing machine interval training protocol
   D) IC treadmill protocol

5. As a CEP, what would your recommendation be regarding aerobic exercise frequency for this particular patient?
   A) 2–4 d · wk^{-1}
   B) 3–5 d · wk^{-1}
   C) 5–7 d · wk^{-1}
   D) None of the above

6. What would Steve's caloric expenditure be if he walked 15 min at his estimated maximal oxygen consumption?
   A) 44 kcal
   B) 63 kcal
   C) 71 kcal
   D) Cannot be determined from data given

7. What was Steve's measured systolic BP in his posterior tibial artery if his ABI was 0.66 at the end of his GXT?
   A) 110 mm Hg
   B) 112 mm Hg
   C) 120 mm Hg
   D) Cannot be determined from the data given

8. What is this patient's pack per year history of smoking?
   A) 40
   B) 75
   C) 100
   D) 125

9. Steve is walking on a treadmill during one of his monitored cardiac rehabilitation sessions and develops bilateral cramping and burning sensation in his calves at minute 6 of his exercise time. He tells the CEP that he has reached a

pain rating of 3 on the IC scale. The CEP should

A) Cease exercise to allow ischemic pain to resolve before resuming exercise.

B) Continue to have Steve walk from the remainder of his exercise time.

C) Switch Steve from the treadmill to the leg cycle ergometer at the point of his reporting of ischemic pain.

D) None of the above.

10. Which of the following is a *primary goal* to effectively treat and manage PAD?

A) Controlling his hypertension through medications and behavior modification

B) Quit smoking

C) Lowering lipids

D) Both A and B

11. Which of the following best describes the benefits of drug-eluting stents as compared to bare-metal stents?

A) Release antibiotics preventing infection.

B) Release anticoagulants preventing clot reformation.

C) Inhibit cell proliferation and inflammation reducing restenosis.

D) Both B and C.

12. Discuss FITT recommendations for aerobic exercise for individuals with PAD.

13. Discuss the importance of using a modified treadmill GXT versus Bruce protocol for this patient.

14. Resistance exercise is recommended to enhance and maintain muscular strength and endurance. Use the FITT principle of exercise prescription to design a resistance exercise regimen for Steve.

15. Identify barriers that may impact exercise compliance for this patient.

16. Explain strategies to overcome these barriers and discuss goals for effective management and treatment of PAD.

CASE STUDY 5: NANCY
Author: Donald M. Cummings, PhD

You are a CEP in a cardiopulmonary rehabilitation department at a medical facility. A new patient, Nancy, a 58-year-old female, has been referred by her physician. Her physician would like her to participate in a 12-week exercise rehabilitation program due to her risk factor profile for cardiovascular disease (CVD) and a positive GXT result that was positive for ST depression. A brief synopsis of Nancy's medical history, fasting blood laboratory report, and recent GXT results is provided in the following section.

Medical History

Nancy is a 58-year-old female who has a height of 5 ft 3 in., weighs 158 lb, (28.05 kg $\cdot$ m^{-2} BMI), and has a WC of 36 in. She reports a family history of CVD on her father's side. She reports him having a three-vessel bypass at the age of 58 years and was deceased at the age of 75 years. Her mother is still living at the age of 75 years with a 20-year history of Type 2 DM. She reports that she has one older sibling, a sister, who underwent a percutaneous coronary intervention (PCI) with a stent in her right coronary artery (RCA) at the age of 60 years. Nancy reports a smoking history of one pack per day for 20 years. She claims that she has not smoked for 15 years. She is currently being treated for hypertension. She has been prescribed a diuretic (spironolactone 50 mg twice a day) and a calcium channel blocker (amlodipine 100 mg once a day). She states that she saw her physician because she desires to lose weight by diet and participation in an exercise program. Nancy denies any other significant medical history. She was referred by her physician for blood analysis and a GXT.

Blood Laboratory Analysis (Fasting)

Glucose	110 mg · dL⁻¹
Urea nitrogen	12 mg · dL⁻¹
Creatinine	1.1 mg · dL⁻¹
Sodium	136 mmol · L⁻¹
Potassium	3.6 mmol · L⁻¹
Chloride	105 mmol · L⁻¹
Carbon dioxide	28 mmol · L⁻¹
Calcium	8.8 mg · dL⁻¹
Cholesterol	184 mg · dL⁻¹
Triglycerides	185 mg · dL⁻¹
HDL-C	46 mg · dL⁻¹
Glycolated hemoglobin (HbA1C)	45 mmol · mol⁻¹
Albumin	3.7 g · dL⁻¹
Aspartate aminotransferase (AST)	36 U · L⁻¹
Alanine aminotransferase (ALT)	42 U · L⁻¹
Alkaline phosphatase (ALKP)	98 U · L⁻¹
Total bilirubin	0.6 mg · dL⁻¹
Unconjugated bilirubin	0.7 mg · dL⁻¹
Direct bilirubin	0 mg · dL⁻¹
LDL	101 mg · dL⁻¹
Very low-density lipoprotein (VLDL)	37 mg · dL⁻¹
Cholesterol/HDL	4.0 mg · dL⁻¹

GXT Results	Name	Nancy
	Age	58 years
	HR$_{rest}$	78 bpm
	Resting electrocardiogram (ECG)	Normal sinus rhythm (NSR)
	Resting BP	
	Supine	138/84 mm Hg
	Standing	140/84 mm Hg

Time (min)	Speed (mph)	Grade (%)	Heart Rate (HR) (bpm)	BP (mm Hg)	Rating of Perceived Exertion (RPE)	Metabolic Equivalent (MET)	Symptoms (scales all out of 4)	ECG
1	1.7	10	88				1+ shortness of breath (SOB)	Sinus rhythm
2	1.7	10	94				1+ SOB	0.5 mm horizontal ST depression
3	1.7	10	107	154/84	14	4.7	2+ SOB	0.5 mm horizontal ST depression
4	2.5	12	125				2+ SOB	1.0 mm horizontal ST depression
5	2.5	12	136				2+ SOB	1.0 mm horizontal ST depression

Time (min)	Speed (mph)	Grade (%)	Heart Rate (HR) (bpm)	BP (mm Hg)	Rating of Perceived Exertion (RPE)	Metabolic Equivalent (MET)	Symptoms (scales all out of 4)	ECG
6	2.5	12	150	176/84	19	7.0	3+ SOB	1.0 mm horizontal ST depression
7	Recovery	Supine	136	182/84			2+ SOB	1.0 mm horizontal ST depression
8	Recovery	Supine	115	166/84			2+ SOB	0.5 mm horizontal ST depression
9	Recovery	Supine	107	148/84			2+ SOB	0.5 mm horizontal ST depression
10	Recovery	Supine	94	136/82			1+ SOB	Normalized ST
11	Recovery	Supine	79	136/80			1+ SOB	NSR
12	Recovery	Supine	68	132/80			SOB resolved	Sinus rhythm

Nancy: Case Study 5 Questions

1. According to the most recent edition of the *ACSM's GETP* and based on Nancy's medical history and GXT results, the approximate maximum "safe" goal-oriented exercise MET level she should exercise would be approximately
   A) 2.5 METs.
   B) 3.5 METs.
   C) 4.5 METs.
   D) 5.5 METs.
   E) 6.5 METs.

2. According to the most recent edition of the *ACSM's GETP* and based on Nancy's GXT results, a good index of exercise intensity would be an exercise RPE on the Borg 6–20 scale of approximately
   A) 12.
   B) 14.
   C) 16.
   D) 18.
   E) 20.

3. According to the most recent edition of the *ACSM's GETP*, which classes of medications prescribed to Nancy may have adverse side effects during exercise?
   A) Diuretics only may have adverse effects during exercise testing or programming.
   B) Dihydropyridine calcium channel blockers only may have adverse effects during exercise testing or programming.

C) Both of Nancy's medications may have adverse effects during exercise testing or programming.
   D) Neither of Nancy's medications have possible reported adverse effects during exercise testing or programming.

4. According to the most recent edition of the *ACSM's GETP*, which classes of medications prescribed to Nancy may have an effect on her HR during exercise?
   A) Diuretic
   B) Dihydropyridine calcium channel blockers
   C) All of the medications that Nancy is prescribed may effect HR during exercise.
   D) None of Nancy's medication classes may have an effect on her HR during exercise.

5. Assuming that the GXT is a true-positive test, the use of ACSM's metabolic calculations for the treadmill would suggest which of the following as a maximal safe workload for Nancy's exercise training?
   A) 2.0 mph and 7.0% grade
   B) 3.0 mph and 3.0% grade
   C) 4.0 mph and 1.0% grade
   D) 5.0 mph and 0.0% grade
   E) Either A or B would be an appropriate treadmill workload for Nancy.

(Continued)

ACSM-CEP

CASE STUDY 5: NANCY (Continued)

6. Assuming that the GXT is a true-positive test, the use of ACSM's metabolic calculations for the cycle ergometer would suggest which of the following as a maximal safe workload for Nancy's exercise training?
   A) 275 Kgm/min
   B) 350 Kgm/min
   C) 550 Kgm/min
   D) 700 Kgm/min
   E) Cannot be determined from the data given

7. Based on Nancy's medical history and according to the most recent edition of the *ACSM's GETP*, what frequency of exercise would you recommend?
   A) $2-3 \text{ d} \cdot \text{wk}^{-1}$
   B) $3-5 \text{ d} \cdot \text{wk}^{-1}$
   C) $3-7 \text{ d} \cdot \text{wk}^{-1}$
   D) $5-7 \text{ d} \cdot \text{wk}^{-1}$

8. According to the most recent edition of the *ACSM's GETP*, a resistance program may be initiated for Nancy incorporating which range of repetitions based on her % 1-RM?
   A) One repetition maximum (1-RM)
   B) 4–6 RM
   C) 6–10 RM
   D) 10–15 RM
   E) Any of the above levels of RM would be appropriate for Nancy.

9. Based the medical history, laboratory report, and GXT, which of the following pathologies would *not* be a consideration when developing and exercise program for Nancy?
   A) Prediabetes
   B) Coronary heart disease (CHD)

   C) Obesity
   D) Hypertension
   E) All of the above pathologies should be a consideration for Nancy's exercise program.

10. Assuming the GXT was a maximum test and based on the maximum exercise MET level as determined in question 1, at what approximate percentage of reserve volume of oxygen consumed per unit of time ($\dot{V}O_2R$) is Nancy working?
    A) 40%
    B) 50%
    C) 60%
    D) 70%
    E) 80%

11. Based upon the information provided in the medical history and the results of the GXT, are there any indications that this may be a false-positive test for obstructive coronary artery disease (CAD)? If you believed the test to be a false-positive test, would you change the exercise prescription you have prescribed for Nancy?

12. The *ACSM's GETP* give guidelines for exercise intensity, duration, frequency, mode, and progression. Based on the information that you have been provided for this client, outline considerations in your development of Nancy's initial exercise program in order to achieve the most favorable outcomes and why?

CASE STUDY 6: JOE
Author: Joselyn M. Rodriguez, MSH

You are a CEP in the cardiopulmonary department of a hospital. Joe is a new patient who has been referred by his physician to participate in your monitored phase II cardiac rehabilitation program. An initial review of his medical history states that he is a 52-year-old male who currently weighs 253 lb and is 72 in. in height ($34.3 \text{ kg} \cdot \text{m}^{-2}$ BMI). He reports a family history of his father having died from a heart attack at the age of 50 years. He quit smoking 4 month ago after having smoked one pack per day for 34 years. During his initial evaluation appointment, his resting vitals were measured as HR$_{rest}$ = 68 bpm, and his resting BP for both right and left arm were 148/84 mm Hg and 142/76 mm Hg, respectively. His WC was 50 in. His body fat (BF) percentage was measured as 34% using a bioelectrical impedance analysis scale. A recent report of his fasting blood values read as follows: Glucose = 110 mg · dL^{-1}, total cholesterol = 203 mg · dL^{-1}, LDL = 137 mg · dL^{-1}, HDL-C = 44 mg · dL^{-1}, and triglycerides = 168 mg · dL^{-1}. He is currently taking metoprolol and atorvastatin to treat his hypertension and dyslipidemia. Joe claims that he attains most of his physical activity through his job as a mover, which is why he has not been exercising regularly. He states that he has been experiencing tightness in his chest on the job for the past several months. His physician referred him to have a GXT (Bruce protocol). A positive GXT indicated a need for a cardiac catheterization, which confirmed a 78% and 75% occlusion of the circumflex and RCAs, both requiring stenting. His ejection fraction (EF) was determined to be 52%. He refrained from taking medication prior to his GXT.

GXT Results:

Name	Joe
Age	52 years
HR$_{rest}$	64 bpm
Resting ECG	NSR
Resting BP	
SUPINE	146/82 mm Hg
STANDING	140/72 mm Hg

Time (min)	Speed (mph)	Grade (%)	HR (bpm)	BP (mm Hg)	RPE	MET	Symptoms (scales are all out of 4)	ECG
1	1.7	10	82					NSR
2	1.7	10	94					NSR
3	1.7	10	114	170/74	11	4.7		NSR
4	2.5	12	126					NSR
5	2.5	12	136					NSR, 2 premature ventricular contraction (PVC)
6	2.5	12	144	182/84	15	7.0	2+ chest pain (CP) 1+ SOB	1.0 mm horizontal ST depression
7	3.4	14	150				2+ CP 1+ SOB	1.0 mm horizontal ST depression, 1 PVC
8	3.4	14	154				2+ CP 1+ SOB	1.5 mm horizontal ST depression
9	3.4	14	158	198/92	18	10.1	3+ CP 2+ SOB	1.5 mm horizontal ST depression, 2 PVC
10	Recovery	Supine	150	184/84			3+ CP 2+ SOB	1.5 mm horizontal ST depression
11	Recovery	Supine	138	178/82			2+ CP 1+ SOB	1.5 mm horizontal ST depression
12	Recovery	Supine	120	164/78			1+ SOB	1.0 mm horizontal ST depression
13	Recovery	Supine	100	156/76				NSR
14	Recovery	Supine	74	148/80				NSR

ACSM-CEP

CASE STUDY 6: JOE (Continued)

Joe: Case Study 6 Questions

1. According to Joe's body fat percentage, calculate his FFM.
   A) 21 kg
   B) 39 kg
   C) 76 kg
   D) None of the above

2. According to Joe's GXT results, which method for prescribing exercise intensity would be most appropriate?
   A) RPE of 11–16 on a scale of 6–20
   B) 40%–80% of HRR
   C) HR below the ischemic threshold (<10 beats)
   D) None of the above

3. Determine an appropriate index of exercise intensity with reference to question 2.
   A) 102–140 bpm
   B) No >134 bpm
   C) 112 bpm
   D) Cannot be determined from the data given

4. According to the most recent edition of the *ACSM's GETP* and Joe's GXT results, what maximal workload would be most suitable for exercise training on a leg cycle ergometer?
   A) 124 W
   B) 157 W
   C) 146 W
   D) Cannot be determined from the data given

5. Joe wants to drop his body fat percentage to 22%. Calculate his target body weight.
   A) 167 lb
   B) 213 lb
   C) 236 lb
   D) Cannot be determined from the data given

6. During Joe's cardiac catheterization, his EF was measured to be 52%. Under which category does his EF fall under?
   A) Normal
   B) Below normal
   C) Congestive heart failure
   D) None of the above

7. According to the table depicting Joe's GXT results, under which circumstance was his test terminated?
   A) Hypertensive response
   B) Excessive ST depression
   C) Development of bundle branch block
   D) Moderately severe angina

8. What would Joe's estimated maximum exercise MET level be based on his GXT results?
   A) 6 METs
   B) 7 METs
   C) 8 METs
   D) 9 METs

9. According to Joe's GXT results, which of the following would be a safe maximal workload for exercising on a treadmill?
   A) 3.0 mph and 2.5% grade
   B) 3.2 mph and 3% grade
   C) 3.6 mph and 4.5% grade
   D) 4.0 mph and 5% grade

10. Estimate Joe's caloric expenditure if he is exercising at his maximal safe workload on a treadmill for a duration of 30 min.
    A) 261 kcal
    B) 288 kcal
    C) 362 kcal
    D) 461 kcal

11. Explain why outpatient cardiopulmonary rehabilitation centers use a multidisciplinary team approach.

12. Sustained weight loss is one of Joe's goals after the completion of monitored phase II cardiac rehabilitation. What adjustments in Joe's exercise prescription are necessary?

13. BMI is a common method of assessing body composition. Discuss the reasons why this method is recommended for Joe's particular case.

14. Explain why the Bruce protocol was chosen as the primary method of GXT for this patient.

15. Joe's job is very physical and involves heavy lifting. Discuss how you would go about prescribing resistance exercise for Joe.

CASE STUDY 7: MR. KYLE
Author: David E. Verrill, MS
Author's Certifications: ACSM-CEP, EIM3

Mr. Kyle, a 63-year-old bank executive, is entering your Phase II cardiac rehabilitation program 3 weeks following an anterior myocardial infarction (STEMI) and stent placements in his left anterior descending (LAD) and left circumflex (LCX) arteries. He also has intermittent periods of atrial fibrillation with slow-to-moderate ventricular rates. A predischarge hospital resting adenosine radionuclide study showed improved areas of myocardial perfusion in the anterior, lateral and apical walls of his left ventricle. He began smoking at age 17 and continues to smoke one and a half packs a day. He was a recreational exerciser until 3 years ago, at which time he had hurt his back when he fell off a ladder at home. Since then, he has gained weight, continued smoking, been diagnosed with hypertension and dyslipidemia, and led a sedentary lifestyle. He is somewhat noncompliant taking his medications. He has a "Type A" personality and refuses to relax at any time (he has an upper level corporate position). The only symptom of exercise intolerance he reports is dyspnea when walking up hills. His brother died of a myocardial infarction at age 60. He also has developed low back pain from a bulging disk compressing a nerve at L-5.

Mr. Kyle's weight is 218 lb and height is 70 in.. His body fast measured by skinfolds was estimated at 35% and his waist circumference is 44 in.. His coronary catheterization report revealed the following information prior to his percutaneous transluminal coronary angioplasty (PTCA) with stent placement procedure: LAD 85% lesion prior to the first diagonal branch; left circumflex 90% proximal lesion; minimal lesions to branches of LAD; nondominant RCA with minimal plaque; ejection fraction = 45%. Upon examination, his resting heart and blood pressure were 76 beats per minute (bpm) and 148/82 mm Hg, respectively. Fasting blood values were measured 2 weeks ago and were as follows: Total cholesterol: 244 mg · dL^{-1} (6.3 mmol/L); low-density lipoprotein cholesterol: 178 mg · dL^{-1} (4.6 mmol/L); high-density lipoprotein cholesterol: 34 mg · dL^{-1} (0.9 mmol/L); triglycerides: 202 mg · dL^{-1} (2.3 mmol/L); glucose: 120 mg · dL^{-1} (6.8 mmol/L). Currently, he is taking the following medications: Diltiazem (Cardizem) 120 mg, twice daily; furosemide (Lasix) 20 mg twice daily; atorvastatin (Lipitor) 20 mg twice daily; nicotinic Acid (Niacin) 500 mg four times daily; aspirin (Ecotrin) 325 mg once daily; digoxin (Lanoxin) 750 mg once daily; Coumadin (warfarin) 2.5 mg once daily; Nitroglycerine spray as needed. Mr. Kyle reports not taking Cardizem or digoxin prior to his graded exercise test per physician request. The following is his cardiac rehabilitation entry Graded Exercise Test (GXT) data (summarized):

Modified Bruce 0% Protocol	Workload	Blood pressure (mm Hg)	Heart rate (b/min)	SaO$_2$ (%)	METS (est.)	Angina (1-4 scale)	Treadmill Time	RPE (6-20 scale)
Rest	—	148/82	72	94%	1.0	None	—	6
PeakExercise	1.7 mph, 10% grade	202/96	142	84%	4.6	1+	9:00	19
Active Recovery	1.5 mph, 2% grade	164/86	118	88%	2.6	None	—	12

Mr. Kyle has been given medical clearance from his physician to begin exercise and education in your cardiac rehabilitation program.

Please answer the following questions pertaining to the previously mentioned case.

Mr. Kyle: Case Study 7 Questions

1. Mr. Kyle takes diltiazem (Cardizem) for his cardiovascular disease. This drug
   A) May reduce resting and exercise heart rate and blood pressure.
   B) Is likely to cause a false-positive ECG during a graded exercise test.
   C) Is a commonly used β-blocker.

CASE STUDY 7: MR. KYLE (Continued)

D) Is a combined calcium channel blocker and α_1 antagonist.

E) Is rarely given for atrial fibrillation.

2. Mr. Kyle had an 85% blockage in his left anterior descending artery prior to his PTCA and stenting procedure. Which region(s) of the heart does this artery supply?

A) The anterior wall of the left ventricle

B) The intraventricular septum

C) The SA node in the right atrium

D) The entire right ventricle

E) Only A and B of the above

3. Mr. Kyle has a resting EF of 45%. According to the most recent edition of the *ACSM's GETP*, what level of cardiovascular risk would he fall under with regard to exercise training?

A) Lowest risk

B) Moderate risk

C) Highest risk

D) None of the above

4. According to the most recent edition of the *ACSM's GETP*, when prescribing his exercise the optimal *initial* intensity of exercise for cardiopulmonary fitness benefits would be set at

A) 10%–<20% HRR or $\dot{V}O_2R$, 1–<2 METS, RPE 7–9, an intensity that causes minimal increases in HR and breathing.

B) 30%–<40% HRR or $\dot{V}O_2R$, 2–<3 METS, RPE 9-11, an intensity that causes slight increases in HR and breathing.

C) 40%–<60% HRR or $\dot{V}O_2R$, 3–<6 METS, RPE 12-13, an intensity that causes noticeable increases in HR and breathing.

D) ≥60% HRR or $\dot{V}O_2R$, ≥6 METS, RPE ≥14, an intensity that causes substantial increases in HR and breathing.

5. Mr. Kyle has a smoking history of _____ pack years.

A) 30

B) 40

C) 50

D) 69

6. During your initial assessment, you give Mr. Kyle various surveys to assess his Quality of Life (QOL), dietary habits and depression. One commonly used survey that assesses QOL in cardiac rehabilitation participants is

A) The Medical Outcomes Study Short Form-36 (SF-36)

B) The Patient Health Questionnaire (PHQ-9)

C) The Physical Activity Readiness Questionnaire (PAR-Q)

D) The Center for Epidemiologic Studies Depression Scale (CES-D)

E) The Zung Depression Survey

7. Mr. Kyle's Body Mass Index (BMI) classifies him as _____ by Expert Panel normative data.

A) Underweight

B) Normal weight

C) Overweight

D) Obese (class I)

E) Obese (class II)

8. An initial exercise prescription for Mr. Kyle would include which of the following recommendations?

A) Level treadmill walking at 2.5 mph at a heart rate of 128–136 bpm and an RPE of 14–17.

B) Rowing ergometer exercise at 15 W at a heart rate of 98–106 bpm and an RPE of 8–11.

C) Cycle ergometer exercise at 0.5 kg (180 kg/min) at a HR of 114-128 and an RPE of 11–16.

D) Stepping on a 5-in. bench, 20 steps/min, at a heart rate of 122–134 at an RPE of 16–18.

9. According to the most recent edition of the *ACSM's GETP*, the recommended frequency of exercise to achieve health benefits for Mr. Kyle would be

A) 1–2 d · wk^{-1}

B) 23 d · wk^{-1}

C) At least 3 d · wk^{-1}, but preferably most days of the week

D) Twice daily, 7 d · wk^{-1}

10. Mr. Kyle currently weighs 218 lb. (99 kg) and has a body fat level of ~35%. He would like to lose weight to achieve a realistic goal % body fat of ~28%. What is Mr. Kyle's goal body weight at this ideal body fat percentage?
    A) 204 lb (92.5 kg)
    B) 197 lb (89.4 kg)
    C) 182 lb (82.6 kg)
    D) 176 lb (79.8 kg)

11. What two undiagnosed diseases (comorbidities) that were not discussed between Mr. Kyle and his physician might Mr. Kyle have at the present time? How would you address these undiagnosed conditions?

12. How would you address Mr. Kyle's noncompliance with his medicines, his continuation of smoking and his level of stress?

13. List at least six purposes for performing graded exercise testing after acute myocardial infarction.

14. Studies show that lack of muscular strength and endurance is of particular concern for the post-MI patient. What type of resistive exercise training regimen and modalities would you recommend for Mr. Kyle during his stay in your cardiac rehabilitation program?

15. Mr. Kyle has intermittent periods of atrial fibrillation. However, this appears to be under control with his current medications. Which three medications is Mr. Kyle taking for his atrial fibrillation? What are some physiologic concerns for the cardiac patient with atrial fibrillation? What are some exercise concerns for the patient with atrial fibrillation?

CASE STUDY 8: SHERYL
Author: Hayden Riley, MS
Author's Certifications: ACSM-CEP

You are a certified clinical exercise physiologist with a new patient starting in your pulmonary rehab class today. As you review her medical records and intake assessment, you gather the following information about the patient:

Sheryl is a 73-year-old female with a past medical history of COPD, pulmonary HTN, Vtach, osteoarthritis, anxiety, depression, and thyroid CA s/p removal and radiation in 2012. Sheryl is currently a "light" cigarette smoker as she reports smoking about 5 CPD. She is on 2 L of continuous flow at night, but she does not require supplemental O_2 at rest or with exercise.

Below are the patient's latest PFT results and baseline 6MWT findings.

Pulmonary Function Laboratory Results: November 1, 2019

Spirometry at BTPS		ATS ✔	Pre Bronchodilator					✔	Post Bronchodilator		
		Actual	Predicted	% Pred	CI Range				Actual	% Pred	% Change
FVC	L	1.95	2.59	75	1.78	3.40	N		2.32	90	19
FEV$_1$	L	1.08	2.03	53	1.39	2.67	A	m	1.35	67	25
FEV$_1$/FVC	%	55	77	71	68	....	A		58	75	5

(Continued)

CASE STUDY 8: SHERYL (Continued)

6MWT: November 20, 2019			
	Rest	Peak Exercise	Recovery
HR	66	113	80
BP	100/60	Not obtained	130/70
SpO$_2$	98% on room air	91% on room air	94% on room air
Distance	1250 with 2 breaks		
MPH	2.4		
METS	2.9		

Prior to initiating any exercise equipment, you ask Sheryl to walk 3 laps around the track to warm up. After a few minutes, you notice that the patients breathing is labored. You have Sheryl sit down so you can do a quick assessment. You ask Sheryl how she is doing and notice that she can barely say "I'm fine." Sheryl reports and RPE of 2 on a 1–10 scale and an RPD of 4/10 (somewhat severe shortness of breath).

HR: 120 bpm, SpO$_2$: 88%, BP: 128/68

Sheryl: Case Study 8 Questions

1. What is Sheryl's GOLD classification of disease severity?
   A) Mild
   B) Moderate
   C) Severe
   D) Very Severe

2. What would be the most appropriate method for prescribing exercise intensity for this patient?
   A) 50%–80% Max HR
   B) 50%–80% HRR
   C) RHR + 30 bpm
   D) Rate of perceived exertion and/or dyspnea

3. What possible modifications would you make to Sheryl's exercise prescription?
   A) Implement 20–30 min of continuous weight-bearing exercise.
   B) Implement 20–30 min of continuous non-weight-bearing exercise.
   C) Accumulate 20–30 min of intermittent weight-bearing exercise.
   D) Accumulate 20–30 min of intermittent non-weight-bearing exercise.

4. This would be an appropriate time to teach the patient about which of the following concepts?
   A) Rating of perceived exertion/dyspnea
   B) The talk test
   C) Pursed lip breathing
   D) All the above

5. How would you best document this encounter?
   A) After several minutes of walking, the patient reported that she was "fine" however, I did not think she was. Patient sat until she stabilized.
   B) Patients heart rate is in the 120-s walking the track. She was walking fast but I do not think this explains the whole reason for the heart rate increase.
   C) Patient experienced increased dyspnea (4/10) with weight-bearing exercise. Exercise prescription modified to reduce rating of perceived dyspnea score to desired range (2–3/10).
   D) Pt had RPD score of 4. SpO$_2$ okay. HR elevated, BP within normal limits.

6. What medication would you ask Sheryl to bring with her to PR in the future?
   A) Nitroglycerin
   B) Metoprolol
   C) Albuterol
   D) Metformin

7. Sheryl tells you that she lives independently but she is struggling with ADL's, specifically stair-climbing while carrying groceries, due to SOB/DOE. Explain how you would develop an exercise program for Sheryl that will help her to meet her goals.

CASE STUDY 9: JIM
Author: Hayden Riley, MS
Author's Certifications: ACSM-CEP

You are a certified clinical exercise physiologist working in cardiac rehab. Today, you are preparing to perform an intake exam on a patient that was referred to your program. The patient, Jim, is a 70-year-old male (DOB July 12, 1946). He is 5'8", 160 lb, with NKDA and a past medical history significant for arthritis, HTN, and a PPM placed in 2016. From the patient's electronic medical record (EMR), you gather that he went to the local ER with chest discomfort on December 30, 2019. Upon arrival, an EKG was performed which showed a paced rhythm at a rate of 63 bpm and evidence of a right bundle-branch-block. Labs were drawn, select results are shown in the following section. Based upon the results, the patient was sent to the cath lab. Per the catheterization report, the patient had 60% occlusion of his mid-LAD, 70% occlusion of his mid RCA, and an estimated ejection fraction (EF) of 55%. Two overlapping drug-eluding stents (DES) were placed in the mid RCA. Following the cath, the patient was asymptomatic and stable (BP: 118/80, HR: 63, SpO_2: 96%). The patient was discharged home the following day.

Jim arrived for his intake with you today, January 13, 2020, and you start the appointment by reconciling his medications in his EMR. The patient reports that he is prescribed: Metoprolol 25 mg extended release and clopidogrel 75 mg; however, he is only taking them one to two times per week as opposed to daily. The patient is also taking lisinopril 2.5 mg/daily, aspirin 81 mg/daily, and one other medication that he cannot recall. Jim is also prescribed a 21 mg nicotine patch for smoking cessation; however, he has told you that he continues to smoke 2 packs of cigarettes per day.

Troponin	10.9
CHO	257
TRIG	207
HDL	36
LDL	181
Ratio	7.1
A1C	5.2

After gathering the patient's medical history, you will establish the patients baseline Individual treatment plan (ITP).

Jim: Case Study 9 Questions

1. Based upon Jim's hospital encounter on December 28, 2019, what do you think is the patients referring diagnosis for cardiac rehab?
   A) STEMI
   B) NSTEMI
   C) CABG
   D) Heart Failure

2. Clopidogrel is a/an
   A) Antiplatelet drug.
   B) β-blocker.
   C) ACE inhibitor.
   D) Antiarrhythmic agent.

3. Based upon the patients' medical history and lab results, the additional medication Jim is taking would most likely be which of the following:
   A) Omeprazole
   B) Metformin
   C) Atorvastatin
   D) Atenolol

4. Jim is scheduled to perform a stress test tomorrow, January 14, 2020. Based upon your assessment, what is the most appropriate course of action?
   A) Perform a TUG test to assess the patient's ability to perform a GXT.
   B) Suggest a modified Bruce protocol considering the patients age and history of arthritis.
   C) Reschedule the patients stress test considering his cardiac event was less than 1 month ago.
   D) Cancel the stress test until the patient is consistently taking his medications as prescribed.

(Continued)

CASE STUDY 9: JIM (Continued)

5. Which of the following is *not* a mandatory component of the cardiac ITP?
   A) Exercise assessment
   B) Nutrition assessment
   C) Risk factor assessment
   D) Oxygen assessment
   E) Psychosocial assessment

6. Part of developing an ITP requires the development of individualized, multidisciplinary goals. At baseline, what goals would you find appropriate for this patient based upon the information given?
   A) Weight loss, smoking cessation, and improved exercise tolerance
   B) Smoking cessation, diabetes management, and lipid management
   C) Lipid management, smoking cessation, and weight loss
   D) Lipid management, smoking cessation, and improved exercise tolerance

7. Considering that the patient is smoking 2 PPD, you decide that you are going to use your motivational interviewing (MI) skills to elicit a conversation about smoking cessation. Which of the following is *not* a component of MI?
   A) Affirmation
   B) Reflective listening
   C) Decisional balance
   D) Open-ended questions

8. What are the five most prescribed classes of medications following an acute cardiac event and/or procedure?

9. Why should you be concerned about Jim's noncompliance with his medication regiment?

CASE STUDY 10: KIMBERLY
DOMAIN IV: LEADERSHIP AND COUNSELING
Author: Shala E. Davis, PhD, FACSM

Kimberly is a 43-year-old woman (65 in. tall and 159 lb), who is an office manager at a large shipping company. She is divorced and has two school-aged children (8 and 11 years old). Kimberly has no known cardiovascular, pulmonary, or metabolic disease but considers herself to be highly deconditioned. Kimberly has been diagnosed with fibromyalgia syndrome (FMS). She works 45 h · wk^{-1} and commutes 30 min each way daily. Her medications are limited to over-the-counter sleep aids and nonsteroidal anti-inflammatory drugs (NSAIDs). Kimberly has initiated multiple exercise programs with little success over the past 2 years and complains of low motivation and depression-like symptoms.

Kimberly: Case Study 10 Questions

1. Which of the following are common symptoms of clients diagnosed with FMS?
   A) Sleep disturbances
   B) Undue fatigue
   C) Diffuse soft tissue pain
   D) Depression
   E) All of the above

2. FMS symptoms may be increased by which of the following?
   A) Emotional stress
   B) Low-intensity exercise
   C) Poor sleep
   D) Both A and B
   E) Both A and C
   F) Both B and C

3. Which of the following theories related to exercise behavior is based on the principle that the person, behavior, and environment all influence future behavior?
   A) Transtheoretical model
   B) Social cognitive theory
   C) Health behavior model
   D) Self-determination model

4. Which of the following is not a strategy or strategies used to increase self-efficacy?
   A) Experiencing successful completion of tasks
   B) Modeling experiences
   C) Social persuasion
   D) Challenging self with difficult goals

5. Which of the following is not part of the SMART principles of goal setting?
   A) Goals should be realistic.
   B) Goals should have a reasonable time frame.
   C) Goals should be challenging.
   D) Goals should be specific.

6. Identify three barriers and elaborate on how each barrier impacts exercise compliance for this client.

7. Provide strategies to address the barriers identified.

8. How would you approach goal setting for this client?

CASE STUDY 11: PATIENT PRIVACY
Author: Mandy J. Van Hofwegen, BS
Author's Certifications: ACSM-CEP

When it comes to health care, protecting patients' privacy is a high priority. Health care providers have access to detailed, personal information about their patients. Keeping this information confidential is important, which is why in 1996, the federal government passed the Health Insurance Portability and Accountability Act (HIPAA). This led to the development of the Privacy Rule in 2000. The Privacy Rule established a set of national standards for the protection, use, and disclosure of certain health information by organizations as well as standards for the privacy rights of individuals.

A central aspect of the Privacy Rule is "minimum necessary" use. Organizations may share health information with others directly involved in the care or treatment of a patient but must only disclose the minimum amount of protected information to accomplish the intended purpose.

Health care organizations must develop policies and procedures to establish privacy practices within their facilities. They must then educate all health care providers in their organization and help them comply with HIPAA regulations. Organizations that violate HIPAA Privacy Rules are subject to monetary fines and civil or criminal charges.

Patient Privacy: Case Study 11 Questions

1. A nurse from a patient's primary care office calls your facility requesting a record of recent BP readings to see if a medication change is necessary for the patient. She also asks for an update on the patient's progress because she knows the patient personally and would like to give an update to her book club tonight. What should you do?
   A) Fax the requested BP readings and give her an updated report on his progress.
   B) Tell the nurse that you cannot give out any of that information.
   C) Fax the BP readings and let the nurse know that you may not give out other personal information on the patient's progress.
   D) Ask the nurse to contact the patient directly for all of the information requested.

2. True or false: The HIPAA Privacy Rule grants individuals the right to access other family member's health information without further consent.

(Continued)

ACSM-CEP

CASE STUDY 11: PATIENT PRIVACY (Continued)

3. A coworker calls you from home and states that he forgot to check for an e-mail from a physician regarding a patient before he left work. He asks you to log on to the computer using his passwords and check for the e-mail. He says it is okay because you know the patient's situation and the information that needs to be communicated from the physician. What should you do?

A) Put him on hold and ask another coworker to take the call.

B) Tell your coworker that you cannot share passwords, but you will call the physician office and obtain the information needed.

C) Log on to the computer using your coworkers passwords, get the information, and then ask your coworker to change his passwords the next time he works.

D) Contact the patient and see if the physician's office possibly contacted them.

4. A physician asks you to pull up a report on a mutual patient. He scans the room and sees that no one else is around. He then asks you to turn the computer toward him, now in public view, so he can see it. When he is finished discussing the report with you, he turns the computer back around.

A) True or false: This is a violation of the patient's privacy.

5. Which of the following information is considered to be protected under the Privacy Rule?

A) Names and addresses

B) Birthdates and social security numbers

C) Past, present, and future medical diagnoses

D) All of the above

6. A patient is graduating from your rehabilitation program today and asks for a photo of himself with your staff to share with his family and friends. Later that night, you check your social media account and see that he has posted this picture with the caption, "Thanks to the rehab facility for the helping me recover after my heart attack."

A) True or false: The patient has violated the Privacy Rule.

7. A coworker knows that she will be running late tomorrow morning and would like to get the patient charts out tonight that will be needed first thing in the morning. She wants to leave them on the desk overnight. This will save 10 extra minutes in the morning, and therefore, it will not matter if she is running late. What should you do?

A) Tell her that you cannot do that and offer to come in earlier to help out.

B) Help her get the charts out and organized for the morning.

C) Leave the charts on the desk with a note on each one stating "Confidential."

D) Tell her you don't think it's a good idea, but she can do what she thinks is best.

CASE STUDY 12: EMERGENCY PREPAREDNESS
Author: Shenelle E. Higbee, MS
Author's Certifications: ACSM-CEP, ACSM-EP

The benefits of regular exercise outweigh the risks. Exercise professionals in clinical and fitness facilities have an obligation to provide the safest possible training and testing environments while minimizing the legal and personal liability associated with adverse outcomes. The best approach to preventing emergencies is through proper screening, selection of appropriate exercise protocols, and supervision and monitoring. Structured participant education, proper placement of exercise equipment, and development of evidence-based exercise prescriptions are additional measures that will enhance the efficacy of patient safety.

Health/fitness facilities should also have policies and procedures to manage medical emergencies. Policy and procedure manuals are an integral part of the day-to-day operations of clinical and wellness facilities. Written emergency plans should list the specific responsibilities of each staff member, emergency equipment, and predetermined contact for emergency response.

Emergency Preparedness: Case Study 12 Questions

1. Which one of the following is not a common piece of emergency equipment or supply for a health/fitness facility?
   A) Cardiopulmonary resuscitation (CPR) barrier masks
   B) Glucometer
   C) First aid kit
   D) Automated external defibrillator (AED) with adult and pediatric attenuator pads (as appropriate)

2. True or false: All health/fitness facilities (levels 1–5) should have an emergency plan in place.

3. A middle-aged man at your fitness facility is currently walking on the treadmill and waves you over to him. He reports that he has suddenly started getting pressure and discomfort in his jaw and upper back. What should you do first?
   A) Check his pulse.
   B) Check his BP.
   C) Have him stop exercising.
   D) Give the patient aspirin.

4. John is attending his third cardiac rehab session today and is exercising on the treadmill without complaint. You are monitoring his ECG, and he starts having ventricular ectopy. You quickly review his chart and note that he has never had ventricular ectopy before. You ask him how he is feeling and he states he feels great. What should you do?
   A) Call a code.
   B) Stop exercise and notify his physician, check and document his vitals, and continue to observe him.
   C) Let him continue at the current workload and finish his exercise session.
   D) Decrease his workload and continue to monitor him for the rest of his exercise session.

5. An individual at your fitness facility waves you over to him while he is resting in a chair. He reports that he just tripped and had severe pain in his wrist from catching himself when he fell. You notice his wrist is extremely bruised and swollen. He states he is unable to move his wrist or put any weight on it. Select the most appropriate acute response to manage this musculoskeletal emergency.
   A) Have the patient rest while you call his physician.
   B) Immediately immobilize his wrist, implement RICE (rest, ice, compress, and elevate), and promptly notify his physician.
   C) Apply ice and ask if the patient if he feels comfortable going home and instruct him to contact his physician if he has any increased in symptoms.
   D) Perform a range of motion test on the patient to see if his pain increases or decreases with different positions. Note any information regarding his pain and relay it to his physician.

6. Jane arrives today at phase III cardiac rehabilitation and states, "I just don't feel right." During your discussion with her, you recognize the signs of a possible transient ischemic attack (TIA) or stroke. What should you do next?
   A) Activate EMS; note the time the symptoms started.
   B) Hook her up to your telemetry system and monitor her ECG.
   C) Call her husband to take her to the emergency room.
   D) Place in a supine position and give administer oxygen.

CASE STUDY 1: ECG
Authors: Dennis Kerrigan (DK), PhD, FACSM
Clinton A. Brawner (CAB), PhD, MS, FACSM
Authors' Certifications: DK: ACSM-CEP; CAB: ACSM-CEP

A 25-year-old male was referred for a clinical exercise stress test following two witnessed episodes of syncope. Both episodes were preceded by vigorous physical activity. The following ECG was recorded at 5 min 11 s postexercise.

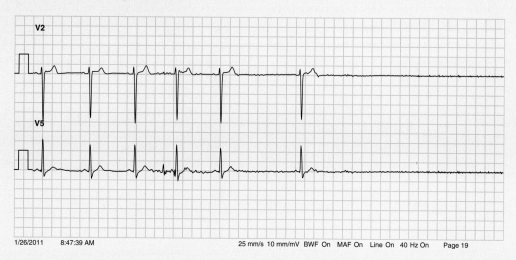

1/26/2011   8:47:39 AM   25 mm/s 10 mm/mV BWF On MAF On Line On 40 Hz On   Page 19

ECG: Case Study 1 Questions

1. What is the disorder? _____

2. What should be the first response to this ECG?
   A) Activate emergency procedures
   B) Defibrillate
   C) Check the BP
   D) Check the patient

3. Which of the following is not true?
   A) A patient can be stable with a sustain presentation of this disorder.
   B) This ECG could be the result of a disconnected lead.

   C) Unless transient, this disorder will cause the patient to become unstable.
   D) If this disorder is sustained and a normal rhythm does not return, cardiopulmonary resuscitation will be necessary.

4. This ECG could also be which of the following?
   A) Fine atrial fibrillation
   B) Course atrial fibrillation
   C) Fine ventricular fibrillation
   D) Course ventricular fibrillation

CASE STUDY 2: ECG
Authors: Dennis Kerrigan (DK), PhD, FACSM
Clinton A. Brawner (CAB), PhD, MS, FACSM
Authors' Certifications: DK: ACSM-CEP; CAB: ACSM-CEP

A 41-year-old male police officer presented to cardiology for a clinical exercise stress test with the following rhythm.

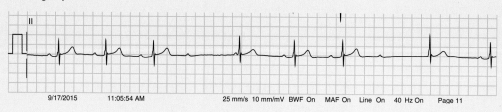

9/17/2015   11:05:54 AM   25 mm/s 10 mm/mV BWF On   MAF On   Line On   40 Hz On   Page 11

ECG: Case Study 2 Questions

1. What is the rhythm? _____

2. What is the disorder? _____

3. What is the ventricular rate? _____

4. What is an important determinant of whether to conduct this test in the presence of this rhythm?
   A) According to the American Heart Association, this is a contraindication to exercise testing.
   B) According to the American Heart Association, a physician should be consulted before conducting the test.
   C) It is okay to perform the test if this is not a new finding.
   D) The patient's medical and symptom history as well as the presence of signs or symptoms of poor perfusion should guide whether the test can be performed.

5. Where is the origin of the impulse that conducts the ventricles?
   A) SA node
   B) Atrioventricular (AV) node
   C) Bundle of His
   D) Ventricles

6. What are the implications if this rhythm was not observed at rest but presented during the exercise test?
   A) According to the American Heart Association, the test should be terminated.
   B) According to the American Heart Association, the test should be terminated if the ventricular rate decreases by 10 beats.
   C) According to the American Heart Association, the test should be terminated if it interferes with maintenance of cardiac output (CO).
   D) According to the American Heart Association, it is not an indication to terminate a test.

CASE STUDY 3: ECG
Authors: Dennis Kerrigan (DK), PhD, FACSM
Clinton A. Brawner (CAB), PhD, MS, FACSM
Authors' Certifications: DK: ACSM-CEP; CAB: ACSM-CEP

A 74-year-old woman presented to phase III (maintenance) cardiac rehabilitation without complaints and resting vitals within normal limits. During exercise, she complained of mid-upper back pain and fatigue. It was also noted that her HR did not increase with exercise. Because of these symptoms, an ECG was obtained (shown in the following section).

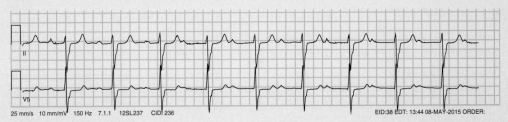

25 mm/s   10 mm/mV   150 Hz   7.1.1   12SL237   CID 236   EID:38 EDT: 13:44 08-MAY-2015 ORDER:

ECG: Case Study 3 Questions

1. What is the disorder?

2. What the atrial rate?

3. What is the ventricular rate?

4. According to the American Heart Association
   A) Presence of this disorder at rest is an absolute contraindication to exercise testing/training.

(Continued)

CASE STUDY 3: ECG (Continued)

B) Presence of this disorder at rest is a relative contraindication to exercise testing/training.

C) If this develops during exercise, it is an absolute indication to end an exercise testing/training.

D) If this develops during exercise, it is a relative indication to end an exercise testing/training.

E) Both A and C are correct.

F) Both B and D are correct.

G) Both A and D are correct.

H) Both B and C are correct.

5. Where is the origin of the impulse that conducts the ventricles?

A) SA node

B) AV node

C) Bundle of His

D) Ventricles

6. Which of the following is not correct?

A) Patients are usually asymptomatic with this disorder.

B) This disorder can compromise CO.

C) This disorder can present due to transient ischemia.

D) This disorder can be an indication for a permanent pacemaker.

CASE STUDY 4: ECG

Authors: Dennis Kerrigan (DK), PhD, FACSM
Clinton A. Brawner (CAB), PhD, MS, FACSM
Authors' Certifications: DK: ACSM-CEP; CAB: ACSM-CEP

A 75-year-old male patient with a recent history (2 months ago) of coronary bypass surgery presents to cardiac rehabilitation for his initial visit with the following rhythm. His vitals are as follows: Weight = 230 lb, BP = 102/84 mm Hg.

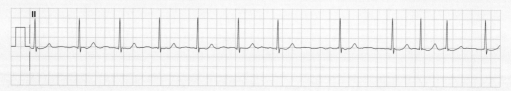

ECG: Case Study 4 Questions

1. What is the rate? _____

2. Regular or irregular? _____

3. Interpret the rhythm. _____

4. Name the medication usually prescribed that prevents a common complication due to this arrhythmia.

A) Lisinopril

B) Warfarin

C) Metoprolol

D) Simvastatin

5. What effect does this arrhythmia typically have on CO?

A) CO is elevated due to the increased contractions in the atria.

B) The "atrial kick" has negligible effect on CO.

C) CO is reduced.

D) None of the above.

6. How should exercise be prescribed in this patient, assuming he performed a sign- and symptom-limited exercise stress test prior to cardiac rehabilitation?

A) RPE

B) An HR 20–30 beats above rest

C) 50%–85% of HRR

D) The patient should not exercise with this arrhythmia.

CASE STUDY 5: ECG
Authors: Dennis Kerrigan (DK), PhD, FACSM
Clinton A. Brawner (CAB), PhD, MS, FACSM
Authors' Certifications: DK: ACSM-CEP; CAB: ACSM-CEP

A patient with a history of cardiac arrest and MI is walking on the treadmill in cardiac rehabilitation when you observe this rhythm.

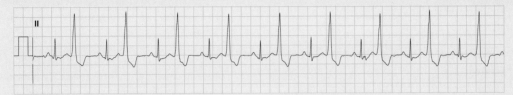

ECG: Case Study 5 Questions

1. What is the underlying rhythm?

   _____

2. What is the dysrhythmia? _____

3. Assuming this patient has a history of this dysrhythmia, what actions should be taken?
   A) Continue to monitor.
   B) Stop the exercise immediately.
   C) Call an emergency code and grab the automatic defibrillator.
   D) Slow treadmill speed and call physician.

4. What might be some potential causes of this dysrhythmia?
   A) Caffeine
   B) Anxiety/stress
   C) Forgetting to take medications
   D) All of the above

CASE STUDY 6: ECG
Authors: Dennis Kerrigan (DK), PhD, FACSM
Clinton A. Brawner (CAB), PhD, MS, FACSM
Authors' Certifications: DK: ACSM-CEP; CAB: ACSM-CEP

A 52-year-old male without a history of heart disease is scheduled in your laboratory for a standard sign- and symptom-limited exercise stress test with ECG to evaluate a recent episode of angina while performing yard work.

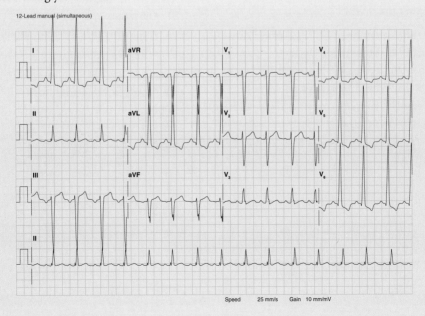

(Continued)

CASE STUDY 6: ECG (Continued)

ECG: Case Study 6 Questions

1. What is the rate? _____

2. Regular or irregular? _____

3. Interpret the ECG. _____

4. Assuming the patient is asymptomatic at rest, what course of action would you follow?
   A) Proceed with the stress test using a low-level treadmill protocol.
   B) Send patient directly to emergency department.
   C) Attempt Valsalva maneuver.
   D) Contact referring physician to verify the test ordered.

5. True or false: If the aforementioned patient presented with the observed ECG abnormality and severe CP, this could indicate an acute MI.

CASE STUDY 7: ECG

Authors: Dennis Kerrigan (DK), PhD, FACSM
Clinton A. Brawner (CAB), PhD, MS, FACSM
Authors' Certifications: DK: ACSM-CEP; CAB: ACSM-CEP

A 42-year-old male with hypertension is undergoing a symptom-limited exercise stress test on a treadmill in response to a recent episode of syncope he experienced while running. The following ECG was taken during stage IV of the Bruce protocol.

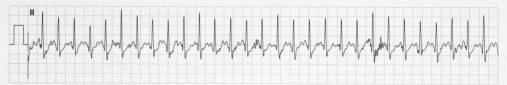

ECG: Case Study 7 Questions

1. What is the rate? _____

2. Regular or irregular? _____

3. Interpret the rhythm. _____

4. If the aforementioned ECG was taken during rest, what might you suspect?
   A) Second-degree AV block, type I
   B) Supraventricular tachycardia (SVT)
   C) Ventricular tachycardia
   D) Both A and B

5. Which of the following medications for hypertension is he likely not taking?
   A) ACE inhibitor
   B) Diuretic
   C) Angiotensin II receptor antagonists
   D) β-blocker

6. Based on the ECG alone and information given earlier, should the stress test be stopped?
   A) Yes
   B) No

CASE STUDY 8: ECG
Authors: Dennis Kerrigan (DK), PhD, FACSM
Clinton A. Brawner (CAB), PhD, MS, FACSM
Authors' Certifications: DK: ACSM-CEP; CAB: ACSM-CEP

A 53-year-old female with ischemic cardiomyopathy is performing a symptom-limited exercise stress test in your laboratory. During stage III of the Naughton protocol, you observe for the first time the following on the ECG.

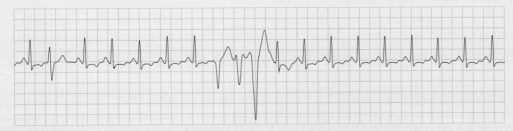

ECG: Case Study 8 Questions

1. What is the rate? _____

2. Regular or irregular? _____

3. Interpret the rhythm. _____

4. What course of action should you take?
   A) Stop the test immediately.
   B) Continue with the test.

C) Take an immediate BP.
D) Administer a sublingual nitroglycerin.

5. What can be said about the ectopic beats?
   A) They are multifocal.
   B) They are unifocal.
   C) They are junctional beats.
   D) They are both ventricular and supraventricular in nature.

CASE STUDY 9: ECG
Authors: Dennis Kerrigan (DK), PhD, FACSM
Clinton A. Brawner (CAB), PhD, MS, FACSM
Authors' Certifications: DK: ACSM-CEP; CAB: ACSM-CEP

A 16-year-old hockey player has an ECG as part of his preparticipation screening. The following is his resting ECG.

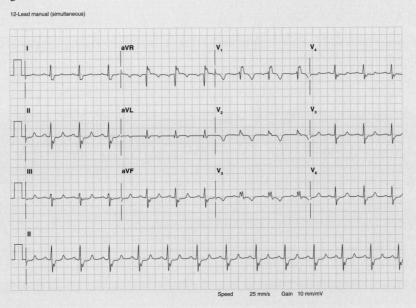

ACSM-CEP

CASE STUDY 9: ECG (Continued)

ECG: Case Study 9 Questions

1. What is the rate? _____

2. Regular or irregular? _____

3. Interpret the ECG. _____

4. Based on the ECG, what will likely happen with this athlete?
   A) The athlete will be cleared to participate without any further workup.

B) The athlete will likely play hockey next year after receiving treatment.

C) The athlete will no longer be able to participate in sports.

D) The athlete will likely undergo additional evaluation before returning to play.

CASE STUDY 10: ECG
Authors: Dennis Kerrigan (DK), PhD, FACSM
Clinton A. Brawner (CAB), PhD, MS, FACSM
Authors' Certifications: DK: ACSM-CEP; CAB: ACSM-CEP

A 32-year-old apparently healthy male cyclist is self-referred for a maximal exercise test to assess his and anaerobic threshold in preparation for an upcoming race. The following is his resting ECG.

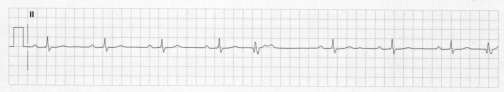

ECG: Case Study 10 Questions

1. What is the rate? _____

2. Regular or irregular? _____

3. Interpret the rhythm. _____

4. True or false: The length of the PR interval is directly responsible for the rate.

5. What are the testing implications of this ECG?
   A) Physician should be notified due to the likelihood of a complete heart block.

B) Due to the decreased CO, O_2 peak will be blunted.

C) This is a benign finding, which will have no effect on the test?

D) There is a slight risk for atrial reentry tachycardia.

ECG CASE STUDY 11
Authors: Dennis Kerrigan (DK), PhD, FACSM
Clinton A. Brawner (CAB), PhD, MS, FACSM
Authors' Certifications: DK: ACSM-CEP; CAB: ACSM-CEP

An 84-year-old female is exercising in cardiac rehabilitation for the first time. While on the recumbent cycle, you see the following on the monitor.

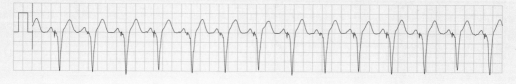

ECG: Case Study 11 Questions

1. What is the rate?

2. Regular or irregular? _____

3. Interpret the rhythm. _____

4. Which of the following conditions might be the reason she received a pacemaker?
   A) Sick sinus syndrome
   B) Ventricular tachycardia
   C) Third-degree AV block
   D) Both A and C

5. During her first three visits, she experiences CP. As a result, her physician sends her for a symptom-limited exercise stress test with nuclear imaging. Why was the nuclear imaging specified?
   A) She is unable to walk very long on a treadmill.
   B) Her pacemaker would interfere with an echocardiogram.
   C) If present, ischemia would not be undetectable by ECG alone due to the pacemaker depolarization.
   D) All of the above.

ECG CASE STUDY 12

Authors: Dennis Kerrigan (DK), PhD, FACSM
Clinton A. Brawner (CAB), PhD, MS, FACSM
Authors' Certifications: DK: ACSM-CEP; CAB: ACSM-CEP

A 64-year-old male with a history of an MI and stent 15 years ago is exercising in your phase III cardiac rehabilitation program. While on the treadmill, he complains of jaw pain and nausea. You place him in a semisupine position with the upper body slightly elevated and attach an ECG.

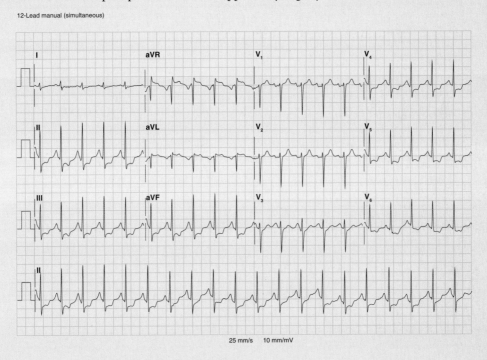

12-Lead manual (simultaneous)

25 mm/s   10 mm/mV

ECG: Case Study 12 Questions

1. What is the rate? _____

2. Regular or irregular? _____

3. Interpret the rhythm. _____

4. Which of the following medications may improve his jaw pain?
   A) Nitroglycerin
   B) Plavix
   C) Epinephrine
   D) Both A and C

(Continued)

ECG CASE STUDY 12 (Continued)

5. Based on the ECG, what regions of the heart are ischemic?
   A) Inferior
   B) Septal
   C) Lateral
   D) Both A and C

ECG CASE STUDY 13

Authors: Dennis Kerrigan (DK), PhD, FACSM
Clinton A. Brawner (CAB), PhD, MS, FACSM
Authors' Certifications: DK: ACSM-CEP; CAB: ACSM-CEP

A 58-year-old female has just completed a low-level exercise test as a predischarge requirement following an STEMI a few days ago. While seated in recovery, you notice a change in the ECG.

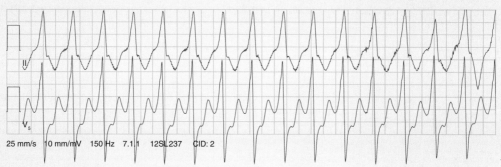

25 mm/s   10 mm/mV   150 Hz   7.1.1   12SL237   CID: 2

ECG: Case Study 13 Questions

1. What is the rate? _____

2. Regular or irregular? _____

3. Interpret the rhythm. _____

4. What actions should you take?
   A) Check the patient.
   B) Notify the physician.
   C) Prepare the crash cart.
   D) All of the above.

5. Your patient suddenly loses consciousness, what was likely the cause of this?
   A) Low blood glucose
   B) Vasovagal response
   C) Seizure
   D) Low CO

GRANT CASE STUDY 1: ANSWERS

1. —B. 33.1 kg · m^{-2}

   250 lb/2.2 = 113.64 kg. 6 ft 1 in. = 73 in.

   73 × 2.54 = 185.42 cm.

   185.42/100 = 1.8524 m.

   113.64 kg/(1.8524)^2 = 33.05 or 33.1 kg · m^{-2}

2. —A. Current lipid values

   The current preparticipation screening guidelines no longer include CVD risk factors as part of the decision-making process for referral to a health care provider prior to initiating a moderate- to vigorous-intensity exercise program. Grant's current lipid values are a CVD risk factor assessment: one that should still be part of an overall cardiovascular and metabolic disease prevention and management program.

   Resource: Liguori G, senior editor. *ACSM's Guidelines for Exercise Testing and Prescription.* 11th ed. Philadelphia (PA): Wolters Kluwer; 2021.

3. —A. Signed informed consent form only

   The preparticipation screening algorithm now takes into account three factors: (1) Current level of physical activity, (2) presence of signs or symptoms and/or known cardiovascular, metabolic, or renal disease, and (3) desired exercise intensity, as these three factors have been identified as important risk modulators of exercise-related cardiovascular events. Grant does not regularly exercise; has no diagnosed cardiovascular, metabolic, or renal disease; and has no sign or symptoms suggestive of such. Medical clearance is not needed for light- to moderate-intensity exercise.

   Resources: James PA, Oparil S, Carter BL et al. 2014 evidence-based guideline for the management of high blood pressure in adults: report from the panel members appointed to the Eighth Joint National Committee (JNC 8). JAMA. 2014;311(5):507–20.

   Liguori G, senior editor. *ACSM's Guidelines for Exercise Testing and Prescription.* 11th ed. Philadelphia (PA): Wolters Kluwer; 2021.

   Resource: Chobanian AV, Bakris GL, Black HR et al. The Seventh Report of the Joint National Committee on Prevention, Detection, Evaluation, and Treatment of High Blood Pressure: the JNC 7 report. JAMA. 2003;289(19):2560–72.

4. —A. Precontemplation

   Resource: Liguori G, senior editor. *ACSM's Guidelines for Exercise Testing and Prescription.* 11th ed. Philadelphia (PA): Wolters Kluwer; 2021.

5. —B. Grant would be classified as having impaired fasting glucose (IFG).

   Resources: Liguori G, senior editor. *ACSM's Guidelines for Exercise Testing and*

GRANT CASE STUDY 1: ANSWERS (Continued)

Prescription. 11th ed. Philadelphia (PA): Wolters Kluwer; 2021.

National Cholesterol Education Program (NCEP) Expert Panel on Detection, Evaluation, and Treatment of High Blood Cholesterol in Adults (Adult Treatment Panel III). Third Report of the National Cholesterol Education Program (NCEP) Expert Panel on Detection, Evaluation, and Treatment of High Blood Cholesterol in Adults (Adult Treatment Panel III) final report. Circulation. 2002;106(25):3143–421.

6. His main goal should be to adopt a more physically active lifestyle, increase his leisure-time physical activity, and exercise to maximize his caloric expenditure. This will benefit Grant in improving all aspects of his risk factor profile. His cardiometabolic risk profile is highly related to his obesity (overall and abdominal) and physical inactivity. By maximizing caloric expenditure and becoming more active, he can improve his body composition, which can aid in improving his blood lipids, glucose levels, and BP.

7. Individuals with metabolic syndrome should continually work toward maximizing energy expenditure; this favorably impacts cardiometabolic profile. Grant should progress to a frequency of $>5\,\text{d}\cdot\text{wk}^{-1}$, gradually increasing his intensity to vigorous ($\geq60\%$ of $\dot{V}O_2R$). Time spent exercising should be between >300 min of moderate-intensity exercise or >150 min of vigorous-intensity exercise per week, or a combination of both. Given his relatively low-current motivation to exercise, modalities chosen should be those Grant enjoys, effectively increasing the likelihood that he will maintain his exercise program.

SEAMUS CASE STUDY 2: ANSWERS

1. —C. Blood glucose control over 2–3 months. (Domain 1A: Patient Assessment)

2. —D. All of the above (Domain IB: Interview)

3. —D. Before, occasionally during, and after exercise (Domain ID Monitoring)

4. —A. Preparation (intending to be regularly active in the next 30 days) (Domain: IE assess physical activity readiness)

5. —C. 9.75–32.5 lb (3%–10% of initial weight) (Domain: IE assess patient goals)

6. —A. Yes (Domain IIC: Symptom-limited exercise testing)

7. —B. SBP ≤220 mm Hg and/or DBP ≤105 mm Hg (Recommendations for individuals with hypertension) (Domain IVC: Monitoring during exercise training)

8. —D. All of the above (Domain IVC: Monitoring during exercise training)

9. —C. (Yes, sulfonylureas increase risk of hypoglycemia and monitoring around exercise is indicated.) (Domain ID: Monitoring)

10. —D. Advise Seamus to report these changes to his physician and inform his physician of his current exercise routine. (Medication changes are not within the scope of practice of CEPs; however, it is important to advise the patient to report this to their physician as increasing exercise levels can lead to dangerous hypoglycemic events in combination with diabetes medications and the dosages may need to be decreased.) (Domain IVG: Reporting symptoms and consulting responsible health care provider)

11. Recommendations for this scenario include the following:
    a. Consume up to 15 g of carbohydrate before beginning exercise.
    b. Follow the "rule of 15" by testing blood glucose 15 min after carbohydrate

ACSM-CEP

consumption and if it is not above 100 mg/dL, consume another 15 g and repeat this process until glucose reaches at least 100 mg/dL.

c. Consider performing either resistance exercise or vigorous-intensity exercise first before moderate-intensity exercise to elicit possible increase in blood glucose at the beginning of the session.

d. Consider interspersing short, higher-intensity intervals during moderate-intensity exercise to lessen chances of exercise-associated hypoglycemia.

e. Monitor blood glucose during and after exercise to be sure it is not dropping to hypoglycemic levels.

f. Monitor for signs and symptoms of hypoglycemia.

g. Educate the patient about the risk of postexercise hypoglycemia up to 12 h or more following exercise and the importance of frequent blood glucose monitoring.

12. Begin with a moderate-intensity load with 10–15 repetitions per set for 1–3 sets at a frequency for 2–3 d $\cdot$ wk^{-1}. Progress when the target number of repetitions per set can be exceeded on a consistent basis. Progression should initially involve increasing the weight/resistance and lowering the number of repetitions to 8-10. Further progression should include increasing the number of sets, and lastly by increasing training frequency.

Resource: Liguori G, senior editor. *ACSM's Guidelines for Exercise Testing and Prescription.* 11th ed. Philadelphia (PA): Wolters Kluwer; 2021.

KEITH CASE STUDY 3: ANSWERS

1. —B. Light to moderate; 30%–<60% of HRR

   Resource: Liguori G, senior editor. *ACSM's Guidelines for Exercise Testing and Prescription.* 11th ed. Philadelphia (PA): Wolters Kluwer; 2021.

2. —D. ≥5 wk^{-1}

   Resource: Liguori G, senior editor. *ACSM's Guidelines for Exercise Testing and Prescription.* 11th ed. Philadelphia (PA): Wolters Kluwer; 2021.

3. —C. Biguanide drug for Type 2 DM

   Resource: Liguori G, senior editor. *ACSM's Guidelines for Exercise Testing and Prescription.* 11th ed. Philadelphia (PA): Wolters Kluwer; 2021.

4. —D. Both B and C

   Resource: Liguori G, senior editor. *ACSM's Guidelines for Exercise Testing and Prescription.* 11th ed. Philadelphia (PA): Wolters Kluwer; 2021.

5. —E. Only A and B of the above

   Resource: Liguori G, senior editor. *ACSM's Guidelines for Exercise Testing and Prescription.* 11th ed. Philadelphia (PA): Wolters Kluwer; 2021.

6. —A. 96–102 bpm

   Resource: Liguori G, senior editor. *ACSM's Guidelines for Exercise Testing and Prescription.* 11th ed. Philadelphia (PA): Wolters Kluwer; 2021.

7. —D. 3.3 mph and 7% grade

   $\dot{V}O_2 = (0.1 \times 3.3 \text{ mph} \times 26.8) + (1.8 \times 3.2 \times 26.8 \times 0.7) + 3.5$

   (Horizontal)　(Vertical)　(Rest)

   $\dot{V}O_2 = (8.84) + (10.8) + 3.5$

   $\dot{V}O_2 = 23.14 \text{ mL} \cdot \text{kg}^{-1} \cdot \text{min}^{-1}$

   METs = 23.14 / 3.5 = 6.61 METs

   Resource: Liguori G, senior editor. *ACSM's Guidelines for Exercise Testing and Prescription.* 11th ed. Philadelphia (PA): Wolters Kluwer; 2021.

ACSM-CEP

(Continued)

KEITH CASE STUDY 3: ANSWERS (Continued)

8. —C. 2–3; moderate

   Resource: Liguori G, senior editor. *ACSM's Guidelines for Exercise Testing and Prescription.* 11th ed. Philadelphia (PA): Wolters Kluwer; 2021.

9. —A. Enhance insulin sensitivity

   Resource: Tresierras MA, Balady GJ. Resistance training in the treatment of diabetes and obesity: mechanisms and outcomes. J Cardiopul Rehabil Prev.2009; 2967-75.

10. —C. ≥500–1,000 MET-min · wk^{-1}

    Resource: Liguori G, senior editor. *ACSM's Guidelines for Exercise Testing and Prescription.* 11th ed. Philadelphia (PA): Wolters Kluwer; 2021.

11. Questions or recommendations include the following:
    a. Ask him about his medication compliance.
    b. Refer him to a smoking cessation program.
    c. Have him schedule a follow-up visit with his physician concerning his abnormal fasting blood values and pulmonary function test values.
    d. Have him talk with the program dietician regarding weight loss strategies.
    e. Ask him about his compliance taking his daily blood glucose measurements.
    f. Ask him if his glucometer works properly.
    g. Ask him if he has a home automatic BP measuring device.
    h. Ask him about the amount of home exercise he is currently performing.
    i. Inquire about any potential orthopedic or musculoskeletal limitations that he may have.

12. Exercise benefits include the following:
    a. Enhanced muscle glucose uptake through improved insulin sensitivity and decreased insulin resistance
    b. Better weight control
    c. Lowered BP
    d. Improved blood lipid and lipoprotein values
    e. Better sleep
    f. Improved mood and outlook on life
    g. Decreased stress level
    h. Decreased fat mass and increased FFM
    i. Stronger bones
    j. Less SOB if he quits smoking
    k. Decreased overall body weight

STEVE CASE STUDY 4: ANSWERS

1. —C. II, III, aVF

   Resource: Dubin D. Rapid Interpretation of EKG's. 6th ed. Tampa (FL): Cover Publishing; 2000.

2. —C. Peripheral arterial disease (PAD)

   Steve displays frequent episodes of IC rated up to a 4 with exertion.

   Resource: Liguori G, senior editor. *ACSM's Guidelines for Exercise Testing and Prescription.* 11th ed. Philadelphia (PA): Wolters Kluwer; 2021

3. —B. 40%–59% HRR or VO$_2$R, allowing him to walk until he reaches an IC pain rating of 3

   Resource: Liguori G, senior editor. *ACSM's Guidelines for Exercise Testing and*

   Prescription. 11th ed. Philadelphia (PA): Wolters Kluwer; 2021

4. —D. IC treadmill protocol

   Leg cycle ergometer may be used as a warm-up but should not be the primary form of aerobic exercise. Weight-bearing exercise such as walking to improve/increase the length of time to ischemic threshold/claudication (patient providing a rating of 3 on IC scale) is recommended.

   Resource: Liguori G, senior editor. *ACSM's Guidelines for Exercise Testing and Prescription.* 11th ed. Philadelphia (PA): Wolters Kluwer; 2021

5. —B. 3–5 d $\cdot$ wk^{-1}

   Resource: Liguori G, senior editor. *ACSM's Guidelines for Exercise Testing and Prescription*. 11th ed. Philadelphia (PA): Wolters Kluwer; 2021

6. —B. 63 kcal

   Estimated maximal oxygen consumption = 3.6

   METs (2.0 mph and 4.0% grade)

   1 MET = 3.5 mL $\cdot$ kg^{-1} $\cdot$ min^{-1}

   $\dot{V}O_2$ Relative = (3.6 METs $\times$ 3.5 mL $\cdot$ kg^{-1} $\cdot$ min^{-1}) = 12.6 mL $\cdot$ kg^{-1} $\cdot$ min^{-1}

   Steve's weight kg = 145 1b / 2.2 = 66 kg

   1 L $\cdot$ min^{-1} = 5 kcal

   Time = 15 min

   $\dot{V}O_2$ Absolute = 12.6 mL $\cdot$ kg^{-1} $\cdot$ min^{-1} $\times$ 66 kg

   $$= \frac{0.8316 \, L \cdot min^{-1}}{1,000 \, mL}$$

   0.8316 L $\cdot$ min^{-1} $\times$ 5 kcal $\times$ 15 min = 6 kcal

   Resource: Liguori G, senior editor. *ACSM's Guidelines for Exercise Testing and Prescription*. 11th ed. Philadelphia (PA): Wolters Kluwer; 2021

7. —C. 120 mm Hg

   ABI = $\frac{\text{Highest ankle systolic pressure}}{\text{Highest brachial systolic pressure}}$ → 0.66 = X

   $\frac{\text{Highest brachial systolic pressure} = (182)}{}$

   0.66 = $\frac{X}{182}$ → (0.66) $\times$ (182 mm Hg) = 120 mm Hg

   Resources: Liguori G, senior editor. *ACSM's Guidelines for Exercise Testing and Prescription*. 11th ed. Philadelphia (PA): Wolters Kluwer; 2021

   Wennberg PW, Rooke TW. Diagnosis and management of diseases of the peripheral arteries and veins. In: Fuster V, Walsh RA, Harrington RA, editors. Hurst's The Heart. 13th ed. New York (NY): McGraw-Hill; 2011. p. 2331–46.

8. —C. 100

   2 packs a day $\times$ 50 years = 100.

   Resource: Liguori G, senior editor. *ACSM's Guidelines for Exercise Testing and Prescription*. 11th ed. Philadelphia (PA): Wolters Kluwer; 2021

9. —A. Cease exercise to allow ischemic pain to resolve before resuming exercise.

   An IC protocol would need to be established for this patient.

   Resource: Liguori G, senior editor. *ACSM's Guidelines for Exercise Testing and Prescription*. 11th ed. Philadelphia (PA): Wolters Kluwer; 2021

10. —D. Both A and B

    Resources: Liguori G, senior editor. *ACSM's Guidelines for Exercise Testing and Prescription*. 11th ed. Philadelphia (PA): Wolters Kluwer; 2021

    Wennberg PW, Rooke TW. Diagnosis and management of diseases of the peripheral arteries and veins. In: Fuster V, Walsh RA, Harrington RA, editors. Hurst's The Heart. 13th ed. New York (NY): McGraw-Hill; 2011. p. 2331–46.

11. —C. Inhibit cell proliferation and inflammation reducing restenosis.

    Drug-eluting stents do not elute antibiotics or anticoagulants.

    Resource: Puranik AS, Dawson ER, Peppas NA. Recent advances in drug eluting stents. Int J Pharm. 2013;441(1):665–79.

12. Individuals with PAD should perform weight-bearing aerobic exercise 3–5 d $\cdot$ wk^{-1}. Patients should exercise at 40%–<60% $\dot{V}O_2R$ that allows the patient to walk until they reach a pain rating of 3 (*i.e.,* intense pain) on the 4-point IC scale. Between bouts of activity, the CEP should allow for the subsiding of ischemic pain by resting prior to resuming exercise. Time for aerobic exercise should be aimed for 30–60 min $\cdot$ d^{-1}. However, someone like Steve may need to start with 10-min bouts and exercise intermittently to accumulate a total of 30–60 min $\cdot$ d^{-1}. Severely deconditioned patients may need to begin the program by accumulating only 15 min $\cdot$ d^{-1}, gradually increasing the time by 5 min $\cdot$ d^{-1} on a biweekly basis. Patients with this clinical history should focus on weight-bearing

(Continued)

STEVE CASE STUDY 4: ANSWERS (Continued)

aerobic exercise in order to increase the length time to ischemic threshold versus a non-weight-bearing exercise such as a leg cycle ergometer (can be used as a warm-up).

13. Steve is a patient who is severely deconditioned. The Bruce protocol is geared toward populations who are younger and physically capable of performing physical activity that involves walking. The Bruce protocol employs relatively large incremental workload adjustments (*i.e.*, 2–3 METs stages) every 3 min. These large incremental workload adjustments would call for an early termination of the GXT had the Bruce protocol been administered to Steve due to possible early onset of IC during the first stage. A ramped treadmill protocol increases the work rate in a constant and continuous manner. Some of the primary advantages of a ramp protocol include the following:
    - Avoidance of large and unequal increments in workload
    - Uniform increase in physiologic and hemodynamic responses
    - Individualized test protocol (ramp rate)
    - More accurate estimates of exercise capacity

    Ramp protocols should be individualized so that the treadmill speed and increments in grade are based on perceived functional capacity of the subject. Increments in work rate should be chosen relative to total test time between 8 and 12 min (assuming the termination point is volitional fatigue). Yet, with severely deconditioned individuals, this is not always the case.

14. There are various types of resistance exercise equipment that can effectively be used to improve muscular strength and endurance. Steve is an older individual who has a chronic condition such as PAD and is deconditioned. He would most likely benefit from using equipment that includes elastic bands, hand weights, and weight machines. Proper techniques such as raising and lowering weights with controlled movements should be demonstrated. He should maintain a regular breathing pattern and avoid holding his breath, straining, and sustained gripping because these factors may induce an excessive BP response.

    - Each major muscle group, at least 8–10 exercises (*i.e.*, chest, shoulders, legs, arms, back, etc.), should be trained between with 48 h separating each resistance exercise session, 2–3 d $\cdot$ wk^{-1}
    - Steve is an older individual and is very deconditioned. The CEP can also apply resistance exercise guidelines that are geared toward older individuals as well.
    - His initial load should begin with 40%–50% of 1-RM, progressing to 60%–70% of 1-RM.
    - The determination of a 1-RM may be deemed inappropriate for individuals with CVD. Therefore, multiple trials using progressively higher loads can be performed until the patient can perform no more than 10 repetitions without straining.
    - If 1-RM is not measured, intensity can be prescribed according to his overall fitness level. Progression can be determined in terms of moderate (5–6) and vigorous (7–8) on an RPE scale of 0–10.
    - One or more sets of 10–15 repetitions exercising each major muscle group should be performed.
    - He should adhere to lower weight and higher repetitions, especially when initiating a resistance exercise regimen.
    - Overall rest periods between sets can range from 2 to 3 min.

15. Those who have PAD may lack motivation in terms of establishing and adhering to an exercise program. Potential barriers regarding the development of a structured exercise regimen include not having the energy, fear of getting hurt, safety issues, and overall concerns with comorbidities. Many patients with PAD tend to have clustering of comorbidities such as diabetes, hypertension, obesity, musculoskeletal conditions, neuropathy, and foot ulcers that may affect exercise tolerance.

16. The CEP should focus on discussing modifications to FITT principles regarding an exercise program. Counseling and motiva-

tional interviewing should be emphasized ("smaller goals, to bigger goals"). Steve's attitude to exercise and lifestyle modifications should be addressed throughout the duration of his monitored phase II cardiac rehabilitation program. Maintenance of lifestyle modification and relapse prevention is highly recommended in this population.

The overall goals of treating PAD include the reduction of symptoms (IC), improvement of QOL, and the prevention of complications. Treatment for Steve is primarily based on his signs and symptoms, risk factors, results from various tests, as well as the outcomes of any interventions or procedures. The lack of aggressive treatment for PAD may lead to complications such as ulcers, sores, and gangrene, which may result in lower-extremity amputation.

Ultimate lifestyle modifications include the cessation of smoking (smoking raises risk for other comorbidities such as stroke, lung cancer, COPD, etc.). Steve should adhere to his regimen of taking his medications as prescribed to control his hypertension and dyslipidemia. His maintenance of an exercise program will further improve the latter comorbidities and general symptoms (IC). A healthy diet plan should be followed as well (monitor sodium intake, trans fat, cholesterol intake, etc.)

Resources: Askew CD, Parmenter B, Leicht AS, Walker PJ, Golledge J. Exercise & Sports Science Australia (ESSA) position statement on exercise prescription for patients with peripheral arterial disease and intermittent claudication. J Sci Med Sport. 2014;17(6):623–9.

Liguori G, senior editor. *ACSM's Guidelines for Exercise Testing and Prescription*. 11th ed. Philadelphia (PA): Wolters Kluwer; 2021

Wennberg PW, Rooke TW. Diagnosis and management of diseases of the peripheral arteries and veins. In: Fuster V, Walsh RA, Harrington RA, editors. Hurst's The Heart. 13th ed. New York (NY): McGraw-Hill; 2011. p. 2331–46.

NANCY CASE STUDY 5: ANSWERS

1. —C. 4.5 METs

   If exercise test data is available, exercise can be prescribed at a workload below the ischemic threshold (~1 MET). Some considerations for this client are as follows:

   Is this a true-positive or false-positive test for CAD?

   Her blood laboratory values indicate that she may have blood glucose control problems (prediabetes).

   The GXT documentation provides real data at workloads that are equivalent to 4.7 and 7.0 METs.

   Based on HR response, the 7 MET workload represents a near maximum test.

   Given all of the aforementioned concerns, a workload equivalent at or near 4.7 METs would seem most appropriate for this client.

   Resource: Liguori G, senior editor. *ACSM's Guidelines for Exercise Testing and Prescription*. 11th ed. Philadelphia (PA): Wolters Kluwer; 2021

2. —B. 14

   If exercise test data is available, exercise can be prescribed at an RPE represented during the stage of testing for that MET level and can act as a calibration of the individual's subjective RPE rating.

   Resource: Liguori G, senior editor. *ACSM's Guidelines for Exercise Testing and Prescription*. 11th ed. Philadelphia (PA): Wolters Kluwer; 2021

3. —C. Both of Nancy's medications may have adverse effects during exercise testing or programming.

   Diuretics may produce hypotension through hypovolemia and therefore result in a higher HR. Caution in interpreting ECG ST-segment depression as representative of an ischemic response must be used due to the possibility of diuretics

(Continued)

ACSM-CEP

NANCY CASE STUDY 5: ANSWERS (Continued)

causing hypokalemia, which can result in a depressed ST segment on the ECG. Dihydropyridine calcium channel blockers commonly used in treating hypertension are an effective vasodilator and may result in a higher HR response due to increased sympathetic compensation.

Resource: Liguori G, senior editor. *ACSM's Guidelines for Exercise Testing and Prescription.* 11th ed. Philadelphia (PA): Wolters Kluwer; 2021

4. —C. All of the medications that Nancy is prescribed may effect HR during exercise.

As previously noted in question 3, the medications that Nancy is taking may result in HR increases during exercise secondarily to potential hypovolemia (diuretics) and/or vasodilation (dihydropyridine calcium channel blockers).

Resource: Liguori G, senior editor. *ACSM's Guidelines for Exercise Testing and Prescription.* 11th ed. Philadelphia (PA): Wolters Kluwer; 2021

5. —E. Either A or B would be an appropriate treadmill workload for Nancy.

Calculations:

Treadmill = 2.0 mph and a 7% grade

Workload Equivalent = 4.5 METs

Resting Component = $3.5 \ mL \cdot kg^{-1} \cdot min$

Walking Horizontal

Component = $0.1 \times speed$
$= 0.1 \times (2.0 \ mph \times 26.8)$
$= 0.1 \times 53.6 \ m \ min$
$= 5.3 \ mL \cdot kg^{-1} \cdot min$

Walking Horizontal

Component = $1.8 \times speed \times grade$
$= 1.8 \times 53.6 \ m \cdot min \times .07$
$= 6.7 \ mL \cdot kg^{-1} \cdot min$

$\dot{V}O_2 \ mL \cdot kg^{-1} \cdot min$ = Resting + Walking Horizontal + Vertical Components

$\dot{V}O_2 \ mL \cdot kg^{-1} \cdot min = 3.5 + 5.3 + 6.7$
$= 15.5 \ mL \cdot kg^{-1} \cdot min$

METs = $\dot{V}O_2 mL \cdot kg^{-1} \cdot min$ / $3.5 mL \cdot kg^{-1} \cdot min$

METs = $15.5 mL \cdot kg^{-1} \cdot min$ / $3.5 mL \cdot kg^{-1} \cdot min$

$= 4.43$ METs

Treadmill = 3.0 mph and a 3% grade

Workload Equivalent = 4.5 METs

Resting Component = $3.5 \ mL \cdot kg^{-1} \cdot min$

Walking Horizontal

Component = $0.1 \times speed$
$= 0.1 \times (3.0 \ mph \times 26.8)$
$= 0.1 \times 80.4 \ m \cdot min$
$= 8.0 \ mL \cdot kg^{-1} \cdot min$

Walking Vertical

Component = $1.8 \times speed \times grade$
$= 1.8 \times 80.4 \ m \cdot min \times .03$
$= 4.3 \ mL \cdot kg^{-1} \cdot min$

$\dot{V}O_2 \ mL \cdot kg^{-1} \cdot min$ = Resting + Walking Horizontal + Vertical Components

$\dot{V}O_2 \ mL \cdot kg^{-1} \cdot min = 3.5 + 8.0 + 4.3$
$= 15.8 \ mL \cdot kg^{-1} \cdot min$

METs = $\dot{V}O_2 \ mL \cdot kg^{-1} \cdot min$ / $3.5 \ mL \cdot kg^{-1} \cdot min$

METs = $15.8 \ mL \cdot kg^{-1} \cdot min$ / $3.5 \ mL \cdot kg^{-1} \cdot min$

$= 4.51$ METs

The ACSM's metabolic equation for walking is most accurate for speeds of 1.9–3.7 mph. All speed units for equations should be in units of meter per minute, which is converted when you multiply miles per hour by the constant 26.8. All grades should be in decimal form, for example, 7% = 0.07.

The vertical component is only valid for estimating the metabolic cost of walking and running on a grade on a treadmill. The vertical component equation is *not* valid for the metabolic cost of ground walking or running on grades.

Resource: Liguori G, senior editor. *ACSM's Guidelines for Exercise Testing and Prescription.* 11th ed. Philadelphia (PA): Wolters Kluwer; 2021

6. —A. $275 \ kg \cdot min^{-1}$

Calculations:

Workload Equivalent

(Treadmill) = 4.5 METs
$= 4.5 \ METs \times 3.5$
$= 15.75 \ mL \cdot kg^{-1} \cdot min$

Workload Equivalent

$$(\text{Cycle Ergometer}) = 15.75 \, \text{mL} \cdot \text{kg}^{-1} \cdot \text{min} \times$$
$$0.90 \, (10\% \, \text{reduction})$$
$$= 14.18 \, \text{mL} \cdot \text{kg}^{-1} \cdot \text{min}$$

Nancy's Body Weight $= 158 \, \text{1b} \times 0.454$
$$= 71.7 \, \text{kg}$$

Resting Component $= 3.5 \, \text{mL} \cdot \text{kg}^{-1} \cdot \text{min}$

Cycle Ergometer Resistance Component
$$= 3.5 \, \text{mL} \cdot \text{kg}^{-1} \cdot \text{min}$$

Cycle Ergometer Resistance Component
$$= (1.8 \times \text{work rate kg} \cdot \text{min}^{-1})/ \, \text{body mass kg}$$

Cycle Ergometer Total Equation mL $\cdot$ kg^{-1} $\cdot$ min $=$ Resistance + Horizontal + Resting

$$14.8 \, \text{mL} \cdot \text{kg}^{-1} \cdot \text{min} = (1.8 \times \text{work rate kg} \cdot \text{min}^{-1})/71.7 \, \text{kg} + 3.5 + 3.5$$

$$7.18 \, \text{mL} \cdot \text{kg}^{-1} \cdot \text{min} = (1.8 \times \text{work rate kg} \cdot \text{min}^{-1})/71.7 \, \text{kg}$$

$$514.8 \, \text{mL} \cdot \text{min}^{-1} = 1.8 \times \text{work rate kg} \cdot \text{min}^{-1}$$

$$286.0 = \text{work rate kg} \cdot \text{min}^{-1}$$

If the initial GXT was completed on a treadmill, then the conversion to similar physiological aerobic stress will be approximately 10%–15% less on a cycle ergometer. Therefore, either the functional capacity or the workload in MET needs to be reduced by 10%–15%. The metabolic equation is most accurate for work rates of 300–1,200 kg $\cdot$ min^{-1}.

Resource: Liguori G, senior editor. *ACSM's Guidelines for Exercise Testing and Prescription*. 11th ed. Philadelphia (PA): Wolters Kluwer; 2021

7. —D. 5–7 d $\cdot$ wk^{-1}

Nancy's medical history indicates that she has low fitness, is overweight, and meets the criteria for both prediabetes and metabolic syndrome. Her stated goal is to exercise to lose weight. Based on all of these criteria, it is recommended that Nancy exercise ≥5 d $\cdot$ wk^{-1}, and preferably she should exercise most days of the week.

Resource: Liguori G, senior editor. *ACSM's Guidelines for Exercise Testing and Prescription*. 11th ed. Philadelphia (PA): Wolters Kluwer; 2021

8. —D. 10–15 RM

Initial loads in beginning a resistance program should allow 10–15 repetitions that can be lifted comfortably (40%–50% of 1-RM, progressing to 60%–70% of 1-RM).

Resource: Liguori G, senior editor. *ACSM's Guidelines for Exercise Testing and Prescription*. 11th ed. Philadelphia (PA): Wolters Kluwer; 2021

9. —C. Obesity

Nancy's BMI was calculated as 28.0 kg $\cdot$ m^{-2}. Although this places her in the "Overweight" category for BMI, her BMI does not achieve the criterion level for "Obesity" (≥30.0 kg $\cdot$ m^{-2}).

Resource: Liguori G, senior editor. *ACSM's Guidelines for Exercise Testing and Prescription*. 11th ed. Philadelphia (PA): Wolters Kluwer; 2021

10. —C. 60%

Calculations:

Maximum Functional Capacity $= 7.0$ METs

$$\dot{V}O_2R = 7.0 \, \text{METs} - 1 \, \text{MET}$$
$$= 6.0 \, \text{METs}$$

Maximum Workload Question
$$1 = 4.5 \, \text{METs}$$

$$\dot{V}O_2R \, \% = [(4.5 \, \text{METs} - 1.0 \, \text{METs})/6.0 \, \text{METs}]$$
$$= 0.583$$
$$= 0.583 \times 100$$
$$= 58.3\%$$

Resource: Liguori G, senior editor. *ACSM's Guidelines for Exercise Testing and Prescription*. 11th ed. Philadelphia (PA): Wolters Kluwer; 2021

11. Considerations of medical history, GXT, and patient goals in developing an exercise program:

(Continued)

NANCY CASE STUDY 5: ANSWERS (Continued)

Medical History

- Risk Factor Profile

1. Family history
2. Hypertension
3. Abnormal fasting blood glucose and HbA1C
4. Dyslipidemia (triglycerides)
5. Fitness level
6. BMI
7. Predicted maximal volume of oxygen consumed per unit time ($\dot{V}O_{2max}$) from GXT
   - Medication Effects on Exercise Testing and Programming

1. Diuretics
2. ST-segment depression (possible)
3. Hypovolemia
4. Hypohydration
5. Calcium channel blockers
6. Dihydropyridine versus nondihydropyridine class effects on exercise
7. Vasodilation compensatory sympathetic response (increased HR)
   - Laboratory Blood Analysis

   Graded Exercise Test as a Basis for Exercise Prescription
   - ECG Changes (ST-Segment Depression) during GXT

1. Causes of abnormal ST changes in the absence of obstructive CAD
   A) Female gender

B) Hypokalemia (diuretic induced)
- Hemodynamic Responses to Exercise
- Subjective RPE
- Predicted $\dot{V}O_{2max}$ from GXT

Patient Goals
- Nancy expressed a desire to lose weight through exercise and diet

12. **Outline of Discussion (II)**
   - Intensity of exercise that minimizes blood lactate accumulation
   - Intensity of exercise that minimizes frustration
   - Intensity/duration of exercise that maximizes caloric expenditure
   - Exercise bout and/or daily interval training
   - Frequency that establishes positive exercise patterns
   - Frequency that aids in blood glucose control
   - Mode in aerobic exercise that involves large muscle mass
   - Mode that minimizes orthopedic joint stress but utilizes bone stress (osteoporosis)
   - Mode in resistance exercise that minimizes delayed onset muscle soreness (DOMS)
   - Progression for a new, low-fit, overweight, middle-aged client with prediabetes

JOE CASE STUDY 6: ANSWERS

1. —B. 39 kg

   Resource: Liguori G, senior editor. *ACSM's Guidelines for Exercise Testing and Prescription.* 11th ed. Philadelphia (PA): Wolters Kluwer; 2021

2. —C. HR below the ischemic threshold (<10 beats)

   Resource: Liguori G, senior editor. *ACSM's Guidelines for Exercise Testing and*

   Prescription. 11th ed. Philadelphia (PA): Wolters Kluwer; 2021

3. —B. No greater than 134 bpm

   If exercise data is provided, exercise should be prescribed at an HR below the ischemic threshold (<10 bpm).

   Resource: Liguori G, senior editor. *ACSM's Guidelines for Exercise Testing and Prescription.* 11th ed. Philadelphia (PA): Wolters Kluwer; 2021

4. —A. 124 W

If GXT is administered on a leg cycle ergometer, there is ~10%–15% less physiological stress than on a treadmill. Functional capacity needs to be reduced by 10%.

$\dot{V}O_2$ Relative = 6 METs $\times$ 3.5 mL $\cdot$ kg^{-1} $\cdot$ min^{-1} = 21.0 mL $\cdot$ kg^{-1} $\cdot$ min^{-1} $\times$ 0.90 = 18.9 mL $\cdot$ kg^{-1} $\cdot$ min^{-1}

Joe's body weight = 253 lb $\times$ 2.2 = 115 kg

1 W = 6.12 kgm

Resting component = 3.5 mL $\cdot$ kg^{-1} $\cdot$ min^{-1}

Leg cycle ergometer horizontal component =

3.5 mL $\cdot$ kg^{-1} $\cdot$ min^{-1}

$\dot{V}O_2$ Relative = $\dfrac{1.8 \times W}{M}$ + 7

18.9 mL $\cdot$ kg^{-1} $\cdot$ min^{-1} = $\dfrac{1.8 \times W}{115 \text{ kg}}$ + 7 $\rightarrow$ 760 kgm/ 6.12 $\rightarrow$ 124 W

Resource: Liguori G, senior editor. *ACSM's Guidelines for Exercise Testing and Prescription*. 11th ed. Philadelphia (PA): Wolters Kluwer; 2021

5. —B. 213 lb

Joe's BF percentage = 34%

Joe's target BF percentage = 22%

Fat mass = 115 kg $\times$ 0.34 = 39 kg

Fat-free mass = 76 kg

Target body weight = Fat-free mass/(1−BF%)

76 kg/(1−0.22) = 97 kg

97 kg $\times$ 2.2 = 213 lb

Resource: Liguori G, senior editor. *ACSM's Guidelines for Exercise Testing and Prescription*. 11th ed. Philadelphia (PA): Wolters Kluwer; 2021

6. —A. Normal

Resting EF of <55% is considered normal.

Resources: Thompson WR, editor. *ACSM's Clinical Exercise Physiology*. 1st ed. Philadelphia (PA): Wolters Kluwer; 2019. Box 3.2.

Liguori G, senior editor. *ACSM's Guidelines for Exercise Testing and Prescription*. 11th ed. Philadelphia (PA): Wolters Kluwer; 2021

7. —D. Moderately severe angina

3+ on a 1–4 scale

Resource: Liguori G, senior editor. *ACSM's Guidelines for Exercise Testing and Prescription*. 11th ed. Philadelphia (PA): Wolters Kluwer; 2021

8. —A. 6 METs

If exercise data is provided, exercise intensity should be prescribed at a workload 1 MET below the ischemic threshold.

Resource: Liguori G, senior editor. *ACSM's Guidelines for Exercise Testing and Prescription*. 11th ed. Philadelphia (PA): Wolters Kluwer; 2021

9. —C. 3.6 mph and 4.5% grade

mph to m $\cdot$ s^{-1} = 3.6 mph $\times$ 26.8 m $\cdot$ s^{-1} = 98.48 m $\cdot$ s^{-1}

Grade % to decimal form = 4.5% = 0.045

Resting component = 3.5 mL $\cdot$ kg^{-1} $\cdot$ min^{-1}

Horizontal component = (0.1 $\times$ speed) = (0.1 $\times$ 98.48 m $\cdot$ s^{-1}) = 9.848 mL $\cdot$ kg^{-1} $\cdot$ min^{-1}

Vertical component = (1.8 $\times$ speed $\times$ grade) = (1.8 $\times$ 98.48 $\times$ 0.045) = 7.976 mL $\cdot$ kg^{-1} $\cdot$ min^{-1}

MET = 21.324 mL $\cdot$ kg^{-1} $\cdot$ min^{-1}/3.5 mL $\cdot$ kg^{-1} $\cdot$ min^{-1} = 6.093 = 6 METs

Resource: Liguori G, senior editor. *ACSM's Guidelines for Exercise Testing and Prescription*. 11th ed. Philadelphia (PA): Wolters Kluwer; 2021

10. —C. 362 kcal

Maximal MET level on treadmill is 6 MET.

$\dot{V}O_2$ Relative = 6 METs $\times$ 3.5 mL $\cdot$ kg^{-1} $\cdot$ min^{-1} = 21 mL $\cdot$ kg^{-1} $\cdot$ min^{-1}

Joe's weight in kg = 115 (253 lb / 2.2)

1 L $\cdot$ min^{-1} = 5 cal

Time = 30 min

ACSM-CEP

JOE CASE STUDY 6: ANSWERS (Continued)

$\dot{V}O_2$ Absoulte $= 21$ mL $\cdot$ kg^{-1} $\cdot$ min^{-1} $\times$ 115 kg $=$

2.415 L $\cdot$ min^{-1}

1,000 mL

2.415 L $\cdot$ min^{-1} $\times$ 5 cal $\times$ 30 min $=$ 362 cal

Resource: Liguori G, senior editor. *ACSM's Guidelines for Exercise Testing and Prescription*. 11th ed. Philadelphia (PA): Wolters Kluwer; 2021

11. Individuals diagnosed with CVD benefit from participation in regular exercise and lifestyle changes. Outpatient cardiopulmonary rehabilitation is commonly encouraged to promote exercise and lifestyle interventions. It generally consists of a coordinated, multifaceted program designed to reduce risk, promote healthy behaviors and compliance, reduce disability, and encourage an active lifestyle for patients with CVD. Taking into account lifestyle modification, a cardiopulmonary rehabilitation program is composed of a medically supervised exercise and education program. The cardiopulmonary team is typically composed of a medical director (physician), program coordinator (registered nurse or CEP), registered nurses, CEPs, registered dieticians, and psychologists among other health care professionals. Individuals who participate in outpatient cardiopulmonary rehabilitation benefit from a multidisciplinary team due to comorbidities or conditions that accompany CVD such as that of obesity, diabetes, dyslipidemia, arthritis, and depression. A multidisciplinary approach assists patients with engaging in a physically active lifestyle, dietary changes, weight loss, smoking cessation, stress management, and overall education about their specific diagnoses.

12. Literature suggests that it may take more than the public health recommendation of 150 min $\cdot$ wk^{-1} or 30 min of physical activity on most days of the week to promote sustained weight loss. Adults such as Joe who bear overweight or obesity are likely to benefit from progression in their exercise routine to approximately >250 min $\cdot$ wk^{-1}, preferably 5–7 d $\cdot$ wk^{-1} of aerobic activity to maximize caloric expenditure. Eventual

progression to more vigorous exercise intensity ($\geq$60% $\dot{V}O_2$R or HRR) is advised and may result in further health benefits. From Joe's medical history and the information provided from his initial evaluation, it is likely that he is one of the individuals who will be encouraged to exercise at a higher than moderate-intensity level. It is important to address Joe's capability and willingness to exercise at higher levels of physical exertion. The key is to enhance the likelihood of the adoption and maintenance of physical activity. This can be achieved by the accumulation of the suggested amount of physical activity in multiple daily bouts of at least 10 min in duration for those previously sedentary individuals. Resistance exercise should also be incorporated into Joe's routine to promote muscular strength and physical function. There may be additional benefits of participating in a resistance exercise routine such as that of improvements in CVD and DM.

13. Excess body mass (measured in kg $\cdot$ m^{-2} [$\geq$30 kg $\cdot$ m^{-2}]), specifically, abdominal adiposity is linked to stroke, hypertension, DM, metabolic syndrome, dyslipidemia, and overall CVD risk. BMI is used to assess weight relative to height. Joe forms part of the general population. That is, Joe is not an athlete such as a body builder, swimmer, or runner. Nevertheless, the rehabilitation center where he is undergoing his cardiac rehabilitation is unlikely have state-of-the-art equipment. This cardiopulmonary rehabilitation center is likely to only treat patients with various CVD and pulmonary issues between the ages of 38 and 90 years; the simplistic approach of assessing BMI is very convenient at the initial and post-program evaluation in terms of obtaining body composition statistics. Athletic population would benefit from having their body composition assessed by hydrodensitometry or air displacement plethysmography as the result of these methods being able to distinguish between fat mass and lean muscle mass unlike BMI.

14. The Bruce protocol is geared toward populations who are younger and physically

capable of performing physical activity that involves walking. It is important to recall Joe's age and his line of work. Joe is fairly young and has a high activity occupational job as a mover. The Bruce protocol employs relatively large incremental workload adjustments (*i.e.*, 2–3 METs per stage) every 3 min. Joe's job as a mover likely elicits MET levels of ≥6 when pushing, pulling, and carrying heavy furniture on a daily basis. The Bruce protocol was the appropriate method of assessing his functional capacity as well as ischemic threshold because he had reported chest tightness/pressure while on the job. A submaximal GXT via leg cycle ergometry would have likely provided an underestimation of results in terms of overall functional capacity and ischemic threshold for this particular patient.

15. Patients who are undergoing cardiac rehabilitation should be considered for a resistance exercise routine geared toward improving ADL and recreational activities. The individual should have no evidence of congestive heart failure, uncontrolled arrhythmias, uncontrolled hypertension, and overall unstable symptoms.

    - Equipment type should consist of elastic bands, hand weights, and weight machines.
    - Proper techniques such as that of raising and lowering weights with controlled movements to full extension should be implemented.
    - Joe is advised to maintain a regular breathing pattern and avoid holding his breath. Nonetheless, it is imperative that he avoids straining and sustained gripping, which may evoke an excessive BP response.
    - An RPE of 11–14 (fairly light to somewhat hard) on a scale of 6–20 may be used as a subjective guide.
    - Resistance exercise should be terminated if abnormal signs or symptoms occur including dizziness, arrhythmias, unusual SOB, or angina.
    - The initial workload should allow for 10–15 repetitions that can be lifted without straining (40%–50% of 1-RM, progressing to 60%–70% of 1-RM).
    - The determination of a 1-RM may be deemed inappropriate for individuals

with CVD. Therefore, multiple trials using progressively higher loads can be performed until the patient can perform no more than 10 repetitions without straining.

- Resistance exercise intensity can be progressed by increasing the resistance, increasing the number of repetitions, or decreasing the rest period between sets or exercises.
- Joe should exercise each major muscle group, with at least 8–10 exercises (chest, shoulders, arms, abdomen, back, hips, and legs).
- Joe's regimen should exercise large muscle groups before small muscle groups and should include multijoint exercises that affect more than one muscle group.
- Joe should participate in resistance exercise 2–3 d · wk^{-1} with at least 48 h separating training sessions for the same muscle group.
- All muscle groups that are trained may be done in the same session or in a split routine.
- Two to four sets are recommended to improve muscular strength and power.
- Rest intervals of 2–3 min between each set provide sufficient recovery.
- Resistance exercise should be performed after the aerobic component of the exercise session allowing for adequate warm-up of the muscles.
- Joe's resistance exercise program progression should be based in slowly increasing (~2–5 lb · wk^{-1}) for upper body and (~5–10 lb · wk^{-1}) for lower body as tolerated.

Resources: American Association of Cardiovascular and Pulmonary Rehabilitation. Guidelines for Cardiac Rehabilitation and Secondary Prevention Programs. 4th ed. Champaign (IL): Human Kinetics; 2004.

Liguori G, senior editor. *ACSM's Guidelines for Exercise Testing and Prescription*. 11th ed. Philadelphia (PA): Wolters Kluwer; 2021

U.S. Department of Health and Human Services. 2018 Physical Activity Guidelines for Americans. Rockville, MD: U.S. Department of Health and Human Services; 2018. Available from: https://health.gov/our-work/physical-activity/current-guidelines

MR. KYLE CASE STUDY 7: ANSWERS

1. —A. May reduce resting and exercise heart rate and blood pressure.

   Resource: Liguori G, senior editor. *ACSM's Guidelines for Exercise Testing and Prescription*. 11th ed. Philadelphia (PA): Wolters Kluwer; 2021

2. —E. Only A. and B. of the above

   Resource: Liguori G, senior editor. *ACSM's Guidelines for Exercise Testing and Prescription*. 11th ed. Philadelphia (PA): Wolters Kluwer; 2021

3. —B. Moderate risk

   Resource: Liguori G, senior editor. *ACSM's Guidelines for Exercise Testing and Prescription*. 11th ed. Philadelphia (PA): Wolters Kluwer; 2021

4. —B. 30–<40% HRR or $\dot{V}O_2R$, 2–<3 METS, RPE 9–11, an intensity that causes slight increases in HR and breathing.

   Resource: Liguori G, senior editor. *ACSM's Guidelines for Exercise Testing and Prescription*. 11th ed. Philadelphia (PA): Wolters Kluwer; 2021

5. —D. 69

   Resource: Verrill D, Graham H, Vitcenda M, Peno-Green L, Kramer V, Corbisiero T.

   Measuring behavioral outcomes in cardiopulmonary rehabilitation—an AACVPR statement.

   Journal of Cardiopulmonary Rehabilitation and Prevention 2009;29:193-203.

6. —E. The Zung Depression survey

   Resource: AACVPR. Guidelines for Cardiac Rehabilitation Programs. 6th ed. Champaign (IL): Human Kinetics; 2021.

7. —E. Obese (class II)

   Resource: Liguori G, senior editor. *ACSM's Guidelines for Exercise Testing and Prescription*. 11th ed. Philadelphia (PA): Wolters Kluwer; 2021

8. —C. Cycle ergometer exercise at 0.5 kg (180 kg/min) at a HR of 114–128 and an RPE of 11–16.

   Resource: Liguori G, senior editor. *ACSM's Guidelines for Exercise Testing and Prescription*. 11th ed. Philadelphia (PA): Wolters Kluwer; 2021

9. —C. At least 3 d · wk^{-1}, but preferably most days of the week

   Resource: Liguori G, senior editor. *ACSM's Guidelines for Exercise Testing and Prescription*. 11th ed. Philadelphia (PA): Wolters Kluwer; 2021

10. —B. 197 lb. (89.4 kg)

    Resource: Swain DP, senior editor. *Resource Manual for ACSM's Guidelines for Exercise Testing and Prescription*, 7th ed. Baltimore (MD): Wolters/Kluwer—Lippincott, Williams & Wilkins, 2014.

11. —Mr. Kyle may have some form of chronic lung disease (*e.g.*, Chronic obstructive pulmonary disease [COPD] or restrictive lung disease) as demonstrated by his oxygen desaturation levels during his rehab entry GXT. He may also have impaired fasting blood glucose (prediabetes mellitus) as demonstrated by a fasting blood glucose level of 120 mg/dL.

    Send the results of the GXT, which shows the oxygen desaturation levels during exercise to the patient's medical office and discuss these results with the physician or the physician's nurse. Also inform his medical office of his elevated fasting glucose values, which may represent prediabetes and require further medical testing and analysis. Chronic obstructive pulmonary disease and diabetes are often comorbid conditions with cardiovascular disease (CVD) due to the common risk factors of smoking, obesity, and poor diet. The presence of COPD in current or former smokers is also an independent predictor of overall cardiovascular events.

    Resources Liguori G, senior editor. *ACSM's Guidelines for Exercise Testing and Prescription*. 11th ed. Philadelphia (PA): Wolters Kluwer; 2021

    de Barros e Silva, PG, Califf, RM, Sun, JL et al., 2014. Chronic obstructive pulmonary disease and cardiovascular risk: insights from the NAVIGATOR trial. International Journal of Cardiology. 176 (3), 1126-1128.

12. —As Mr. Kyle may not be compliant with his medications at the present time, you should inform his medical office (*e.g.*, physician) of potential noncompliance issues with regard to his medication usage. You should talk to Mr. Kyle about the purpose and importance of taking each medication as prescribed in a one-on-one consultation. Discuss barriers that he encounters when taking his medications (*e.g.*, undesirable side effects, inconvenience, difficulty swallowing pills). You should also discuss potential side effects for each of his medications and whether or not he is experiencing any associated side effects should be discussed with him. Finally, you should record Mr. Kyle's daily medication compliance at rehab entry and at each follow-up evaluation with established medication compliance surveys.

You should inform Mr. Kyle's medical office (*e.g.*, physician) of his current smoking status. His physician may want to consider some form of nicotine replacement therapy or medications such as Bupropion to help Mr. Kyle with his tobacco cravings. You should also suggest that Mr. Kyle see the staff rehab psychologist (with permission from his personal physician) to address the barriers to smoking cessation that currently exist. You should monitor and record his number of cigarettes smoked daily at rehab entry and at each follow-up evaluation to demonstrate progress or regression in his smoking cessation efforts. Finally, you should recommend the hospital's smoking cessation program to Mr. Kyle and check on his smoking status during each cardiac rehabilitation visit.

You should inform Mr. Kyle's medical office (*e.g.*, physician) of his current level of high stress status. His physician may want to consider some form of anti-anxiety or antidepressant medication, as well as professional counseling. He should take an established depression or anxiety survey (*e.g.*, Beck Depression Inventory II) at rehab entry and at each follow-up evaluation to help determine if he is suffering from clinical depression and/or anxiety. You should also suggest that he see the staff rehab psychologist (with permission from his personal physician) to discuss stress management techniques. He should also attend the cardiac rehab educational classes on stress management and participate in the relaxation sessions offered weekly during the exercise sessions. Mr. Kyle may also want to pursue Tai Chi, yoga, or other form of relaxation-inducing exercise program that you present to him.

Resource: Verrill D, Graham H, Vitcenda M, Peno-Green L, Kramer V, Corbisiero T. Measuring behavioral outcomes in cardiopulmonary rehabilitation—an AACVPR statement. Journal of Cardiopulmonary Rehabilitation and Prevention 2009;29: 193-203.

13. —At least six purposes are as follows:

1. To evaluate signs, symptoms, and potential myocardial ischemia.

2. To determine the need for coronary angiography in patients treated initially with a noninvasive strategy.

3. To determine the effectiveness of medical therapy.

4. To assess future level of cardiovascular risk and prognosis.

5. To develop the initial exercise prescription for cardiac rehabilitation participation with regard to training HR and MET level.

6. To objectively determine the patient's functional capacity for return to work, vocational, and avocational activities.

Resource: Thompson WR, editor. *ACSM's Clinical Exercise Physiology*. 1st ed. Philadelphia (PA): Wolters Kluwer; 2019. Chapter 8, pg. 349–364.

14. —The following resistive exercise training regimen and modalities could be recommended:

- **Modalities:** Free weights, dumbbells, elastic bands, wall or weight machine pulleys, stability balls, weighted wands, machines (*i.e.*, resistive machines specific to avoid further injury to Mr. Kyle's lower back). Light dumbbell weights (2–5 lb.) or moderate resistance elastic bands performed during each rehab session during his early rehabilitation sessions.

(Continued)

MR. KYLE CASE STUDY 7: ANSWERS (Continued)

- **Frequency:** 2–3 d · wk^{-1} with at least 48-h separating training sessions for the same muscle group.
- **Intensity:**
  - Initial workloads of 10–15 repetitions at an RPE of 11–14 (6–20 scale).
  - Initial workloads of 40%–50% of 1-RM (if 1-RM testing performed).
  - If 1–RM technique is not used, multiple trials using progressively higher workloads performed until the patient can perform >10 repetitions without straining.
  - One to three sets of resistive exercises, increasing up to four sets over time if indicated.
- **Progression:** Increase weight slowly as the patient adapts to the program (*e.g.*, ~2–5 lb · wk^{-1} for the upper body and 5–10 lb · wk^{-1} for the lower body).
- Resistance exercises for each major muscle group of the upper and lower body.
- Exercise large muscle groups before small muscle groups.
- Circuit weight training may be incorporated with low-level resistance stations to better prepare Mr. Kyle to perform his occupational and leisure time activities.

Resource: Liguori G, senior editor. *ACSM's Guidelines for Exercise Testing and Prescription*. 11th ed. Philadelphia (PA): Wolters Kluwer; 2021

15. —The following:
  a. **Medications:** Diltiazem (Cardizem), digoxin (Lanoxin), Coumadin (warfarin)
  b. **Physiologic Concerns:**
    - Increased risk of thromboembolic events
    - Rapid ventricular rates when the AV-node is inadequately suppressed
    - Incomplete ventricular filling causing reduced cardiac output
    - Decreased functional capacity
    - Fatigue
    - Arrhythmic symptoms (*e.g.*, palpitations, rapid HR, slow HR)
  c. **Exercise Concerns:**
    - Decreased exercise tolerance
    - Difficult to determine systolic BP due to variability in diastolic filling
    - Difficult to determine pulse due to rapid, irregular ventricular response
    - Marked variability in maximal HR response—age-predicted maximal HR targets not valid
    - Longer sampling of pulse may be needed for reliable target HR determination
    - May need to be on continuous electrocardiographic monitoring

Resource: Durstine JL, Moore GE, Painter PL, Roberts SO. ACSM's Exercise Management for Patients with Chronic Disease and Disabilities. Champaign, IL: Human Kinetics, 2009, pp. 73–78.

SHERYL CASE STUDY 8: ANSWERS

1. —B. Moderate

   FEV1 is 50%–79%

2. —D. Rate of Perceived Exertion and/or Dyspnea

   6MWTs are usually performed for pulmonary patients prior to starting PR, therefore a THR would not be calculated for this population. As a result, we would prescribe exercise based upon their RPE and dyspnea rating.

3. —D. Accumulate 20–30 min of intermittent non-weight-bearing exercise.

   Sheryl should start with intermittent bouts of non-weight-bearing activity to build strength and endurance. Non-weight-bearing activity should help to keep her SpO$_2$ within a desired range.

4. —D. All the above.

   We can tell by the patient's heart rate response, SpO$_2$, and difficulty breathing, that the patient is exhibiting difficulty with the exercise; however, the patient reported the exercise as "light" on the RPE scale. With a pulmonary patient, it would be beneficial to discuss how and why the RPE and RPD scales are used, the ease in which a person should be able to talk while exercising, and how to use pursed lip breathing to maintain SpO_2 levels and reduce RPD scores.

5. —C. Patient experienced increased dyspnea (4/10) with weight-bearing exercise. Exercise prescription modified to reduce rating of perceived dyspnea score to desired range (2–3/10).

   A and B include subjective information—when writing a note, you want to avoid saying things such as "I think." Option C is appropriate because it explains the issue at hand, provides factual information using scales for exercise intensity, and provides a solution. Option D lacks important, specific, information.

6. —C. Albuterol

   Albuterol is a bronchodilator that helps to increase exercise capacity by limiting bronchospasm. Albuterol can increase HR, which is important to be aware of.

7. Teach Sheryl about pursed lip breathing, pacing, and energy conservation. Establish a program for Sheryl that specifically trains her for tasks she finds difficult. Start with simple chair exercises progress to activity simulation.

   Chair exercises can include sit to stand, leg extension, standing leg curl (using the chair for balance), over head reaching, should press, front raises, etc.

   Standing exercises can include hip hinge, weight shifts (for vacuuming), squatting and bending (for laundry), step-ups (stair climbing), etc.

   Teach the patient when and how to breathe during the various movements and eventually progress to ADL simulation.

Domains Covered:

Domain IA

Domain IIA

Domain III: A, B, C, D

Domain IV: D, E

JIM CASE STUDY 9: ANSWERS

1. —B. NSTEMI.

   EKG did not show evidence of infarction (STEMI); however, the patient's troponin levels were elevated.

2. —A. Antiplatelet drug

   Commonly prescribed for 12 months following PCI to prevent adverse outcomes.

3. —C. Atorvastatin

   Jim has hyperlipidemia based upon the labs provided. A statin would help to control this risk factor. In addition, statins are routinely prescribed following an ACS event/procedure.

4. —D. Cancel the stress test until the patient is consistently taking his medications as prescribed.

You would not want to perform a stress test until the patient is taking his β-blocker and antiplatelet drug routinely/as prescribed. Exercising the patient may cause an adverse outcome otherwise.

5. —D. Oxygen assessment

   This is mandatory for pulmonary rehab but no cardiac rehab.

6. —D. Lipid management, smoking cessation, and improved exercise tolerance.

   Managing these modifiable risk factors will help reduce the rate of an additional event/procedure in the future. Weight loss would not necessarily be a goal because the patient has a BMI of 24. Diabetes management would not be a goal because the patient is not a diabetic and his A1C is within normal limits.

(Continued)

ACSM-CEP

JIM CASE STUDY 9: ANSWERS (Continued)

7. —C. Decisional balance

   Decisional balance may be used in MI; however, it is not a part of the fundamental techniques included in the acronym OARS: open-ended questions, affirmation, reflective listening, summary reflections.

8. —The five most prescribed are as follows:

   1. Aspirin
   2. Anti-platelet therapy (clopidogrel)
   3. β-blocker (metoprolol)
   4. ACE inhibitors (lisinopril)
   5. Statins (atorvastatin)

9. Jim is not regularly taking clopidogrel, an antiplatelet therapy. Noncompliance with clopidogrel can lead to the formation of clots, which poses an increased risk for MI following PCI placement. Considering that Jim continues to smoke as well, his risk for subsequent MI is further increased due to the fact that cigarette smoking causes increased platelet aggregation. In addition, Jim is not taking his β-blocker regularly. β-blockers are important following an MI to help alleviate the workload placed on the heart by reducing heart rate and blood pressure.

Domains Covered:

Domain I: A, B, C

Domain II: C

Domain V: C, D

KIMBERLY CASE STUDY 10: ANSWERS

1. —E. All of the above
2. —E. Both A and C
3. —B. Social cognitive theory
4. —D. Challenging self with difficult goals
5. —C. Goals should be challenging.

   Resource: Swain D, senior editor. *ACSM's Resource Manual for Guidelines for Exercise Testing and Prescription*. 7th ed. Baltimore (MD): Lippincott Williams & Wilkins; 2014. 896 p.

6. The following are the three barriers and its impact on exercise compliance:

   a. Time: A full-time job and primary child care responsibilities place a time crunch on the client. Discontinuous bouts of activity with a focus on walking may alleviate the burden of time as a significant barrier. In addition, this mode of activity can be completed in various convenient settings, thereby matching the work and commuter schedule.

   b. Fatigue/pain: Patients with FMS often complain of multiple tender points, undue fatigue, and morning stiffness. In addition, the client's sleep disturbances coupled with chronic soft tissue discomfort may make some exercise intensities and types of exercise difficulty. Consideration of using low-intensity exercise with shorter bouts may reduce the fatigue and pain response. Remind the client that discomfort during exercise may occur, but that pain may require exercise termination or selection of various modalities of exercise.

   c. Depression/motivation: Due to the primary symptoms associated with FMS and life demands currently placed on Kimberly, it is not uncommon to see a significant reduction in motivation toward physical activity. In addition, the incidence of depression is higher in patients with FMS as compared to their apparently healthy counterparts.

7. Selecting types of exercise that Kimberly enjoys and has easy access to may alleviate some of the barriers that she presents. Little skill and equipment (good walking shoes, pedometer, polar heart monitor) are necessary to implement an effective exercise program.

In addition, shorter, discontinuous bouts of exercise may be warranted considering the numerous demands on Kimberly's time. Suggestions to include her children in the exercise plan (biking alongside) would

increase her social support, which has been demonstrated to increase adherence.

8. The client should be part of the goal-setting process with the health care team to develop realistic goals, timeline for implementation, periodic measures, and revisions to goals as warranted. Developing a goal-setting contract with signature for client and CEP provides a public proclamation, which often may enhance the effectiveness of the goal-setting plan. In addition, both short- and long-term goals should be included with regular assessment to allow for new strategies if necessary.

PATIENT PRIVACY CASE STUDY 11: ANSWERS

1. —C. Fax the BP readings and let the nurse know that you may not give out other personal information on the patient's progress.

You may fax the requested BP readings to the patient's primary care office because this is a continuation of care and necessary for treatment of the patient. You may not give out a status update to the nurse who is planning to share this information with others and which is not directly related to the care of this patient. Follow the "minimum necessary" use guidelines when sharing information with others involved in the care of the patient.

2. —False

Unless the individual has legal authority to make decisions for the patient, they do not have access to other family member's health information without written consent from the patient. In some states, even minors have certain rights to privacy from their parents. Be familiar with your state laws regarding release of health information to others.

3. —B. Tell your coworker that you cannot share passwords, but you will call the phy-

sician office and obtain the information needed.

Sharing computer passwords or posting them in a public place is a HIPAA violation. When individuals share passwords, they pose a direct threat to patient privacy. The recipient, even if a coworker, can use your passwords to access confidential information in an unauthorized way, for which you will be held responsible.

4. —False

The physician scanned the room first to make sure that no unauthorized individuals would hear or see confidential patient information. Turning the screen to view it in a public location is acceptable when only authorized individuals are in the room. If others were present who should not hear or see this information, the physician would need to go behind the desk to view the information.

5. —D. All of the above

All information that identifies an individual is protected under the Privacy Rule. This includes, but is not limited to, name, address, e-mail address, date of birth, social security numbers, phone and fax

(Continued)

PATIENT PRIVACY CASE STUDY 11: ANSWERS (Continued)

numbers, medical record number, and photographs. It also includes past, present, and future medical records as well as billing information.

6. —False

A patient has the right to disclose their own personal health information and diagnosis to anyone they want. A patient sharing information about themselves is not a violation of the Privacy Rule.

7. —A. Tell her that you cannot do that and offer to come in earlier to help out.

Under the Privacy Rule, organizations are required to have reasonable safeguards in place for the protection of confidential patient information. This includes storing patient records in a locked file cabinet or record room. Leaving the charts out on the desk at night, even if they are labeled confidential, is allowing for the potential of unauthorized access to private patient information. There may be other individuals that enter your facility when you are not there, including housekeeping staff, maintenance workers, and security staff. These individuals may be authorized to access your work area but not the confidential information on patients that is stored there. The safest place for medical records is safely locked in a storage file or records room.

Resource:

Health Insurance Portability and Accountability Act of 1996 Web site [Internet]. Washington, DC: U.S. Department of Health and Human Services; [cited 2016 Jan 28]. Available from: http://www.hhs.gov/hipaa/for-professionals/index.html

EMERGENCY PREPAREDNESS CASE STUDY 12: ANSWERS

1. —B. Glucometer

A glucometer is not a common piece of emergency equipment or supply found in a health/fitness facility.

2. —True.

All health/fitness facilities should have emergency plans in place regardless of their level.

3. —C. Have him stop exercising

The first action when an individual reports possible angina for the first time is to stop activity.

4. —B. Stop exercise and notify his physician, check and document his vitals, and continue to observe him

The patient is asymptomatic, but the ventricular ectopy is new and needs to be treated.

5. —B. Immediately immobilize his wrist, implement RICE (rest, ice, compress, and elevate), and promptly notify his physician.

The correct response is to immediately immobilize this type of injury, implement RICE, and notify the individual's physician. Promptly dealing musculoskeletal injury is extremely important to decrease pain and stabilize the individual.

6. —A. Activate EMS; note time the symptoms started.

The acute action that should be taken is to notify EMS and note the time the symptoms started.

Resources: Sanders ME, senior editor. ACSM's Health/Fitness Facility Standards and Guidelines. 5th ed. Champaign (IL): Human Kinetics; 2018.

ECG CASE STUDY 1: ANSWERS

1. Asystole

2. —D. Check the patient.

3. —A. A patient can be stable with a sustain presentation of this disorder.

4. —C. Fine ventricular fibrillation.

   Teaching points: Syncope is a common diagnosis, occurring at least once in a lifetime in approximately 40% of individuals. The majority of syncopal episodes are vasovagal related, which can lead to sudden drops in both BP and HR. Often, if the individual is monitored during the syncopal event, the presenting rhythm can be pronounced bradycardia, an advanced AV block (type 2 or 3), or transient asystole, as defined as a ventricular pause of >3 s (*i.e.*, 75 mm at 25 mm $\cdot$ s^{-1}). Typically, such syncopal episodes carry a low-mortality rate and are considered benign. However, such events can reoccur, which can impact QOL and possibly lead to trauma. In some individuals, the placement of a permanent pacemaker has helped to reduce recurrence. Other treatments include adequate fluids and sodium as well as medications such as β-blockers, selective serotonin reuptake inhibitors, and fludrocortisone. Although the case presented here was benign, prolonged asystole is the most grave rhythm indicating end of life. Often, the latter is precipitated by ventricular tachycardia and/or fibrillation and could be mistaken for fine ventricular fibrillation.

   Resource: Ganzeboom KS, Mairuhu G, Reitsma JB, Linzer M, Wieling W, van Dijk N. Lifetime cumulative incidence of syncope in the general population: a study of 549 Dutch subjects aged 35–60 yrs. J Cardiovasc Electrophysiol. 2006;17:1172–6.

ECG CASE STUDY 2: ANSWERS

1. Sinus

2. Second-degree AV block (Mobitz type I)

3. 45–50 bpm

4. —D. The patient's medical and symptom history as well as the presence of signs or symptoms of poor perfusion should guide whether the test can be performed.

5. —A. SA node

6. —C. According to the American Heart Association, the test should be terminated if it interferes with maintenance of cardiac output (CO).

   Teaching points: Unlike a second-degree type II AV block, a second-degree type I AV block generally does not progress to a complete heart block (*i.e.*, third-degree AV block). Therefore, unless an individual with a second-degree type I AV block (also known as Wenckebach) becomes symptomatic due to bradycardia, a pacemaker is not usually indicated. When the ventricular rhythm is irregular, as in second-degree AV block or atrial fibrillation, the ventricular rate can be estimated by counting the number of ventricular complexes that appear over a given time. As displayed on this ECG, the standard ECG paper speed is 25 mm $\cdot$ s^{-1}. That results in 50 large (5 mm) boxes (starting after the calibration mark) across a standard ECG for 10 s of time (50 × 5 mm = 250 mm/ 25 mm $\cdot$ s^{-1} = 10 s). In this example, there are eight ventricular complexes during this 10-s period for an estimated ventricular rate of 48 bpm. The clinician could also use a millimeter ruler to measure 150 mm (30 large boxes) across an ECG, which would represent 6 s (count the complexes and multiple by 10 for the rate). A standard Bic pen with the cap on can be a useful estimate of 150 mm.

ECG CASE STUDY 3: ANSWERS

1. Third-degree AV block

2. 60 bpm

3. 60–65 bpm

4. —H. Options B and C are correct.

5. —B. AV node

6. —A. Patients are usually asymptomatic with this disorder.

   Teaching points: Often, patients with a third-degree AV block (*e.g.*, complete heart block) are symptomatic with pronounced hypotension and bradycardia. However, on occasion, patients may be hemodynamically stable at rest and present as asymptomatic or with mild complaints of fatigue or light-headedness. The defining characteristics of third-degree AV block are a regular atrial rhythm and a regular (but dissociated) ventricular rhythm, which is very slow (*e.g.*, 30–60 bpm). P waves can be hidden within the QRS complex and/or T waves but still should "march out" to show an underlying regular sinus rhythm. Additionally, the QRS complex can be wide; however, the width of the QRS complex depends on where the escape rhythm originates (*e.g.*, AV node vs. ventricles). The treatment for a third-degree AV block is a permanent pacemaker.

ECG CASE STUDY 4: ANSWERS

1. Rate is approximately 70 bpm.

2. Irregular rhythm

3. Atrial fibrillation

4. —B. Warfarin

5. —D. None of the above

6. —A. RPE

   Teaching points: Warfarin is often prescribed in patients with atrial fibrillation to prevent the formation of and to treat existing thrombi that result due to the unorganized and weak contractions of the atria. It is important to confirm that the patient is on some type of anticoagulation therapy. Patients presenting with new onset atrial fibrillation should see a physician before resuming cardiac rehabilitation. Regarding exercise training, while compromised with this condition because of the reduced "atrial kick," patients can still improve fitness. Although HR does increase with exercise, the HR method is not reliable because of the irregular nature of this arrhythmia. Because of the irregular rhythm, when measuring the HR with atrial fibrillation, the number of cardiac cycles should be counted from a 6- or 10-s strip.

ECG CASE STUDY 5: ANSWERS

1. Sinus

2. Ventricular bigeminy

3. —A. Continue to monitor.

4. —D. All of the above

   Teaching points: Ventricular bigeminy is a stable and non-life-threatening dysrhythmia. Patients with this may or may not report feeling "skipped beats." Regardless, as with any new-onset arrhythmias, the referring physician should be notified, but this does not warrant withholding exercise. Although emotional distress and stimulants, such as caffeine, can lead to increased rates and ectopic beats, some patients may regularly have frequent ventricular activity without precipitating factors. Regardless, the clinician should first "rule out" medication noncompliance before considering secondary causes in a new onset.

ECG CASE STUDY 6: ANSWERS

1. 98 bpm

2. Regular

3. Sinus rhythm with left ventricular hypertrophy (LVH) and a left bundle-branch block (LBBB)

4. —D. Contact referring physician to verify the test ordered.

5. —True

Teaching points: Both LVH as well as LBBB can mask changes due to myocardial ischemia that are typically seen on a standard 12-lead ECG. Therefore, a symptom-limited exercise stress test with ECG only is typically not administered due to the inability to diagnose ischemia. However, new-onset LBBB in the presence of angina may indicate an acute coronary event. Regardless of the presence (or lack) of angina, a new occurrence of LBBB should be reported to a physician to determine the underlying cause.

ECG CASE STUDY 7: ANSWERS

1. 176 bpm

2. Regular

3. Sinus tachycardia

4. —B. Supraventricular tachycardia (SVT)

5. —D. β-blocker

6. —B. No

Teaching points: The HR response in the earlier ECG is normal for someone during stage IV of the Bruce protocol. Although his HR is close to his age-predicted maximum, percentage of age-predicted maximum HR is not a criterion for stopping at test. If this ECG were obtained at rest, it would be abnormal and likely an SVT, not emanating from the SA node. Finally, because of the normal HR response during exercise, if this individual was on antihypertensive medications, it would likely not be a type of β-blocker because they attenuate the chronotropic response to exercise.

ECG CASE STUDY 8: ANSWERS

1. 115 bpm

2. Irregular

3. Sinus tachycardia with a premature ventricular contraction (PVC) and a ventricular triplet

4. —B. Continue with the test.

5. —A. They are multifocal.

Teaching points: An isolated ventricular triplet, although associated with a greater likelihood of ventricular tachycardia, is not by itself dangerous. Therefore, although an isolated triplet should be noted, it is not an indication for stopping a test, according to *ACSM's GETP*. The fact that these are multifocal PVC, thus originating at different ventricular areas does not change these guidelines. More than one observed ventricular triplet, however, is listed as a relative contraindication for stopping a stress test.

ACSM-CEP

ECG CASE STUDY 9: ANSWERS

1. 78 bpm

2. Regular

3. Sinus rhythm with a right bundle-branch block (RBBB)

4. —D. The athlete will likely undergo additional evaluation before returning to play.

   Teaching points: RBBB is not an uncommon finding in athletes. As long as there is no underlying structural heart disease, most athletes are cleared to return to play.

ECG CASE STUDY 10: ANSWERS

1. 50 bpm

2. Regular

3. Sinus bradycardia with a first-degree AV block and premature ventricular contraction (PVC)

4. —False

5. —D. There is a slight risk for atrial reentry tachycardia.

Teaching points: First-degree AV block is a benign finding in healthy individuals. There is no known risk for individuals who have a first-degree AV block to develop more severe AV nodal disruptions that necessitate a pacemaker. The bradycardia is caused by enhanced vagal tone (*i.e.*, parasympathetic influence), which is common in endurance athletes. Isolated PVCs are also benign.

ECG CASE STUDY 11: ANSWERS

1. 83 bpm

2. Regular

3. Sinus with ventricular-paced rhythm (notice pacemaker spike before QRS complex)

4. —C. Third-degree AV block

5. —C. If present, ischemia would not be undetectable by ECG alone due to the pacemaker depolarization.

   Teaching points: Pacemakers are indicated when the heart's natural pacemaker (*i.e.*, SA node) does not depolarize properly, as in sick sinus syndrome, or complete AV nodal block (*i.e.*, third-degree block). Due to the fact that this ECG is only ventricular paced, the cause was likely not sick sinus syndrome; otherwise, there would also be a pacer spike before the P wave. Similar to LVH and LBBB, ventricular pacemakers can hide ECG changes due to myocardial ischemia.

ECG CASE STUDY 12: ANSWERS

1. 120 bpm

2. Regular

3. Sinus tachycardia with 2 mm of ST-segment depression in the inferior and lateral leads

4. —A. Nitroglycerin

5. —D. Both A and C

Teaching points: This is an example of classic ST-segment depression due to myocardial ischemia. The ECG reveals 2 mm of ST-segment depression in both the inferior leads (II, III, and aVF) and the lateral leads (VL, V5, and V6). Although left-sided chest pressure along with concomitant left arm pain is considered classic angina by many, pain in the jaw, between the shoulder blades, indigestion-type sensation, or just excessive SOB can be anginal equivalents. If discontinuing exercise and rest do not relieve the angina, then the drug of choice would be nitroglycerin. Typically, given sublingually for rapid absorption, the main mechanism of nitroglycerin in reducing the ischemic burden is the reduction of preload on the heart from dilation of the veins.

ECG CASE STUDY 13: ANSWERS

1. 125 bpm

2. Regular

3. Ventricular tachycardia

4. —D. All of the above

5. —D. Low CO

Teaching points: Ventricular tachycardia can be a lethal arrhythmia and is an indication for stopping a stress test. When a patient loses consciousness and a pulse cannot be obtained, immediate defibrillation is indicated. Although transient changes leading to wide QRS complexes are also seen with rate-dependent bundle-branch blocks and aberrancies, the clinician should always rule out ventricular tachycardia first because of its serious implications.

Editors for the Previous Two Editions*

EDITORS FOR THE FIFTH EDITION

Senior Editor

James R. Churilla, PhD, MPH, MS, FACSM, ACSM-PD, ACSM-RCEP, ACSM-CEP, ACSM EP-C
Brooks College of Health
University of North Florida
Jacksonville, Florida

Associate Editors

Andrew Bosak, PhD, ACSM EP-C
Liberty University
Lynchburg, Virginia

Brittany Montes, MSH, ACSM-CEP, ACSM EP-C
Brooks College of Health
University of North Florida
Jacksonville, Florida

Paul Sorace, MS, FACSM, ACSM-RCEP
Hackensack University Medical Center
Hackensack, New Jersey

EDITORS FOR THE FOURTH EDITION

Senior Editor

Gregory B. Dwyer, PhD, FACSM, ACSM-ETT, ACSM-CES, ACSM-RCEP, ACSM-PD
East Stroudsburg University
East Stroudsburg, Pennsylvania

Associate Editors

Nancy J. Belli, MA, ACSM-HFS
Asphalt Green
New York, New York

Meir Magal, PhD, FACSM, ACSM-CES
North Carolina Wesleyan College
Rocky Mount, North Carolina

Paul Sorace, MS, ACSM-RCEP
Hackensack University Medical Center
Hackensack, New Jersey

*Degrees, certifications, and affiliations current at time of editor contributions.

B Contributors to the Previous Two Editions*

CONTRIBUTING AUTHORS TO THE FIFTH EDITION

Clinton A. Brawner, PhD, MS, FACSM, ACSM-RCEP, ACSM-CEP
Henry Ford Hospital
Detroit, Michigan
Cases: Domain of Patient/Client Assessment for CEP (Electrocardiograms)

Melissa Conway-Hartman, MEd, LAT, ATC, ACSM EP-C
Brooks College of Health
University of North Florida
Jacksonville, Florida
Cases: Domain on Exercise Leadership and Client Education of CPT, Domain on Legal, Professional, Business, and Marketing of CPT, Domain on Exercise Counseling and Behavioral Strategies of EP-C

Donald M. Cummings, PhD
East Stroudsburg University
East Stroudsburg, Pennsylvania
Cases: Domain of Exercise Prescription for CEP

Shala E. Davis, PhD, FACSM
East Stroudsburg University
East Stroudsburg, Pennsylvania
Cases: Domain of Leadership and Counseling for CEP

Shawn Drake, PT, PhD, ACSM-RCEP, ACSM-PD, ACSM-CEP
Arkansas State University
Jonesboro, Arkansas
Cases: Domain of Exercise Prescription and Implementation for EP-C

Trent A. Hargens, PhD, FACSM, ACSM-CEP
James Madison University
Harrisonburg, Virginia
Cases: Domain of Patient/Client Assessment for CEP

Shenelle E. Higbee, MS, ACSM-RCEP, ACSM-CEP, ACSM EP-C
PeaceHealth St. Joseph Medical Center
Bellingham, Washington
Cases: Domain of Legal and Professional Considerations of CEP

Dennis Kerrigan, PhD, ACSM-CEP
Henry Ford Hospital
Detroit, Michigan
Cases: Domain of Patient/Client Assessment for CEP (Electrocardiograms)

Frederick Klinge, MBA, ACSM EP-C
Ochsner Health System/Varsity Sports
New Orleans, Louisiana
Cases: Domain of Management for EP-C

Angela Kvies, BS, ACSM-CEP
Cardiac/Pulmonary Rehabilitation
Baptist Medical Center Beaches
Jacksonville, Florida
Cases: Domain on Exercise Leadership and Client Education of CPT

Brittany C. Montes, MSH, ACSM-CEP, ACSM EP-C
Brooks College of Health
University of North Florida
Jacksonville, Florida
Cases: Domain on Exercise Programming and Implementation of CPT

Matthew W. Parrott, PhD, ACSM EP-C
H-P Fitness, LLC
Kansas City, Missouri
Cases: Domain of Legal and Professional for EP-C

Will Peveler, PhD
Northern Kentucky University
Highland Heights, Kentucky
Cases: Domain on Health and Fitness Assessment of EP-C

M. Ryan Richardson, MSH, ACSM EP-C
Brooks College of Health
University of North Florida
Jacksonville, Florida
Cases: Domain of Initial Client Consultation
and Assessment of CPT

Joselyn M. Rodriguez, MSH, ACSM EP-C
Cardiopulmonary Rehabilitation and
H.E.A.R.T. Fitness
Memorial Hospital
Jacksonville, Florida
Cases: Domain on Exercise Prescription of CEP

Peter Ronai, MS, FACSM, ACSM-RCEP, ACSM-CEP
Sacred Heart University

Fairfield, Connecticut
Cases: Domain on Exercise Programming and
Implementation of CPT

Mandy J. Van Hofwegen, BS, ACSM-RCEP, ACSM-CEP
PeaceHealth St. Joseph Medical Center
Bellingham, Washington
Cases: Domain of Legal and Professional
Considerations of CEP

David E. Verrill, MS, FAACVPR
University of North Carolina at Charlotte
Charlotte, North Carolina
Cases: Domain of Program Implementation
and Ongoing Support for CEP, Domain on
Exercise Prescription of CEP

Review Question Contributors to the Fifth Edition

Travis Armstrong, BS, ACSM-CEP, ACSM EP-C, ACSM EIM II
HealthLink Fitness & Wellness Center
Baptist Health System
San Antonio, Texas

Robert Berry MS, ACSM-CEP, ACSM-RCEP
Henry Ford Health System
Detroit, Michigan

Melissa Conway-Hartman, MEd, LAT, ATC, ACSM EP-C
Brooks College of Health
University of North Florida
Jacksonville, Florida

Gregory B. Dwyer, PhD, ACSM-CEP, RCEP, ETT, PD, EIMIII, FACSM
East Stroudsburg University
East Stroudsburg, Pennsylvania

Michael A. Figueroa, EdD
William Paterson University
Wayne, New Jersey

Amanda K. Hovey, BS, ACSM-CEP, ACSM EP-C
Olmsted Medical Center
Rochester, Minnesota

Kevin Huet, MS, EP-C, CSCS
Kennesaw State University
Kennesaw, Georgia

Dana Killefer, MS, ACSM-RCEP
Touro Infirmary Cardiac and Pulmonary
Rehabilitation and Wellness Center
New Orleans, Louisiana

Thomas P. Mahady, MS, CSCS
Center for Cardiac Prevention and
Rehabilitation
Hackensack University Medical Center
Hackensack, New Jersey

Joseph A. Mychalczuk, MS, ACSM-RCEP
Sacred Heart University
Fairfield, Connecticut

Matthew Owens, MS, ACSM-CEP
East Stroudsburg University
East Stroudsburg, Pennsylvania

Will Peveler, PhD
Northern Kentucky University
Highland Heights, Kentucky

Greg Ryan, PhD, CSCS
Georgia Southern University
Statesboro, Georgia

Natalie Santillo, BS, MS
Precision Sports Performance
East Hanover, New Jersey

Brianna Trump, MS, ACSM-CEP
East Stroudsburg University
East Stroudsburg, Pennsylvania

David E. Verrill, MS, FAACVPR
University of North Carolina at Charlotte
Charlotte, North Carolina

Brianna Wells, MS, CSCS
Henry Mayo Fitness and Health
Valencia, California

CONTRIBUTING AUTHORS TO THE FOURTH EDITION

Nancy J. Belli, MA, ACSM-HFS
Asphalt Green
New York, New York
Cases: Domain of Legal, Professional, Business,
and Marketing for CPT

**Clinton Brawner, MS, FACSM, ACSM-RCEP,
ACSM-CES**
Henry Ford Hospital
Detroit, Michigan
Cases: Domain of Patient/Client Assessment for
CES (Electrocardiograms)

Nikki Carosone Russo, MS, ACSM-CPT
Long Island University
Brooklyn, New York
Cases: Domain of Exercise Programming and
Implementation for CPT

**Brian Coyne, MEd, ACSM-RCEP,
ACSM/NCPAD-CIFT**
Duke University Health System
Durham, North Carolina
Cases: Domain of Exercise Counseling and
Behavioral Strategies for HFS

**Donald M. Cummings, PhD,
ACSM-CES**
East Stroudsburg University
East Stroudsburg, Pennsylvania
Cases: Domain of Exercise Prescription
for CES

**Shala E. Davis, PhD, FACSM, ACSM-ETT,
ACSM-CES, ACSM-PD**
East Stroudsburg University
East Stroudsburg, Pennsylvania
Cases: Domain of Leadership and
Counseling for CES

Kimberly DeLeo, BS, PTA, ACSM-CPT
Health and Exercise Connections, LLC
Middleboro, Massachusetts
Cases: Domain of Legal, Professional,
Business, and Marketing for CPT

**Julie J. Downing, PhD, FACSM, ACSM-CPT,
ACSM-HFS**
Central Oregon Community College
Bend, Oregon
Cases: Domain of Health and Fitness
Assessment for HFS

**Shawn Drake, PT, PhD, ACSM-RCEP,
ACSM-PD**
Arkansas State University
Jonesboro, Arkansas
Cases: Domain of Exercise Prescription and
Implementation for EP-C

Trent A. Hargens, PhD, ACSM-CES
James Madison University
Harrisonburg, Virginia
Cases: Domain of Patient/Client Assessment
for CES

Dennis Kerrigan, PhD, ACSM-CES
Henry Ford Hospital
Detroit, Michigan
Cases: Domain of Patient/Client Assessment for
CES (Electrocardiograms)

Frederick Klinge, MBA, ACSM-HFS
Ochsner Health System/Varsity Sports
New Orleans, Louisiana
Cases: Domain of Management for HFS

Timothy S. Maynard, MS, ACSM-PD
Providence Hospital
Mobile, Alabama
Cases: Domain of Legal and Professional
Considerations for CES

Matthew W. Parrott, PhD, ACSM-HFS
H-P Fitness, LLC
Kansas City, Missouri
Cases: Domain of Legal/Professional for HFS

James H. Ross, MS, ACSM-RCEP, ACSM-CES
Wake Forest University
Winston-Salem, North Carolina
Cases: Domain of Exercise Prescription for CES

**Tom Spring, MS, FAACVPR, ACSM-CPT,
ACSM-HFS, ACSM-CES**
WebMD Health Services
Detroit, Michigan
Cases: Domain of Initial Client Consultation
and Assessment for CPT

**David E. Verrill, MS, FAACVPR,
ACSM-RCEP, ACSM-CES**
University of North Carolina at Charlotte
Charlotte, North Carolina
Cases: Domain of Program Implementation and
Ongoing Support for CES

**Janet P. Wallace, PhD, FACSM, ACSM-CES,
ACSM-PD**
Indiana University
Bloomington, Indiana
Cases: Domain of Exercise Prescription for CES

Michael J. Webster, PhD, FACSM, ACSM-CES
University of Southern Mississippi
Hattiesburg, Mississippi
Cases: Domain of Exercise Leadership and
Client Education for CPT

*Degrees, certifications, and affiliations current at time of author contributions.

Index